Traumatic Brain Injury Rehabilitation for Speech-Language Pathologists

Traumatic Brain Injury Rehabilitation for Speech-Language Pathologists

Rita J. Gillis, PhD
Consultant, Gillis and Pierce Associates, Pensacola, Florida

With contributions by
Jeffrey N. Pierce, MD
Director, Brain Injury Program, The Rehabilitation Institute, Department of Physical Medicine and Rehabilitation, West Florida Regional Medical Center, Pensacola, Florida

Monica McHenry, PhD
Adjunct Assistant Professor of Internal Medicine, Pulmonary Division, University of Texas Medical Branch; Speech Scientist, Department of Speech-Language Pathology, Galveston Institute of Human Communication, Transitional Learning Community, Galveston, Texas

Butterworth-Heinemann

Boston   Oxford   Johannesburg   Melbourne
New   Dehli   Singapore

Midtown

Every effort has been made to ensure that the drug
dosage schedules within this text are accurate and
conform to standards accepted at time of publication.
However, as treatment recommendations vary in the light
of continuing research and clinical experience, the reader
is advised to verify drug dosage schedules herein with
information found on product information sheets. This is
especially true in cases of new or infrequently used
drugs.

Recognizing the importance of preserving what has been
written, Butterworth-Heinemann prints its books on
acid-free paper whenever possible.

Library of Congress Cataloging-in-Publication Data

Gillis, Rita J., 1955–
  Traumatic brain injury rehabilitation for speech-language
pathologists/Rita J. Gillis; with contributions by Monica
McHenry, Jeffrey N. Pierce.
    p.   cm.
  Includes bibliographical references and index.
  ISBN 0-7506-9650-8 (hardcover)
  1. Brain damage—Patients—Rehabilitation. 2. Speech therapy.
3. Cognitive therapy. I. McHenry, Monica. II. Pierce, Jeffrey N.
III. Title.
  [DNLM: 1. Brain Injuries—complications. 2. Cognition Disorders—
rehabilitation. 3. Speech Disorders—rehabilitation. WL 354
G481t 1996]
RC387.5.G54   1996
616.8′046—dc20
DNLM/DLC
for Library of Congress   96-15261
                                                           CIP

British Library Cataloguing-in-Publication Data
A catalogue record for this book is available from the British Library.

The publisher offers special discounts on bulk orders of this book.
For information, please contact:
Manager of Special Sales
Butterworth-Heinemann
313 Washington Street
Newton, MA 02158-1626
Tel: 617-928-2500
Fax: 617-928-2620

For information on all medical publications available, contact our World Wide Web home page at:
http://www.bh.com/bh/

10 9 8 7 6 5 4 3 2 1

Printed in the United States of America

4/14/99 – A.S.

Contents

Preface

Although numerous comprehensive works have been written in the area of traumatic brain injury rehabilitation, few are intended to guide new clinicians entering the field, specifically in the area of cognitive-communicative rehabilitation. This text is written in such a manner that the information is accessible to graduate students who have completed their primary course work, to practicing clinicians entering the field of traumatic brain injury, and to those who wish to have a more thorough understanding of this complicated field of study. The book is somewhat unusual in that it is not a compilation of material from many different authors, but is coordinated and predominantly written by a single author. This provides cohesion from one section to another and allows information to be presented in detail, because one chapter builds upon another.

In part, the field of traumatic brain injury is complex because it draws expertise from a broad arena of diverse specialties that includes philosophy, law, ethics, social work, psychology, education, medicine, surgery, and rehabilitation. Few texts have attempted to synthesize or explain this comprehensive information in a manner that guides the new clinician struggling with concepts and terminology. Therefore, every attempt has been made to define terms and avoid the excessive use of acronyms so common to the medical field today. Although this lengthens the text, reading comprehension should be enhanced. A glossary of acronyms is provided in Appendix A to give clinicians an easy guide when reading medical reports. Chapter One, which provides an introduction to the field, discusses problems in terminology. Terminology in the field of communication disorders is discussed in Chapter Five as well.

Although various texts do address the medical issues of traumatic brain injury, terminology can be overwhelming, particularly to the inexperienced clinician. In Chapters Three and Four, Pierce provides a discussion of the mechanisms of brain injury, neurologic sequelae, and the medical complications most pertinent to speech-language pathologists—a discussion that explains the complicated aspects of traumatic brain injury in understandable terms.

The nature of cognitive-communicative impairments and their rehabilitation is explained from both theoretical and clinical perspectives in Chapters Five and Six. In order to provide effective treatment, clinicians must have a rationale for treatment. This requires a background in cognitive and behavioral psychology that many clinicians do not obtain from their academic training. Numerous theoretical and clinical models of intervention are presented, to provide clinicians with a strong foundation from which to develop an individualized approach. Although every possible setting in which a clinician might work cannot be reviewed, the differences between acute rehabilitation and postacute rehabilitation are delineated, and the nature of clinical intervention during these different phases of recovery and rehabilitation is discussed in Chapters Seven and Eight.

In the field, it is often easy for clinicians, speech-language pathologists in particular, to concentrate on the cognitive aspects of impairment, yet motor speech disorders are common sequelae. In Chapter Nine, McHenry provides a thorough discussion of motor speech disorders from a systems perspective, and provides an overview of relevant advances in the areas of respiration, phonation, resonance, and articulation. Particular attention is given to instrumentation.

In this text, the reader will detect a strong commitment from the primary author to helping clinicians develop a philosophy of rehabilitation and patient care. Although it is true the population with traumatic brain injury is unique, as clinicians, researchers, and policymakers we must not fail to include those with traumatic brain injury among the larger population of persons with disabilities who have similar needs and struggles. Chapter Two addresses traumatic brain injury rehabilitation in the broader context of health care, disability, and handicap. In a similar vein, the framework for ethics in rehabilitation is based on work conducted with other types of disease and disability. Ethics in health care is of a critical concern to providers and consumers alike. Chapter Ten provides clinicians with a framework from which to consider ethical dilemmas that arise in traumatic brain injury rehabilitation, a topic seldom addressed in academic training programs.

In rehabilitation, the importance of the support network for any individual should not be overlooked. Clinicians new to their fields of practice often feel armed with all the answers and right decisions for family members. Yet, as clinicians we, unlike the families, do not have the lifetime responsibility of caring for an individual with a traumatic brain injury. Chapter Eleven explores traumatic brain injury as something that occurs to families; it is written to help clinicians remember to place each individual in the context of a family or support system.

In the Appendices the reader will find the aforementioned glossary of acronyms, a list of selected readings, and a list of commonly referenced assessment scales. The reading list, although extensive, is not intended to be exhaustive, but rather to provide clinicians with easy access to references for specific topics in the field. Similarly, all possible acronyms and scales cannot be included, but those commonly used and referenced are listed for easy referral.

In summary, this book will be of use to a wide range of clinicians who are either entering the field of traumatic brain injury rehabilitation for the first time or are practicing within the field and wish to expand their knowledge. It is written, however, in a manner that defines terms and provides examples, so as to make it a useful teaching text as well. In such a broad field as traumatic brain injury, it is impossible for a text to cover all topics in sufficient detail. Numerous topics, therefore, have been omitted intentionally, in order to provide adequate detail in the areas addressed. It is hoped this text will encourage all clinicians to evaluate the complexity of traumatic brain injury and to understand the uniqueness of each individual.

RJG

1

Introduction

Traumatic brain injury rehabilitation as a subspecialty of rehabilitation, and as an industry, is relatively new. The treatment of head injuries, on the other hand, is not new to medicine or society, and it has been a human concern since antiquity. Head injuries are known to have been treated in Egyptian societies from as early as 3000 B.C.[1,2] There have always been head injuries, of course, as may be seen from archaeological finds of prehistoric human skulls with fractures and holes. In general, the earliest causes of head injury—blows, falls, and projectiles—have not changed. New causes, however, have been added, such as high-speed motor vehicle accidents and high-velocity weapons.[1] With these new causal agents have come more fatal and severe injuries than were known previously. Head injuries have, however, provided medicine and its many allied services with a wealth of information about the brain. Much of what has been learned about brain-behavior relationships has come from early studies conducted on individuals who sustained missile injuries during war times. Even as early as the 1860s, a number of studies investigated brain injuries received during railway collisions. These injuries came to be known as "railway brain."[3]

Survival from head injuries has increased dramatically, particularly since World War II, when systemic antibiotic medications came into use. Further improvements in early medical management came with the rapid transfer of patients to hospitals and better resuscitation techniques.[1] Improved emergency medical care has paralleled other technological and economic advancements, such as the development of the automobile and a massive highway system. Motor vehicle travel is a way of life and the predominant cause of head injuries in industrialized nations during peace times. As technology has continued to improve, so has the survival rate from previously fatal injuries sustained in motor vehicle accidents. Since the early to mid-1970s, the entity of head injuries that has provoked the greatest amount of interest and concern has been that of nonmissile origin.

TERMINOLOGY

In the area of head injury, terminology has been an issue of confusion for some time. In 1966, in an attempt to improve consistency in use, an ad hoc committee of the Congress of Neurological Surgeons[4] was appointed to prepare a glossary of head injury terms to be used in clinical neurosurgery. Many of the terms had, as part of the definition, qualifying comments such as "an imprecise term." One such term, *coma*, remains imprecise in definition today.

The term *head injury* itself is problematic in that it encompasses a range of injuries that includes simple bumps on the head, scalp lacerations, facial injuries, and injuries that result in severe brain damage.[5] Within the field of brain injury rehabilitation, terms have been used without consistency or precision. In reviewing a recent text, which had been edited, the author found four different labels used, apparently to refer to the same entity or population. These included *traumatic closed head injury, head trauma, closed head trauma,* and *nonfocal brain damage.* Vogenthaler[6] has defined head injury as "damage to living brain tissue that is caused by an external mechanical force," and he further adds that it is usually accompanied by altered consciousness. Although this definition does little to delineate a specific condition, it was one of the few that were offered in hundreds of articles reviewed.

Prior to the mid- to late eighties, *closed head injury* appeared to be used most often to refer to nonpenetrating injuries to the head. The distinction being made is between "open" head injuries, in which the skull has been penetrated by some external object, such as a bullet or knife, and "closed" head injuries, in which there was no opening of the skull. This distinction has come to have great significance because of the implications of focal (common to open injuries) versus diffuse damage to the underlying brain.[6] (Focal and diffuse damage are discussed in greater detail in Chapter Two.) *Closed head injury* has been used most often to refer to injuries produced by "blunt" trauma, as differentiated from "sharp" or penetrating trauma. There are several problems with this dichotomy. Skull fractures may be considered open head injuries and can be the result of nonpenetrating forces (for example, a fall, an automobile accident, or a direct blow), in which case diffuse brain damage may result. Further, other injuries that are considered to be primarily "within the head," such as hematomas, have been labeled closed head injuries, without any particular reference to the cause or the nature of the brain damage. A review of the literature suggests the origin of this distinction is unknown. In a 1945 study, Denny-Brown[7] noted the difficulty in studying a population that was poorly defined, and placed the term *closed head injury* in quotation marks, indicating that it was used for lack of a more precise term. Although used for some time, the open/closed classification system may have developed in part from the *International Classification of Diseases (ICD)*[8] used by most medical facilities. A variety of codes (categories) is available to use in the classification of head injury, but fractures to the skull are divided into closed and open. Either classification can include other aspects of the injury, such as hematoma, cerebral laceration, contusion, or intracranial injury, if present and detected. However, the nature of brain injury is not clearly delineated by the terms *closed* and *open* unless additional criteria are included.

These confusions have more serious implications than mere mislabeling, or complicating communication in clinical practice. Many of the research studies that have investigated the nature of language impairment following head injury have included patients with focal and diffuse brain damage[9,10,11,12] or have failed to describe the population adequately.[13,14,15,16,17] Therefore, discussions regarding specific consequences or sequelae of the injuries have little meaning if the intention is to relate sequelae to a particular type of brain injury, as is usually the case. Additionally, as will be discussed in the next section, imprecision in diagnostic terminology and classification greatly affects the accuracy of incidence studies.

The term *acquired brain damage*, or *acquired brain injury*, is sometimes used to refer to brain damage that did not occur prior to or during birth.[18,19] The term typically includes brain damage resulting from traumatic brain injuries, stroke, tumors, infectious processes, metabolic disturbances, or other causes, but does not usually include Alzheimer's disease and other progressive neurologic conditions. It is a term often used to differentiate these conditions from congenital or developmental disabilities.

In recent years, attempts have been made to standardize terminology to the extent possible. In the words of renowned neurosurgeon Bryan Jennett,[5] "What matters in a head injury is brain damage." *Traumatic brain injury (TBI)* appears to be the preferred term, at least in rehabilitation, because it accurately reflects the structure injured and, to some extent, the cause. It differentiates brain damage that occurs as a result of trauma (also commonly referred to as mechanical forces) from that which occurs secondary to cerebrovascular disease, tumor, infection, progressive neurologic disease, and metabolic or neurochemical disturbances, although some have interpreted the term to include brain damage resulting from or in any *traumatic event* in the broadest sense. Parker,[20] for example, has included brain damage resulting from shock, drowning, fires, strangulation, birth injuries, neurotoxins, and so on. This author, however, does not think that the scope of the term *traumatic brain injury* is meant to be quite so broad.

More specifically, "Traumatic brain injury is defined as a blow to the head that results in diminished abilities subsequent to the injury and that requires rehabilitation intervention . . . [and] is primarily caused by motor vehicle accidents and violent crimes."[21] A key and clarifying point to this definition is that the injury results in diminished abilities indicative of brain damage, as distinguished from an injury to the head that may or may not result in brain damage. Brooke et al.[22] have indicated that "traumatic brain injury is used to describe the injury to the brain caused primarily by physical trauma," and then refer to *closed head injury* as "one of the most common types of traumatic brain injury." Although it is recognized that traumatic brain injury includes penetrating injuries, in the literature, these injuries are virtually always defined as such, typically including the cause as well (for example, gunshot wound).

Traumatic brain injury is used throughout this text, except when information from other works is presented. Then, the original terminology is preserved. Penetrating injuries are not the focus of this text, although many of the topics discussed are pertinent to brain damage in general.

EPIDEMIOLOGY

Epidemiology is a field of medical science that investigates "the frequency and patterns of distribution of disease, impairment and disability in a defined geographic region and population."[23] Epidemiologic studies provide information that is often used in planning health care services and allocating resources. Thus, data from epidemiologic studies can impact public policy. Although it is now considered a major health concern, there are no reported descriptive epidemiologic studies on traumatic brain injury prior to 1980. This imprecision in definition makes it difficult to ascertain the incidence of traumatic brain injury per se.[2,23,24,25] In order for researchers to accurately study a population and make predictions, there must be clear inclusion criteria.[24]

The incidence of "head injury" is frequently cited in the literature, although a relatively small number of epidemiologic studies have been conducted. The results from most studies conducted to date are summarized in Table 1.1. These studies represent findings based on incidence, not prevalence, and include all injuries: mild, moderate, and severe. The classification of injuries is discussed by Pierce in Chapter Two. However, to assist the reader, at this point the following general distinction is made: a mild head injury is typically considered as one in which there has been a loss of consciousness of less than 30 minutes,[6] and severe injuries are classified by a loss of consciousness of six hours or more.[26] Other criteria are used to determine the extent of injury (discussed later); loss of consciousness is seldom used alone.

Incidence refers to the number of new cases during a specified period, and *prevalence* refers to the total number of cases with a specific disease or disability at a particular point in time.[23] Prevalence is often estimated from incidence figures; therefore, if one is over- or underestimated, so is the other. Since the diagnosis of traumatic brain injury may be difficult, the exact incidence of the injury is contingent upon the diagnostic criteria. Incidence statistics generally are taken from hospital admissions or discharges. In the hospital setting, the type of problem for which the individual is seeking medical attention is assigned a diagnostic code (usually from the International Classification of Diseases). Typically, coding is not performed by the clinicians who have examined the patient, but rather by medical

Table 1.1
Studies of Incidence of Head Injury.

Reference	Occurrence per 100,00	Year(s) Studied	Region
Kalsbeek et al.[27]	200	1970–1974	National
Caveness[28]	3,486	1976	National
Klauber et al.[29]	285	1978	San Diego County
Jagger et al.*[30]	208	1978	Rural Virginia
Annegers et al.*[31]	195	1935–1974	Omsted County, MN
Fife et al.[32]	152	1979–1980	Rhode Island
Whitman et al.*[33]	403 inner-city black 394 suburban white 196 suburban black	1979–1980	Chicago (inner-city) and Evantson, IL
Cooper et al.[34]	277 black 261 Hispanic 209 white	1980–1981	Bronx, NY
Kraus et al.*[35]	180	1983	San Diego County

* Notes studies that separated injuries by severity.

records personnel, who must ascertain the condition from medical reports.[23] In severe accidents, conditions other than a brain injury may be more obvious, and hence may be coded as the primary condition. If persons are not treated in a hospital setting (for example, in an emergency medical clinic), they are not counted by this method. Both of these problems can result in underestimation of the population.

Another point of consideration, when statistics are taken from hospital admission or discharge numbers, is the medical criteria used by the hospital for admitting mild traumatic brain injuries. Emergency room visits are not necessarily included as admission/discharge cases. Because the majority of traumatic brain injuries are mild and often seen through the emergency department, some researchers think there is an underestimation of the incidence.[2] A similar underestimation occurs for severe injuries that become fatalities prior to hospital admission and are therefore not counted.[24,36]

In the International Classification of Diseases,[8] there are over thirty diagnostic codes that can be used to classify open and closed skull fractures alone, and another twenty-five or more that can be used to classify intracranial injury without skull fractures. It is important to note that none of the classifications that appear in the manual includes the terminology *head injury* or *traumatic brain injury*. Some epidemiology studies have included a number of diagnoses that do not necessarily indicate brain damage (for example, facial fractures and scalp lacerations).[23] Further, incidence figures typically are collected for a specified time period, such as one year or five years. When hospital admission and discharge statistics are used to determine incidence, persons with the same condition may be counted multiple times if admitted to the hospital more than once during the specified period. The problems of overinclusion of related diagnoses and repeat entries in data collection result in overestimation of the condition.[23]

Finally, traumatic brain injury occurs along a continuum of injury within subpopulations. The majority of injuries included in incidence studies are mild head injuries, but data have been gathered in such a way that subgrouping was not done. Four of the reported studies (noted in Table 1.1 by an asterisk) classified injuries by severity. These have been reviewed by Kraus and Arzemanian.[37] However, the diagnostic criteria used to group cases by severity varied among the studies. Because there are a number of variations in the way data have been collected in all of the studies listed, comparisons between studies are difficult to make. Depending upon the criteria applied when evaluating epidemiologic studies, some authors think there has been a tendency for the incidence of traumatic brain injury to be underestimated,[2] and others think the tendency has been toward overestimation.[23]

Regardless of the problems in methodology in epidemiologic studies, a number of statistics remain constant. Traumatic brain injuries occur in males more than in females (two to one); the population distribution is bimodal, most frequently affecting the young (15–24 years of age), followed by the elderly (65–75 years of age); approximately fifty percent of all injuries are the result of a motor vehicle accident; and, alcohol is a significant factor in cause and recovery.[25,26,38] The costs associated with a severe traumatic brain injury are enormous.[2,23] We have only begun to examine the costs of long-term disability and the effects of rehabilitation in reducing those costs.

REHABILITATION

As stated earlier, much of what we know about brain injuries and brain functions comes from studies conducted on veterans. Certainly this is true in the case of aphasia. It is of interest to the speech-language pathologist that some of the earliest attempts to provide specialized brain injury rehabilitation were focused on the communication impairments resulting from brain injuries sustained in War World I. The following is an excerpt from the *Berlin Letter*, February 15, 1916, which appeared in the *Journal of the American Medical Association*:[39]

> . . . Speech disturbances of various kinds practically make invalids of these patients, and they become unfitted for various occupations . . . some of the patients can be reeducated, especially if they are young, so that a sort of

compensation for lost function can be established. They must be taught to speak just as children are; but they will be found to be much more backward . . . A special school should be established, and the reeducation treatment must be begun early before the surgical treatment is completed . . . The schools should be established in hospitals, and special institutions for further treatment provided so that the patients can remain separated from the usual run of "nervous" patients. The results obtained thus far are very promising. It probably will not be possible, however, to restore these patients so that they can return to their former places in the community, but every effort should be made to influence them psychically to a degree which will permit any one of them to return to his family.

This passage reflects some of the thoughts about brain injury rehabilitation in Germany, where the field was quite advanced, in comparison to the work done in the United States. According to Boake,[40,41] during World War I, only one United States hospital provided specialized services for brain injury which included a Section of Defections of Hearing and Speech. During World War II, brain injury units were present in the United States, Britain, and the Soviet Union, the latter's being noted for the contributions of Alexandria Luria[42,43] to the field of cognitive rehabilitation.

Following the war, interest in brain injury rehabilitation declined, and many of the specialized units closed.[40,41] In the 1970s, brain injury rehabilitation took a new course with a new focus: nonmissile traumatic brain injuries. Not surprisingly, this has coincided with increased survival rates from motor vehicle accidents and other forms of blunt trauma (for example, falls, blows, et cetera). Since the mid-1970s, an entire continuum of specialized brain injury rehabilitation programs has developed. Yet, brain injury rehabilitation owes its growth to more than professional interest. The treatment of traumatic brain injury, like that of other disabilities, was a cause promoted by someone personally affected. That individual was Marilyn Price Spivack, cofounder, with her husband, of the National Head Injury Foundation (now called the Brain Injury Association). On April 19, 1980, the Spivacks,[44] along with a few other families and professionals, met to form the organization that has since grown into a national presence with membership in the thousands. This organization has been responsible for developing and sponsoring numerous large multidisciplinary educational conferences that have drawn international speakers and audiences. It has served as a resource and distribution center, supplying educational materials to professionals, families, and individuals with injuries, and it has facilitated the development of state organizations. Its members have successfully lobbied federal and state governments for changes in policy and allocation of financial resources for improved services to individuals with traumatic brain injuries. Although certainly not solely responsible for the advances made in traumatic brain injury rehabilitation, the Brain Injury Association has made many contributions to the field.

SPECIAL POPULATIONS

Because the author believes that clinicians concerned with, and interested in, traumatic brain injury must also concern themselves with larger issues, this text addresses a number of rehabilitation issues that may be considered pertinent to all disability groups. Regarding evaluation and treatment issues, the information presented is largely concerned with individuals with severe traumatic brain injury, although a number of suggestions are applicable to other groups. The author recognizes there are subpopulations within the broader classification of traumatic brain injury. These warrant mentioning, but only as an introduction to the subject, and with the recognition that no single text can address all of the dimensions of traumatic brain injury. Each of the subpopulations introduced below has been addressed in other works, to which the reader is referred. A list of topic-specific readings is provided in Appendix B.

Pediatric Traumatic Brain Injury Rehabilitation

It may seem self-evident that children with brain injuries are not merely "little adults" with brain injuries, yet many programs approach the pediatric population from an adult rehabilitation model. Oftentimes, this occurs because only a few children are in the program, and it may be considered too expensive to offer specialized services or provide staff training to meet their needs. In the author's opinion, in most cases, children should return to their homes as soon as possible and receive services in nonresidential settings. This is consistent with a general move, in traumatic brain injury rehabilitation, toward community-based services. Families must be actively involved in the rehabilitation program, and program designs should begin with this in mind. Educational and counseling services should be available to siblings, who often feel neglected when a brother or sister becomes the focal point of parental concern.

When children are treated in settings with a disproportionate number of adults, the children often become the focus of attention of staff and the other patients and families. Although this may be unintentional, and may seem harmless, it can bring about behavioral problems. Children learn from their peers, who range in personality and ability, in the normal school setting. Therefore, it is logical that children be treated with a group of peers if at all possible.

School re-entry is inevitable and essential; therefore, networks to facilitate school re-entry must be developed. This requires that staff be committed to developing relationships with school personnel and district officials. Clinicians must be well trained in the stages of physical, cognitive, linguistic, and social development of children. It is as inappropriate to adapt adult treatment materials to children as it is to use childlike materials with adults.

Resources must be allocated for age-appropriate furnishings, therapy equipment, and supplies.

Neurobehavioral Rehabilitation

Behavioral intervention is a part of all traumatic brain injury rehabilitation. However, individuals who have severe behavior problems as a result of the traumatic brain injury, or preexisting problems exacerbated by the injury, can often disrupt the rehabilitation program of other participants. Severe behavioral disorders can present an enormous challenge to the clinical staff as well, particularly when staff are unprepared for them. Programming and facility restraints (for example, entrances/exits that can be secured, calming rooms with low stimulation, high staff/patient ratio, removal of harmful objects) must be more carefully attended to than in other types of rehabilitation programs. Staff must be trained in behavioral intervention before patients are admitted, and the organization must make a commitment to ongoing training. A neuropsychiatrist should be readily available to the program. Although a number of behavioral problems may be managed in a nonspecialized traumatic brain injury rehabilitation program, the author's experience suggests that severe behavioral problems require specialized programming with staff who are well trained in behavior modification theory and principles.

Mild Traumatic Brain Injury Rehabilitation

In recent years, numerous articles[45,46,47,48,49,50,51,52] and texts[53,54] have appeared that address the unique needs of the mildly injured population. Although at a programmatic level the needs and the commitment of resources are not as great as with the other two subpopulations mentioned, a number of issues are unique and must be addressed. Physical appearance is generally unchanged in the mildly injured person, and therefore, validation of the significance of the injury may be lacking.[50] Reassurance becomes a major focus of the therapeutic relationship and the program. Staff need to have ample personal resources to provide the continual reassurance that is often required. Counseling services should be an essential part of the program. A support group of peers with injuries can provide an important source of reassurance, and programs should be prepared to develop and assist such groups.

Program staff need to develop strong relationships with emergency room personnel by providing education and a system for referrals. Like other subpopulations, patients with mild traumatic brain injury need to be treated by staff who are well trained and prepared to regard them as a population distinct from those with severe injuries. Comprehensive neuropsychological assessment should be provided, with repeated assessments throughout the course of recovery.[50] Return to work or school is often of primary concern. In some cases, individuals who return to work will be struggling, or will fail altogether. Cognitive rehabilitation may be indicated, but it should be geared toward the demands of the job, living situation, and/or academic pursuits, as indicated.

SUMMARY

Head injuries have been of interest throughout recorded history. Yet, despite this long history, terminology remains imprecise and often unclear. *Traumatic brain injury* is the preferred term today, although many of the problems associated with other terms, such as *closed head injury*, remain. Because of the imprecision and variability among diagnostic criteria, definitive studies of the magnitude of the health problem posed by traumatic brain injury are yet to be done. However, with the most recent investigations in the area of mild brain injuries, criteria are being refined, and will be further refined as interest in treatment outcome and cost grows.

Brain injury rehabilitation is not new, but a renewed interest has arisen, following changes in the population. In the earlier part of the twentieth century, war injuries were of primary concern; today, brain injuries resulting from motor vehicle accidents, falls, and assaults are of greater concern. Although traumatic brian injuries occur along a continuum of injury and disability, the scope of this text is limited to the population of moderate and severe injuries most often seen by the speech-language pathologist.

REFERENCES

1. Gurdjian ES. *Head Injury from Antiquity to the Present with Special Reference to Penetrating Head Wounds.* Springfield, IL: Charles C Thomas; 1973.
2. Levin HS, Benton AL, Grossman RG. *Neurobehavioral Consequences of Closed Head Injury.* New York, NY: Oxford University Press; 1982:3–48.
3. Evans RW. The postconcussion syndrome: 130 years of controversy. *Seminars in Neurology.* 1994;14:32–39.
4. Cook AW et al. Report of ad hoc committee to study head injury nomenclature. *Clinical Neurosurgical Journal.* 1966;12:386–394.
5. Jennett B. Assessment of the severity of head injury. *Journal of Neurology, Neurosurgery, and Psychiatry.* 1976;39:647–655.
6. Vogenthaler DR. An overview of head injury: its consequences and rehabilitation. *Brain Injury.* 1987;1:113–127.
7. Denny-Brown D. Disability arising from closed head injury. *Journal of the American Medical Association.* 1945;127:429–436.
8. *International Classification of Diseases, 9th rev-Clinical Modification, 4th rev, Vol 1.* Los Angeles, CA: Practice Management Information Corporation; 1995.

9. Arseni C et al. Considerations on posttraumatic aphasia in peace time. *Psychiatria, Neurologia, Neurochirurgia.* 1970;73:105–112.

10. Kriendler A et al. Aphasia following non-missile injury of the brain. *Reviews in Romanian Medicine-Neurology and Psychiatry.* 1975;13:247–254.

11. Levin HS et al. Aphasic disorder in patients with closed head injury. *Journal of Neurology, Neurosurgery, and Psychiatry.* 1976;39:1062–1070.

12. Levin HS et al. Linguistic recovery after closed head injury. *Brain and Language.* 1981;12:360–374.

13. Groher M. Language and memory disorders following closed head trauma. *Journal of Speech and Hearing Research.* 1977;20:212–223.

14. Thompsen IV. Verbal learning in aphasic and non-aphasic patients with severe head injuries. *Scandinavian Journal of Rehabilitation Medicine.* 1977;9:73–77.

15. Sarno MT, Buonaguar A, Levita E. Characteristics of verbal impairment in closed head injured patients. *Archives of Physical Medicine and Rehabilitation.* 1986;67:400–405.

16. Sarno MT. The nature of verbal impairment after closed head injury. *Journal of Nervous and Mental Disease.* 1980;168:685–692.

17. Crosson B et al. California Verbal Learning Test (CVLT) performance in severely head-injured and neurologically normal adult males. *Journal of Clinical and Experimental Neuropsychology.* 1988;10:754–768.

18. Goldstein G, Ruthven L. *Rehabilitation of the Brain-Damaged Adult.* New York, NY: Plenum Press; 1983:3–43.

19. *Standards Manual and Interpretative Guidelines for Medical Rehabilitation.* Tucson, AZ: Commission on Accreditation of Rehabilitation Facilities; 1995:107–124.

20. Parker RS. *Traumatic Brain Injury and Neuropsychological Impairment.* New York, NY: Springer-Verlag; 1990:1–10.

21. Ellis DW, Christensen AL. Introduction. In Ellis DW, Christensen AL (eds). *Neuropsychological Treatment after Brain Injury.* Boston, MA: Kluwer Academic Publishers; 1989:1–11.

22. Brooke M et al. In Beukelman DR, Yorkston KM (eds). *Communication Disorders Following Traumatic Brain Injury: Management of Cognitive, Language and Motor Impairments.* Austin, TX: Pro-Ed; 1991:15–45.

23. Willer B, Abosch S, Dahmer E. Epidemiology of disability from traumatic brain injury. In Wood RL (ed). *Neurobehavioural Sequelae of Traumatic Brain Injury.* New York, NY: Taylor and Francis; 1989:18–33.

24. Frankowski RF, Annegers JF, Whitman S. Epidemiological and descriptive studies part I: epidemiology of head trauma in the United States. In Becker DP, Povlishock JT (eds). *Central Nervous System Trauma Status Report.* Bethesda, MD: National Institute of Neurologic and Communicative Disorders and Sciences; 1985:33–43.

25. Cope DN. The rehabilitation of traumatic brain injury. In Kottke FJ, Lehmann JF (eds). *Krusen's Handbook of Physical Medicine and Rehabilitation 4th ed.* Philadelphia, PA: WB Saunders; 1990:1217–1251.

26. Whyte J, Rosenthal M. Rehabilitation of the patient with head injury. In DeLisa J (ed). *Rehabilitation Medicine: Principles and Practices.* Philadelphia, PA: JB Lippincott; 1988:585–611.

27. Kalsbeek WD et al. The national head and spinal cord injury survey: major findings. *Journal of Neurosurgery.* 1980;53:S19–S31.

28. Caveness, WF. Incidence of craniocerebral trauma in the United States in 1976, and trend from 1970–1975. In Thompson RA, Green JR (eds). *Advances in Neurology.* New York, NY: Raven Press; 1979:1–3.

29. Klauber MR et al. The epidemiology of head injury: a prospective study for an entire community—San Diego County, California, 1978. *American Journal of Epidemiology.* 1981;113:500–509.

30. Jagger J et al. Epidemiologic features of head injury in a predominantly rural population. *Journal of Trauma.* 1984;24:40–44.

31. Annegers JF et al. The incidence, causes, and secular trends of head trauma in Olmsted County, Minnesota 1935–1974. *Neurology.* 1980;30:912–919.

32. Fife D et al. Incidence and outcome of hospital-treated head injury in Rhode Island. *American Journal of Public Health.* 1986;76:773–778.

33. Whitman S, Coonley-Hoganson R, Desai BR. Comparative head trauma experience in two socioeconomically different Chicago-area communities: a population study. *American Journal of Epidemiology.* 1984;4:570–580.

34. Cooper KD et al. The epidemiology of head injury in the Bronx. *Neuroepidemiology.* 1983;2:70–88.

35. Kraus JF et al. The incidence of acute brain injury and serious impairment in a defined population. *American Journal of Epidemiology.* 1984;2:186–201.

36. Kraus JF. Injury to the head and spinal cord: the epidemiological relevance of the medical literature published from 1960–1978. *Journal of Neurosurgery.* 1980;53:S3–S9.

37. Kraus JF, Arzemanian S. Epidemiologic features of mild and moderate brain injury. In Hoff J, Anderson T, Cole T (eds). *Contemporary Issues in Neurological Surgery: Mild to Moderate Head Injury, Vol. 1.* Boston, MA: Blackwell Scientific Publications. 1989:9–28.

38. Alves WM et al. Understanding posttraumatic symptoms after minor head injury. *Journal of Head Trauma Rehabilitation.* 1986;1:1–12.

39. Berlin Letter. Schools for soldiers with brain injuries. *Medical News, Journal of the American Medical Association.* 1916;66:968–969.

40. Boake C. A history of cognitive rehabilitation of head-injured patients, 1915 to 1980. *Journal of Head Trauma Rehabilitation.* 1989;4:1–8.

41. Boake C. History of cognitive rehabilitation following head injury. In Kreutzer JS, Wehman PH (eds). *Cognitive Rehabilitation for Persons with Traumatic Brain Injury: A Functional Approach.* Baltimore, MD: Paul H Brookes Publishing; 1991:3–12.

42. Luria AR. *Traumatic Aphasia: Its Syndromes, Psychology and Treatment.* Bowden D (trans). The Hague, The Netherlands: Mouton; 1970.

43. Luria, AR. *Restoration of Function after Brain Injury.* Haigh B (trans). London, England: Pergamon Press; 1963.

44. Spivack MP. Pathways to policy: a personal perspective. *Journal of Head Trauma Rehabilitation.* 1994;9:82–83.

45. Gronwall D, Wrightson P. Delayed recovery of intellectual function after minor head injury. *Lancet.* 1974;2:605–609.

46. Rimel RW et al. Disability caused by minor head injury. *Neurosurgery.* 1981;9:221–228.

47. Barth JT et al. Neuropsychological sequelae of minor head injury. *Neurosurgery.* 1983;13:529–533.

48. Colohan ART et al. Neurologic and neurosurgical implications of mild head injury. *Journal of Head Trauma Rehabilitation.* 1986;1:13–21.
49. Ruff RM, Levin HS, Marshal LF. Neurobehavioral methods of assessment and the study of outcome in minor head injury. *Journal of Head Trauma Rehabilitation.* 1986;1:43–52.
50. Barth JT et al. Forensic aspects of mild head trauma. *Journal of Head Trauma Rehabilitation.* 1986;1:63–70.
51. Gronwall D. Rehabilitation programs for patients with mild head injury: components, problems, and evaluation. *Journal of Head Trauma Rehabilitation.* 1986;1:53–62.
52. Levin HS et al. Neurobehavioral outcome following minor head injury: a three-center study. *Journal of Neurosurgery.* 1987;66:234–243.
53. Levin HS, Eisenberg HM, Benton AL (eds). *Mild Head Injury.* New York, NY: Oxford University Press; 1989.
54. Hoff J, Anderson T, Cole T (eds). *Contemporary Issues in Neurological Surgery: Mild to Moderate Head Injury, Vol. 1.* Boston, MA: Blackwell Scientific Publications; 1989.

2

Models of Rehabilitation and Types of Programs

Medicine makes use of numerous models, approaches, and programs to characterize current practices, provide structure for service delivery, and propose methods for future improvement. A variety of models, programs, and approaches, with which the clinician should become familiar, exists in rehabilitation as well. This chapter is intended to provide the clinician with a framework from which to consider traumatic brain injury within the larger context of health and disability. It is placed at the beginning of the text so as to introduce a philosophical perspective that can be used to evaluate the many theoretical and clinical views presented in the remainder of the book. Readers are challenged to consider these models in relation to their own clinical practice. A description of the different types of programs is also provided, in order to delineate the scope of traumatic brain injury rehabilitation. The application of the different models and treatment approaches discussed in later chapters will depend, in part, upon the setting in which one works. Readers should bear this in mind as well.

A *model* can be defined as an example of something to be imitated or followed in practice, or as a way to conceptualize complex ideas. From a sociological perspective, it is a "complex, integrated system of meaning used to view, interpret, and understand a part of reality."[1] The reality discussed here is illness and disability.

An *approach* is a manner or method used to deal with a particular subject, which may be a person, thing, or purpose (for example, to rehabilitate, to evaluate, or to communicate). A *program* is a specific plan with defined components, procedures, activities, et cetera, designed to accomplish a goal; it may be so precise as to include timetables, schedules, and criteria. These terms are often used interchangeably, and it may be accurate to do so, in some instances. For instance, a particular approach to a problem may become a model to emulate. Likewise, a program may become a model. However, for clarity, one should attempt to determine the exact usage, in clinical practice. A clinician may be asked to explore a particular treatment approach, which is quite different from being asked to follow a specific model, or to participate in a program with defined goals.

It is important to understand some of the views, represented as models, approaches, and programs, that have shaped the field of traumatic brain injury rehabilitation. Those who are aware of these views and practices can make better choices and can alter practices. They can propose models, develop approaches, and design programs that can lead to further improvement in the field.

MODELS IN HEALTH CARE

The Medical Models

The *medical model* is a term that is used to label a variety of aspects of health care, ranging from the way in which society views illness to the relationship between health care providers and patients. Sometimes it is used so loosely as to refer to any intervention practices that occur within a medical setting, inaccurate as this may be. In traumatic brain injury rehabilitation, it is a label bandied frequently among lay persons and professionals in verbal contexts such as "We don't practice the medical model here," or "Larry would have done much better if his program had not been so entrenched in the medical model." Without knowing the frame of reference of the speaker, and the concept that the label was intended to impart, *medical model* means very little in either of those examples.

From a sociological perspective, the medical model is a system that allows society to view illness as a form of social deviancy, that is, a varying from the norm. As such, it may be thought of as a normative model, in which the goal of medicine (rehabilitation included) is to return the patient to a "normal" state. According to Veatch,[1] in our society, illness or sickness constitutes a new role for the individual afflicted, the sick role, and with it the individual assumes certain characteristics, exemptions, and responsibilities. Included in the sick role is the assumption that the sickness is undesirable and negatively evaluated by society. The person in the sick role is exempt from normal social responsibilities, from responsibility for the condition, and from the act of getting well by will or decision (that is, exercising one's personal choice and control to become well). Further, the individual has an obligation to seek competent help. The person in the sick role comes to the professional to obtain expert advice and, ultimately, a cure. It is within this context that disease is evaluated and treated in our society. The patient, if legitimately sick, can have no responsibility, and the clinician, as expert, assumes all responsibility.

In writing about the meaning of illness from the perspective of a multiple sclerosis patient, Toombs[2] describes the expectations of modern medicine:

> Since technology and science have been extremely successful in eradicating or ameliorating many diseases, not only is illness perceived as an unwarranted

intrusion but the person who is ill expects medical intervention to provide him with nothing less than a complete restoration of health.

Because this is a societal view, *medical model* in this context has the broadest application. Veatch[1] considers it to be an extremely dominant model in our society, with an enormous tendency to make illnesses out of a range of social abnormalities, such as unwanted pregnancy, alcoholism, drug abuse, and various criminal behaviors.

A great deal has been written about the nature of mental illness,[1,3,4] and whether or not it is best viewed within the medical model. The motivation to find an organic basis to mental illness stems, in part, from the question of how it should be managed—as a medical problem or as a social issue similar to socioeconomic disadvantage. This distinction may seem of little concern to the practicing clinician, but the fact is that financial resources come into consideration in a large way. The establishment of a medical basis to an illness has often been a prerequisite for receiving reimbursement for rehabilitation services. Only within recent years has this begun to change. Speech-language pathologists who work with children with developmental learning disabilities are quite aware of this distinction as a factor in obtaining reimbursement for therapy.

The controversy over how mental illness and social abnormalities should be conceptualized is in fact relevant to traumatic brain injury, but not because an organic (medical) basis is difficult to establish. Typically, with the exception of mild injuries and injuries that occurred in childhood with no clear recorded history, organicity is not an issue in traumatic brain injury. Rather, the way the clinician, organization, or society views mental illness is relevant because of the large number of individuals with traumatic brain injury who also have drug and alcohol abuse patterns[5] and preinjury mental illnesses. Are individuals with addictions exempt from responsibility, as suggested by the medical model? Should they continue to receive treatment when such addictions interfere with the rehabilitation program? Should drug and alcohol addictions be treated in the rehabilitation center or in a different setting? When resources are limited, as they generally are, who should be treated first: the person with a traumatic brain injury and drug addiction, or the person who has only a traumatic brain injury? Regardless of organizational policies and criteria, these questions often are answered at the level of the clinician, as they arise. Consequently, clinicians need to be aware of their own views and attitudes, and how they can affect the manner of service delivery. Additionally, the conceptualization of mental illness is pertinent to the way in which clinicians view postinjury psychological impairments, which may be seen as having a primary organic basis, as attributable to premorbid personality characteristics, or as reactive in nature.

Although Veatch suggests that society is entrenched in the medical model, he also recognizes the movement toward individual responsibility for health.[6] This trend is evidenced by the number of health clubs and spas that have appeared in recent years, and by the so-called "fitness craze." No doubt if this movement continues, as it probably will, persons who sustain brain injuries as a result of driving while intoxicated, driving motorcycles without helmets, or from other high risk activities, may come under greater scrutiny for services than in the past.

Closely related to the medical model described above is the *traditional model* of medical decision making.[7] The traditional model is a term used to label the relationship between patients and their physicians, as well as their other health care providers. In this context, the clinician is considered "all knowing" and makes decisions for the patient, generally with the patient's implied permission. As such, the clinician is *paternalistic* toward the patient in delivering treatment; hence, the model is also referred to as the *paternalistic model*.[8] This model is discussed further in Chapter Ten. The term often is used interchangeably with *medical model*, but in the author's opinion, it has less social implication. *Paternalistic model* is the more accurate label to use when describing a provider-patient relationship that is paternal, parental, or authoritarian. The medical model, as described, is more than a model of the provider-patient relationship; it represents societal views of health and illness.

The term *medical model* also has been used to refer to the manner in which disease or illness is viewed as a biologic (scientific) versus social phenomenon.[9] The *scientific* or *biomedical model* must be viewed from the perspective of the historical development of medicine, as it has moved from the practices of the Middle Ages and Renaissance, when the body was conceptualized abstractly, to the early modern era of medicine (beginning in the seventeenth century), which has taken a concrete approach to the body.[10] Modern medicine views the patient from a very mechanistic and analytic perspective. (The field of communication disorders and sciences has witnessed a similar course of development with the increasing use of instrumentation to delineate speech and language characteristics in normal and pathological states.)

Under the scientific or biomedical model, the diagnostic process moves in a linear manner from the level of system to cellular structures, until the cause of the disease is determined, and appropriate intervention can be applied.[11] The body is seen as a "totality of discretely functioning parts,"[10] somewhat analogous to a car or other machine. From this perspective, the patient (body) is viewed as being "self-contained and self-sufficient," distinct from the external environment.[10] The biomedical model is an important model to understand, as it is applied in a variety of rehabilitation settings in which different specialists/disciplines claim separate aspects of the patient, often dividing and subdividing skills and functions. Stanczak and Hutcherson[11] have argued that the model or approach most often used in brain injury rehabilitation is the biomedical model, whereby physical beings are viewed as "constituent parts explained with physical laws." Accordingly, under this model, rehabilitation moves in a linear fashion and

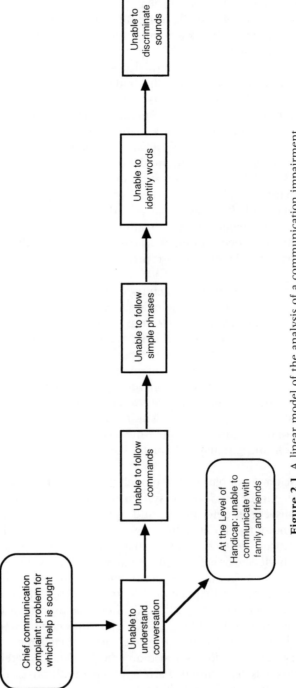

Figure 2.1 A linear model of the analysis of a communication impairment representing a reductionistic approach to disability.

assumes an "organismic locus of dysfunction" (that is, within the patient).[11] Figure 2.1 illustrates how an analytical process might be applied to the evaluation of a communication disability. The biomedical model is viewed as reductionistic. Whitman[12] has noted that:

> A rehabilitation model based on this philosophical framework focuses on discrete disciplines, segregated departments, and distinct demarcations in resources allocation and utilization. This approach is better suited to conditions such as a well-localized stroke, uncomplicated orthopedic injuries, or minor sports injuries [in contrast to traumatic brain injury] where disease entities are well defined, treatment regimes clearly established, and prognosis and recovery highly predictable.

In rehabilitation, the biomedical model has also been referred to as the *physical disability model*[13] As characterized by these models, the locus of control for health care rests with the provider. Many are critical of rehabilitation that has followed the medical model, because of its failure to view the patient in the larger context of society, as a person with the full rights of decision making afforded the nondisabled.[11,14,15]

Alternative Models

The *contractual model* also has been used to refer to the provider-patient relationship and its role in medical decision making.[7,16] Under this model, the patient and provider share in the decision making, and care is provided only to the extent that it is desired by the patient. Critical care is the exception, and the authority to decide on behalf of the patient is assumed by the provider, in order to preserve life. Although in theory the contractual relationship can be established on the basis of verbal agreement, in practice, the informed consent document has emerged as the contract indicating agreement.[7,16] (Informed consent is discussed in greater detail in Chapter Ten.) Contracts are used frequently in rehabilitation settings and range from program participation agreements to behavior modification contracts. The problem with the contractual model, as it is applied in the rehabilitation setting, is that there must be an assumption of mental competence on the part of both parties, if the contract is to be legitimate. In traumatic brain injury rehabilitation, the extent of cognitive impairment, as it relates to the decision-making abilities of the individual, must be carefully considered, under the contractual model.

The *educational model* has been proposed[16,17,18] as an alternative to the paternalistic model. Under the educational model, the relationship between the provider and the patient is one "that is centered around guidance and cooperation, and geared towards mutual participation."[18] Further, "the health care team has an obligation to act in ways that encourage patients to participate in their own care, not simply to present options."[16] Some have argued that this is the model followed by rehabilitation.[18] Anderson[17] reinforces the notion that rehabilitation is about teaching the patient skills, and that it is largely an educational process:

> The aim of patient education is to help the person who is or has been a patient to assimilate information, learn skills, and develop attitudes that will encourage behavior likely to result in achieving or maintaining health and the highest potential for quality of life.

Education assumes some desire and willingness to learn. Thus, under the educational model, there is a level of responsibility placed on the patient, as is not the case under the medical model.

Medicine at large, rehabilitation specialties included, has begun to appreciate that a person is more than discretely functioning parts. According to Levin and Solomon,[10] late modern medicine has:

> . . . tried to see the body as a self-regulatory system whose functioning is dependent on, and inseparable from, the larger world, and which consequently can exist only in continuous, psychologically mediated interaction with a complex field of social, cultural, historical, and environmental conditions.

This sentiment parallels the independent living movement in rehabilitation that began in the 1970s, a societal movement initiated primarily by persons with disabilities.[19] The movement has brought attention to the fact that persons with disabilities are more than a combination of impairments that need to be treated (that is, normalized); they, like all of us, are interdependent members of society. Many[9,11,15,20] think that rehabilitation efforts focused exclusively at the disease level, with a goal to "fix" or cure, will always fall short of the more important goal of rehabilitation: improving quality of life. The medical model does not lend itself to this goal because it fails to share responsibility with the patient.

Consequently, clinicians are being challenged to adopt a different model or paradigm. The *interdependent* or *empowerment model* proposed by Condeluci[15] offers one such alternative. In this model, the problem of disability is placed in a broader context than the individual who has the disability. It is placed in the context of society or community, as a problem caused by poor attitudes and a lack of supports. As an example, unemployment is not so much caused by a person's disability, as by a lack of available employment opportunities. The challenge is to change the system and attitudes in the direction not only of acceptance but of welcoming persons with disabilities.

O'Hara and Harrell[20] have proposed the "Empowerment Rehabilitation Model" as the preferred model for traumatic brain injury rehabilitation. They subscribe to the "belief that all persons who have sustained traumatic brain injury, their families, and treatment providers have needs for empowerment." Their model includes five basic components, each of which is assessed and addressed at three integrated levels: the patient, the family, and the provider. The components of the model are structure, internal and external; motivation; information; acceptance; and skills (to extend beyond the cognitive and physical to include the interpersonal and emotional). In this model, clinicians need to be empowered as "empathic, motivated, well-informed, highly skilled professionals" who are prepared to meet the unmet needs of families and survivors of traumatic brain injury.[20] Condeluci[15] captures the essence of the difference between the medical paradigm and the interdependent/empowerment paradigm in the following questions: "Are we responsible for, or to, the people we serve?" "Should people be in or of communities?" "Do we want caring little communities, or communities that care?"

MODELS OF IMPAIRMENT, DISABILITY, AND HANDICAP

Up until this point, the models presented, for the most part, have dealt with disease. Disability, as a consequence of disease, is not distinct under these models and, as such, is poorly addressed. The following definitions by Halbertsma[21] provide some clarification:

Disease is a *theoretical concept* developed to *explain* health problems of medical science, and devised primarily for diagnostic and epidemiological purposes. Disease stands for the medical model of illness, the relationship between a specific pathogen and a specific set of illness phenomena by means of a specific pathological process. Thus disease refers to a process, to a development in time. Impairment, disability and handicap are *empirical concepts*, in the sense that they are closer to direct observation. They describe health problems at a particular point in time, which they do in medical terms as well as in terms of the daily-life aspects of health problems.

The International Classification of Impairments, Disabilities, and Handicaps (ICIDH) is a model for classifying the consequences of disease within the context of health[22]; in other words, handicaps related to socioeconomic status, sex, or race are not part of the classification system. Originally published in 1980 by the World Health Organization (WHO), it was intended to complement the *International Classification of Diseases (ICD).*[23] All clinicians should become familiar with the International Classification of Diseases[24], as it is used almost exclusively for coding diseases and disorders on insurance, Medicare, and Medicaid claims. Codes are typically required for reimbursement of services provided by third party payers, which demonstrates the importance that classification systems can come to have.

The goal of the International Classification of Impairments, Disabilities, and Handicaps was to clarify and establish consistent terminology to be used internationally to refer to the consequences of diseases. Yet, the distinction between handicap, impairment, and disability has occasioned controversy.[22] Under this classification system, they are defined in the following manner:[23]

In the context of health experience, an *impairment* (italics added) is any loss or abnormality of psychological, physiological or anatomical structure or function. (Note: "Impairment" is more inclusive than 'disorder' in that it covers losses, e.g. the loss of a leg is an impairment but not a disorder.) . . . a *disability* is any restriction or lack (resulting from an impairment) of ability to perform an activity in the manner or within the range considered normal for a human being . . . a *handicap* is a disadvantage for a given individual resulting from an impairment or a disability, that limits or prevents the fulfillment of a role that is normal (depending on age, sex and social and cultural factors) for that individual.

Although these are important distinctions to understand, the terms often are used interchangeably, even within the field of rehabilitation.[19] In practice, handicap may be the most difficult of the three to distinguish, and conceptually it has caused the most controversy.[22] Disability is an objectifying of impairment that is observable. Handicap may be thought of as the interaction between the observable impairment (disability) and the environment in which the individual must function (live), with all of its physical, social, and psychological barriers. Although disability may vary over time, it is relatively stable in contrast to handicap, which is more dependent upon the situation.[9] According to Williams,[9] "handicap . . . describes the burden imposed by an objective and social world upon those with disabilities."

Even though the terms *impairment, disability,* and *handicap* are meant to conceptualize a condition relative to different points in time, they should not necessarily be considered on a continuum. An impairment does not always lead to disability, and not all disabilities are handicaps. Further, there is not necessarily a one-to-one relationship among the three. That is to say, one impairment does not necessarily result in only one disability or one handicap. For example, the individual with a traumatic brain injury—the pathology—may have numerous impairments leading to a communication disability. Depending upon the context of the evaluation and the intention of the clinician, the nature of impairment could be viewed as one impairment (language) or many (decreased auditory comprehension, word finding difficulties, paraphasias, et cetera). Such impairments may result in a communication *disability* whereby the individual has difficulty conveying thoughts, and probably would result in a *handicap* if the individual could no longer work, participate in recreational activities, or have a meaningful conversation with the family.

As previously discussed, many have criticized rehabilitation efforts for focusing primarily or exclusively on the level of impairment and disability, in both assessment and treatment. Gray and Dean[25] have suggested that speech-language pathologists most often evaluate at the level of impairment and only sometimes at the level of disability, as is the case with Holland's[26] *Communicative Activities of Daily Living (CADL)*. Gray and Dean's[25] implications are that most clinicians use only formal language batteries to assess communication abilities. Clinicians who limit testing to formal batteries do, in fact, assess primarily at the level of impairment. Yet, the distinction is not that straightforward. As another example, the individual with a traumatic brain injury frequently will have a memory impairment. Most clinicians will test the person's ability to remember the clinician's name, the office, and even perhaps the ability to remember a strategy for finding the office at the next appointment. These are daily activities requiring memory. In the clinical setting, the distinction is often made between testing deficits (impairment level) and testing functional skills (disability level).

There is a strong movement in the field of traumatic brain injury rehabilitation towards assessing and promoting what are termed functional skills—functional communication being one such skill.[27] (Functional skills and rehabilitation are discussed in greater depth in the chapters that specifically address intervention.) Occupational therapy is one rehabilitation discipline noted for addressing functional skills in daily activities, for example, dressing, bathing, and eating. Therefore, occupational therapists often assess and treat at the level of disability. Functional status measures,[19] or functional assessment scales, are designed to assess "a person's ability to perform daily life activities for the purpose of determining appropriate treatment and services." They are used widely in rehabilitation (for example, the Functional Independence Measure).[28,29,30,31] Anyone who has been involved in the design of such scales knows the difficulty many clinicians have in distinguishing between impairment and disability. Clinicians (the author included) who are accustomed to using objective measurements in assessment and treatment (such as frequency counts, measurements of length, time, or complexity, et cetera) often have difficulty translating these measures into functional scales. Whether or not scales of this nature are the best measures of accountability and outcome has yet to be determined, but to judge from the literature,[32,33,34,35,36] their use is not likely to diminish.

Further, the impairment, disability, and handicap controversy is more than an issue of conceptualization and terminology. In the past, reimbursement for rehabilitation services has been closely tied to impairment. It has often been necessary for clinicians to demonstrate severe levels of impairment (that is, numerous deficits) in order to obtain reimbursement for rehabilitation services. "Medical necessity" is a familiar term to seasoned clinicians who have written letters to insurance companies and Medicare intermediaries in order to obtain services for their patients. It is not expected that this requirement will change in the near future, given the current emphasis on managed care. These are not reasons to defend a model that focuses on impairment versus handicap; rather, the discussion is intended to highlight to the reader some of the complexity of the issues in rehabilitation practice.

It should be apparent to the reader, at this point, that the models presented do not encompass a unitary concept of health care. Rather, they are models that represent different aspects of health care and reflect some of the dominant ideas in rehabilitation. Most practicing clinicians apply components of the different models, and often apply them simultaneously. Because of the interpersonal nature of rehabilitation, decisions are usually dictated by the personalities of the clinicians and the patients treated, rather than by a particular model. However, clinicians who do not make a conscientious effort to understand their own model of operation may find themselves without a clear framework for making decisions and providing treatment. Scofield[18] provides useful advice in the following:

> Professional self-awareness is the flip side of respecting patients as persons . . . Professionals owe it to themselves, their patients, and colleagues to know what motivations, concerns, fears, strengths, and weaknesses they bring to the clinical encounter . . . and [they] need to be aware of and sensitive to how their attitudes, expectations, and feelings influence their interactions with patients, families, and colleagues.

APPROACHES TO REHABILITATION

Although there are numerous approaches to traumatic brain injury rehabilitation specific to each discipline, this section is intended to address team approaches. In virtually all settings, with the exception of private practice, the speech-language pathologist will be a member of a larger team composed of multiple specialties. The team concept did not originate with traumatic brain injury rehabilitation. In health care, it is a concept of service delivery that "evolved as a compromise between the benefits of specialization and the need for continuity and comprehensiveness of care."[37] In traumatic brain injury rehabilitation, the team may be composed of any of the following members: patient, family, physiatrist, physician assistant or nurse practitioner, nurse, dietitian, speech-language pathologist, physical therapist, psychologist, neuropsychologist, social worker, occupational therapist, vocational evaluator or specialist, recreational or leisure therapist, music therapist, special educator, team leader, case manager, community liaison, discharge planner, and so on. It is often the organization, its needs and the expertise of the various staff, versus the professional credentials (licensing and certification) of a clinician, that determines the role an individual assumes on the team. Social workers may function as discharge planners, admissions coordinators, family counselors, case managers, community liaisons, or a combination of all of these. Psychologists may perform neuropsychological assessments and provide psychotherapy and family counseling. An occupational therapist may perform vocational evaluations and job skills training. A speech-language pathologist may be team leader or case manager, and so on. However, it is extremely important that clinicians understand the scope of their professional practice when delivering therapies and educating families. A speech-language pathologist is not qualified to interpret the results of a nerve conduction study of the arm, to make medication recommendations, or to evaluate the severity of a decubitis ulcer, for example.

Team Approaches Used in Rehabilitation

Although there may be other team approaches used in health care, the three typically discussed in rehabilitation circles are the multidisciplinary, interdisciplinary, and transdisciplinary approaches. As described by Melvin,[38] the multidisciplinary approach:

> ... refers to activities which involve the efforts of individuals from a number of disciplines. These efforts are disciplinary-oriented and, although they may impinge upon clients or activities dealt with by other disciplines, they approach them primarily through each discipline relating to its own activities ... and through these efforts [of each discipline] experience results representing the sum of each discipline providing its own unique activity, rather than an outcome which represents more than this simple sum.

The interdisciplinary approach also requires the efforts of multiple disciplines. In the interdisciplinary approach, clinicians from the various disciplines may overlap in their activities, and all share the responsibility for achieving treatment goals,[14] which ideally are the goals of the patient, and hence of the comprehensive rehabilitation program. Using this approach, clinicians must:

> ... [apply] the skills of their own discipline, but also have the added responsibility of the group effort on behalf of the activity or client involved. This effort requires the skills necessary for effective group interaction and the knowledge of how to transfer integrated group activities into a result which is greater than the simple sum of the activities of each individual discipline. The group activity of an interdisciplinary program is synergistic, producing more than each individually and separately could accomplish.[38]

In the multidisciplinary approach, the contributions of each discipline (to the rehabilitation program) are able to stand on their own.[39] As an approach, it is consistent with the scientific or biomedical model, in which patients are perceived as being composed of parts or distinguishable functions. This is viewed as counterproductive in the interdisciplinary approach, where team members work together to achieve outcome goals. The multidisciplinary approach is considered to be less well coordinated and focused toward a common goal than is the interdisciplinary approach. Even in the multidisciplinary approach, however, team members typically meet as a group to discuss progress, patient and family needs, and discharge plans. This effort is usually coordinated by a team leader, case manager, physician, or some other team member. The approach is more patient-oriented than if there were not a team, and clinicians did not communicate with one another, as is often the case in outpatient clinics or acute care facilities. Fordyce[39] has argued that the distinction between interdisciplinary and multidisciplinary approaches should not be of primary concern, for "the essence of the matter is that each of the participating professions needs the others to accomplish what, collectively, they have agreed are their objectives."

Although the differences between multi- and interdisciplinary approaches to rehabilitation have been described and are fairly well differentiated by rehabilitation professionals, the transdisciplinary approach is less common. It has also been referred to as a "blending" approach,[13] and some use *transdisciplinary* and *interdisciplinary* interchangeably.[40] At a semantic level, the prefix "inter" means "between." Conceptually, in an interdisciplinary approach, responsibilities are shared between disciplines with a shared responsibility for treatment goals. The prefix "trans" means "across," "beyond," or "through," and in rehabilitation it connotes going "beyond" or "through" the barriers established by one's professional training, to deliver treatment as determined by the goal (that is, the patient's needs), not by one's particular discipline.

The attempt to truly actualize this approach, of course, makes licensed professionals a bit unsure. There is potential for reduced accountability if clinicians are held responsible only for goals, not for the direct intervention most likely to achieve the goals. For example, Mary has a goal to use longer sentences with correct grammatical structures (*syntax*, in professional jargon). The occupational therapy assistant has the best rapport with Mary and sees her in treatment most often; therefore, she designs strategies to improve Mary's sentence length and structure. The speech-language pathologist provides guidance for Mary's program but has less direct responsibility for the progress, simply because of the time factor. In this scenario, how accountable is the speech-language pathologist?

An additional problem of accountability exists if treatment services are billed as "fee for service" or by discipline, as they typically are in the United States.[14] There is a level of increased ethical and legal risk if clinicians are required to bill for a service delivered by someone in a different discipline. Using the above example, under fee for service, how should the hypothetical occupational therapy assistant bill for a language treatment session?

Theoretically, the transdisciplinary approach has great merit, but accountability may be an issue. Because of accountability and billing issues, it is quite difficult to implement a transdisciplinary team approach. The author has worked in a traumatic brain injury rehabilitation center (in the United States) where a transdisciplinary approach was attempted. In the role of program director, the author interviewed staff regarding the success of the transdisciplinary approach. The consensus of the team's opinion was that professional expertise was not utilized in the best manner, the quality of treatment was diluted, and time was wasted with inefficient treatment. Therefore, it was not considered to be a cost-effective approach. This is not to say that a transdisciplinary approach is not to be preferred, only that attitudes, reimbursement mechanisms, and the training needs of the team must be evaluated carefully prior to the implementation of any approach. In the author's opinion, a strong commitment from the organization, extending beyond financial consideration, is needed for the transdisciplinary approach to be successful.

In many settings, the same can be said of the interdisciplinary approach. Although the interdisciplinary team approach has been used in brain injury rehabilitation for at least a decade, its success in producing better outcomes than can be accomplished with a multidisciplinary team has not been established. Further, most interdisciplinary teams are managed by placing additional responsibilities on team members, who, in most settings, have other responsibilities to their departments (discipline specific) that may or may not support the team effort. Most organizations allocate resources (clinical and support personnel, space, equipment, et cetera) according to the productivity of the individual departments, not according to the productivity of a particular team. Under this type of organizational structure, the interdisciplinary team is expensive.[41] Regardless of the specific approach, for the team to be effective there must be a great deal of communication among team members. This typically translates into time spent in meetings, resulting in lost revenues.

In recent years, the author has witnessed a change in the organizational structure of many health care facilities, from discipline-specific departments to program teams, much like the change seen in the manufacturing industry (especially the computer field) in the 1970s and 1980s. (This is also known as the movement to "do away with middle management.") According to personal communication with a number of clinicians who have worked in settings that have implemented program-based organizational structures, there appears to be a loss of professional identity, when departments are abolished, and a perceived lack of support for the unique role of the discipline. As students, clinicians are seldom taught the skills needed to be successful members of a team, and instead are quite focused on professional identity.[41] Organizations that are not sensitive to this, and do not allocate the resources for training clinicians in team dynamics and group interaction, will fail to meet the goals of increased efficiency and improved quality of care. Clinicians can help themselves be better contributors to the team by taking continuing education courses in team leadership and team dynamics, and by taking courses in communication—such as group dynamics—while still enrolled in their academic programs.

TYPES OF REHABILITATION PROGRAMS

Terms Used and Regulation Requirements

Terms used to refer to types of traumatic brain injury rehabilitation can be confusing, as some refer to the type of facility, and others refer to programs. In this section, both facility types and program types are discussed. Although most types are included, new programs and terms appear

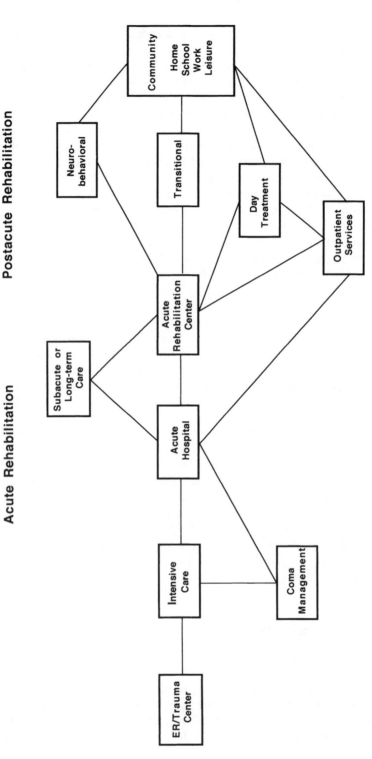

Figure 2.2 The continuum of traumatic brain injury rehabilitation services.

frequently. For the most part, the terms used to refer to programs are not standardized in any way. Moreover, this section is provided only as an overview of the types of programs, and does not provide sufficient detail to develop programs, but it should provide clinicians with an understanding of the differences among programs and the types of services that can be expected in each. Figure 2.2 depicts the continuum of traumatic brain injury rehabilitation services.

Finally, facilities that provide inpatient health care services are regulated by state licensing agencies (usually under the Department of Health and Human Services), and therefore must legally meet certain standards. The detail of the standards depends upon the nature of the services provided, with hospitals probably having to meet the largest number of standards. Organizations that participate in the Medicare program (inpatient and outpatient) must also meet certain federal standards in order to receive reimbursement from Medicare. Programs, on the other hand, are not necessarily regulated in any manner. The *Commission on Accreditation of Rehabilitation Facilities (CARF)*[42] is an independent (nongovernmental) agency that establishes and promotes standards for rehabilitation facilities and evaluates programs according to these standards. However, organizations choose voluntarily to comply with these standards and to become "accredited." Consequently, the Commission has no regulatory power over the organizations it surveys. For these reasons, rehabilitation programs that occur outside of state licensing bodies are, for the most part, self-regulatory.

In recent years fraud and abuse have been widely reported within the field of brain injury rehabilitation,[43] and in 1992 a federal investigation was conducted. Among the many findings of the Human Resources and Intergovernmental Relations Subcommittee[44] that led to the "oversight investigation of the rehabilitation industry serving Americans with head injuries," were poor regulation by state authorities, overcharging and failure to deliver services, and abuse of patient rights. Unfortunately, it is often up to the consumer—and in the case of employment, the clinician—to investigate the legal and ethical practices of rehabilitation facilities. Clinicians are provided some guidelines for evaluating programs at the end of this chapter.

Critical Care

Rehabilitation, typically, is not an aspect of emergency room treatment, with the possible exception of consultation services. Yet, this is the point at which most persons with traumatic brain injury enter into the rehabilitation continuum. Programs that exist at this level are largely educational aimed at families and the trauma center/emergency room personnel.

After leaving the emergency room, persons with severe injuries typically move into intensive care units, most often neurosurgical intensive care. At this point, acute rehabilitation teams evaluate patients at most hospitals, and begin family education programs.[45] Sometimes the services are well coordinated, but typically each discipline treats patients independently of the other disciplines.

Coma stimulation programs may be offered in the intensive care setting. These programs are aimed at the earliest possible intervention, with a goal of providing sensory stimulation to facilitate emergence from coma. Preventive measures should be an important aspect of coma management programs (for example, reducing the risk of decubitus ulcers, pulmonary infections, contractures). Coma stimulation programs were quite popular in the eighties and developed at a rapid rate inside and outside of hospital settings. They are also referred to as *coma management programs.* Coma management programs may exist in a variety of settings, including acute hospitalization (following intensive care), acute and subacute rehabilitation, and nursing homes. The nature of these programs is discussed in detail in Chapter Seven.

Because of the expense of the heavily staffed intensive care units, patients are transferred to other units or floors of hospitals once they have stabilized and no longer require frequent monitoring. At this point, when the patient is no longer in a life and death situation, programs may be considered *acute rehabilitation,* but they are also referred to as *acute hospitalization with rehabilitation services.* Services provided in the acute hospital setting may or may not be interdisciplinary in approach. Large hospitals usually have an acute care rehabilitation team, but most often clinicians on the team provide services to a variety of patients and not just to those with traumatic brain injuries.

Acute and Subacute Rehabilitation Programs

The majority of urban areas in the United States have one or more hospitals with rehabilitation centers. *Acute rehabilitation centers* may be freestanding (separate from, although often attached to, the hospital), or they may be limited to a unit, floor, or wing within the hospital. Freestanding rehabilitation centers, and even units within hospitals, frequently will have (and should have) designated beds for patients with traumatic brain injury. In these settings, therapies typically are provided in discipline-specific areas, although in facilities committed to a team approach, an entire team may work together in a designated area. The distinction between acute rehabilitation centers and acute hospitalization with rehabilitation services is usually the level of medical care required by the patient and the extent of nursing and physician support provided.

Subacute generally refers to the level of care required by the patient as well, and implies that the level of acuteness (that is, requiring aggressive, intensive, and comprehensive medical management) is lower than that seen in an acute hospital or rehabilitation center. One might interpret this to mean that patients in subacute settings have progressed well and require little intervention, but this is generally not the case. These patients usually have a low activity level and cannot tolerate a great deal of therapy, but they do not require the level of medical services provided in an intensive care or acute hospital unit. A coma management program might be offered in a subacute unit, depending upon the nature of the particular facility.

Subacute rehabilitation units have become increasingly popular in recent years, as rehabilitation services have grown in *skilled nursing facilities (SNFs)*.[46] (*Skilled nursing facility* is a classification under the Medicare program.) Often, in acute rehabilitation/hospital settings, patients who have slowed in their progress are transferred to a subacute program as a temporary arrangement in hopes that their status and tolerance for activity may improve to the extent that they can be transferred to an acute rehabilitation program. Because of the rapid growth of subacute programs, standards have been developed by the Commission on the Accreditation of Rehabilitation Facilities and the Joint Commission on the Accreditation of Healthcare Organizations.[46]

Postacute Rehabilitation Programs

Postacute rehabilitation can occur in any number of settings, including hospitals, freestanding rehabilitation centers, psychiatric hospitals, outpatient clinics, office space, vocational centers, renovated homes and schools, and churches. The setting or facility is not what defines the type of program(s) so much as the nature and focus of the services provided. As with coma management programs, the 1980s witnessed the rapid growth of a variety of residential programs aimed at the postacute level of rehabilitation. These are often called *transitional programs,* as they are not intended to be an end point but rather a "transition" to returning to the community. Such programs may focus on the activities of daily living, school, or work, or they may offer some other type of specialized service, such as behavioral management. The hallmark of transitional programs is that they are intended to facilitate the return of the individual to the community, and to prepare the individual for that return. Unfortunately, a number of these programs were developed in isolated areas outside of any urban district, which brings into question their real ability to offer programming at the level of community re-entry. The programs with good financial resources were (and many still are) quite self-contained, complete with work opportunities, stores, apartments, and recreational facilities. Since the majority of persons with traumatic brain injury do not have the resources to remain in such self-contained facilities for their entire life, one might also question the suitability and ecological validity of these "simulated" real life experiences. In some instances, however, the cities near these facilities have become the community or home for individuals in the program.

A number of postacute programs are situated within urban areas and do utilize these real communities. Programs that are provided on an outpatient basis typically offer services to persons from the local community, or at least to those in an area that is within driving distance; hence, they utilize the community in which the patients actually live. The focus of the facility may be such that programs are simply an array of multidisciplinary services (therapies) provided at an intensive level (several hours per day), or for only a few hours per week. The intensive daily programs are usually referred to as *day treatment* and the weekly programs as *outpatient.* Technically, both are outpatient programs, because the individuals receiving services reside in a place other than the facility.

Often, the distinguishing feature between outpatient and day treatment is only the intensity of the therapy offered. Ideally, however, day treatment programs should be well coordinated and interdisciplinary in approach[47] with the aim of preparing the patient for school, work, and community re-entry. Programs of this nature should have the flexibility to truly individualize each patient's services. Within a day treatment center, there may actually be several programs: school re-entry (college included), work re-entry (or entry, given the number of persons with traumatic brain injury who do not have an established work history), and community living, for individuals who may not return to school or work, but who can live more independently in their community than would be possible without the services.

Other Programs

In addition to the above, there are programs and facilities that provide services to subpopulations of patients with traumatic brain injury. Two of these are: *pediatric programs* and *neurobehavioral programs.* Again, in the 1980s, specialized programs were advertised frequently at conferences and in publications on traumatic brain injury rehabilitation. The underlying concept behind specialized programs is that treating persons with similar disabilities together, in programs specifically geared to their unique needs, is better than treating them in general programs. As stated in the introductory chapter, most would agree that children should not be treated as adults, or in settings with a majority of adults. Therefore, pediatric programs are necessary, whether inpatient or outpatient.

On the other hand, neurobehavioral programs are almost always conducted on an inpatient or residential basis, because the behavioral disabilities are severe, requiring 24 hour programming, and the individuals require a great deal of supervision. These programs are often provided in psychiatric facilities or in psychiatric facilities with a rehabilitation "branch." Clinicians working in these settings must be well trained in behavioral management techniques, including the management of physically aggressive behaviors—something most rehabilitation professionals are not trained to manage.

Evaluating Programs as a Clinician/Employee

It is unfortunate, but true, that many of the decisions regarding rehabilitation programming and approaches are based on financial considerations. The eighties experienced an amazing growth in facilities and program types because funding was available and traumatic brain injury rehabilitation was a profitable industry.[48] Few of these program types have been evaluated for their effectiveness.[49] Nonetheless, by recognizing the range of programs that has been developed, clinicians can improve their understanding of the diversity of the needs of this population—a factor that has not changed with funding, and is not likely to change in the near future. Additionally, this overview should provide clinicians with a basis for comparison regarding the type of setting in which they might wish to work. The guidelines listed below, in the form of questions and suggestions, can be used to evaluate programs as a clinician and potential employee of an organization. Failure to obtain complete answers to all the questions does not, in and of itself, reflect negatively on the program. Newly established programs may not have a complete policy and procedure manual, inservice education programs, or a large staff with whom to interview. The intentions of the program to develop procedures and systems, and to refine organizational structure, are important. Evasiveness in answers, conflicting answers, disorganization, or a lack of organizational and program expectations may be cause for concern.

Questions to Consider When Evaluating Programs as a Clinician/Employee

- What is the management structure of the organization?
- What regulatory agencies oversee the services?
- Are criteria for admission applied consistently?
- When exceptions are made to criteria, what are the bases for these decisions?
- What are the organization's policies on charitable care?
- How is the organization supported (for example, by profits, grants, charitable contributions, endowment)?
- Does the organization have a quality improvement program?
- Does the brain injury program have a program evaluation system?
- How are patients' rights protected?
- How are patients and families involved in the program?
- What is the typical staff/patient ratio?
- What is the staff turnover rate?
- Is there an employee grievance policy and procedure?
- Is there a consumer grievance policy and/or procedure?
- Are there provisions for continuing education and inservice training?
- Ask to review marketing materials and outcome data.

- Ask to examine the policy and procedure manual, although many organizations protect this information.
- Ask to interview with more than one person, but always interview with the person who will be the clinical and/or administrative supervisor.

Additionally the following should be observed:

- The general appearance of the facility, interior and exterior.
  Is it safe?
  Is it accessible?
  Is it clean?
  Are there enough restrooms for staff and patients?
  Are escape routes posted?
  Are credentials and licenses posted?
  Is a mission statement of the organization posted?
  Does the physical environment support the mission of the program (for example, if it is a community re-entry program, is it in the community or in a hospital)?
- The general appearance and attitude of the staff.
- The general appearance and attitude of the patients.

SUMMARY

Medicine and rehabilitation employ a number of models, approaches, and programs, with which clinicians should become familiar. These are not merely theoretical; they operationally define the manner in which services are delivered. This chapter has presented a global view of how disease and disability are conceptualized in society, as a framework from which to consider traumatic brain injury as more than a unique diagnostic label.

The *medical model* (traditional, paternalistic, and biomedical or scientific), *contractual model, educational model,* and *empowerment model* are some of the predominant models followed in rehabilitation. In general, these models delineate the conceptualization of disease and disability within the context of the provider-patient relationship. A description and critique of each has been provided. The *International Classification of Impairments, Disabilities, and Handicaps* was introduced as the predominant classification system used to describe the consequences of disease. *Impairment* refers to the psychological, anatomical or physiological loss or abnormality of structure or function (for example, loss of a leg). *Disability* is the restriction in activity (for example, walking) that results from the impairment. *Handicap* is the disadvantage to or limits placed on the individual because of an impairment or disability (for example, the inability to work, if work requires the use of the leg or requires the ability to walk). A common criticism leveled against rehabilitation is that its efforts are largely focused at the level of impairment, when it is the level of handicap that impacts quality of life the most.

The approach to rehabilitation most often observed in traumatic brain injury rehabilitation is the team approach. The differences among the *multidisciplinary, interdisciplinary,* and *transdisciplinary* approaches have been discussed, along with the financial and ethical considerations that affect them. The need for clinician training in team communication and dynamics was emphasized.

The scope of rehabilitation services in the field of traumatic brain injury rehabilitation is considerably larger today than it was in the 1970s, and clinicians have a wide choice of settings in which to work. A continuum of rehabilitation programs exists, ranging from intensive care and coma stimulation programs to transitional and day treatment programs. A brief description of each has been provided, along with a discussion of the regulation of rehabilitation programs and a list of questions and suggestions to serve as guidelines to the clinician seeking employment.

REFERENCES

1. Veatch RM. The medical model: its nature and problems. *Hastings Centers Studies.* 1973;1:59–76.
2. Toombs SK. The meaning of illness: a phenomenological approach to the patient-physician relationship. *Journal of Medicine and Philosophy.* 1987;12: 219–240.
3. Sedgwick P. Illness—mental and otherwise. *Hastings Center Studies.* 1973;1:19–40.
4. Szasz T. The myth of mental illness. *American Psychologist.* 1960;15:113–118.
5. Sparedo FR, Gill D. Effects of prior alcohol use in head injury recovery. *Journal of Head Trauma Rehabilitation.* 1989;4:75–82.
6. Veatch RM. *The Patient-Physician Relationship.* Bloomington, IN: University Press; 1991:196–210.
7. Caplan AL, Callahan D, Haas J. Ethical and policy issues in rehabilitation medicine. *Hastings Center Report.* 1987;17:1–20.
8. Emanuel EJ, Emanuel LL. Four models of the physician-patient relationship. *Journal of the American Medical Association.* 1992;267:2221–2226.
9. Williams RS. Ability, dis-ability and rehabilitation: a phenomenological description. *Journal of Medicine and Philosophy.* 1984;9:93–112.
10. Levin DM, Solomon GF. The discursive formation of the body in the history of medicine. *Journal of Medicine and Philosophy.* 1990;15:515–537.
11. Stanczak DE, Hutcherson WL. Acute rehabilitation of the head-injured individual: toward a neuropsychological paradigm of treatment. In Long CJ, Ross LK (eds). *Handbook of Head Trauma: Acute Care to Recovery.* New York, NY: Plenum Press; 1992:125–136.
12. Whitman M. Case management in head injury rehabilitation. *Rehabilitation Nursing.* 1991;16:19–22.
13. Goldstein G, Ruthven L. *Rehabilitation of the Brain-Damaged Adult.* New York, NY: Plenum Press; 1983:44–92.

14. Wood RL. A salient factors approach to brain injury rehabilitation. In Wood RL, Eames PG (eds). *Models of Brain Injury Rehabilitation*. Baltimore, MD. Johns Hopkins University Press;1989:75–99.
15. Condeluci A. Brain injury rehabilitation: the need to bridge paradigms. *Brain Injury*. 1992;6:543–551.
16. Caplan AL. Informed consent and provider-patient relationships in rehabilitation medicine. *Archives of Physical Medicine and Rehabilitation*. 1988;69:312–317.
17. Anderson TP. Educational frame of reference: an additional model for rehabilitation. *Archives of Physical Medicine and Rehabilitation*. 1978;59:203–206.
18. Scofield GR. Ethical considerations in rehabilitation medicine. *Archives of Physical Medicine and Rehabilitation*. 1993;74:341–346.
19. Batavia AI. Assessing the function of functional assessment: a consumer perspective. *Disability and Rehabilitation*. 1992;14:156–160.
20. O'Hara CC, Harrell M. The empowerment rehabilitation model: meeting the unmet needs of survivors, families, and treatment providers. *Journal of Cognitive Rehabilitation*. 1991;9:14–21.
21. Halbertsma J. The ICIDH: health problems in a medical and social perspective. *Disability and Rehabilitation*. 1995;17:128–134.
22. Badley EM. The genesis of handicap: definition, models of disablement, and role of external factors. *Disability and Rehabilitation*. 1995;17:53–62.
23. de Kleijn-de Vrankrijker MW. The international classification of impairments, disabilities, and handicaps (ICIDH): perspectives and developments (Part I). *Disability and Rehabilitation*. 1995;17:109–111.
24. Practice Management Information Corporation. *International Classification of Diseases, 9th rev-Clinical Modification, 4th rev, Vol 1*. Los Angeles, CA: Practice Management Information Corporation, 1995.
25. Gray J, Dean E. Functional aspects of communication disorders. In Greenwood R, Barnes MP, McMillan TM, Ward CD (eds). *Neurological Rehabilitation*. Edinburgh, Scotland: Churchill Livingstone; 1993:355–362.
26. Holland AL. *Communicative Abilities in Daily Living*. Baltimore, MD: University Park Press; 1980.
27. Hartley LL. *Cognitive-Communicative Abilities Following Brain Injury: A Functional Approach*. San Diego, CA: Singular Publishing Group; 1995.
28. Granger CV, Greer DS. Functional status measurement and medical rehabilitation outcomes. *Archives of Physical Medicine and Rehabilitation*. 1976;57:103–109.
29. Heinemann AW et al. Relationships between impairment and physical disability as measured by the Functional Independence Measure. *Archives of Physical Medicine and Rehabilitation*. 1993;74:566–573.
30. Dodds TA et al. A validation of the Functional Independence Measurement and its performance among rehabilitation inpatients. *Archives of Physical Medicine and Rehabilitation*. 1993;74:531–536.
31. Kaplan CP, Corrigan JD. The relationship between cognition and functional independence in adults with traumatic brain injury. *Archives of Physical Medicine and Rehabilitation*. 1994;75:643–647.
32. Johnston MV, Keith RA, Hinderer SR. Measurement standards for interdisciplinary medical rehabilitation. *Archives of Physical Medicine and Rehabilitation*. 1992;73:S3–S23.

33. Stineman MG et al. Four methods for characterizing disability in the formation of function related groups. *Archives of Physical Medicine and Rehabilitation.* 1994;75:1277–1283.

34. Cook L, Smith DS, Truman G. Using functional independence measure profiles as an index of outcome in the rehabilitation of brain-injured patients. *Archives of Physical Medicine and Rehabilitation.* 1994;75:390–393.

35. Johnston MV, Hall KM. Outcomes evaluation in traumatic brain injury rehabilitation part I: overview and system principles. *Archives of Physical Medicine and Rehabilitation.* 1994;75:SC2–SC9.

36. Fuhrer MJ. An agenda for medical rehabilitation outcomes research. *American Journal of Physical Medicine and Rehabilitation.* 1995;74:243–248.

37. Rothberg JS. The rehabilitation team: future direction. *Archives of Physical Medicine and Rehabilitation.* 1981;62:407–410.

38. Melvin JL. Interdisciplinary and multidisciplinary activities and the ACRM. *Archives of Physical Medicine and Rehabilitation.* 1980;61:379–380.

39. Fordyce WE. On interdisciplinary peers. *Archives of Physical Medicine and Rehabilitation.* 1981;62:51–53.

40. Giles GM, Clark-Wilson J. *Brain Injury Rehabilitation : A Neurofunctional Approach.* London, England: Chapman and Hall; 1993.

41. Melvin JL. Status report on interdisciplinary medical rehabilitation. *Archives of Physical Medicine and Rehabilitation.* 1989;70:273–276.

42. Commission on Accreditation of Rehabilitation Facilities. *Standards Manual and Interpretative Guidelines for Medical Rehabilitation.* Tucson, AZ: Commission on Accreditation of Rehabilitation Facilities; 1995:107–124.

43. Kerr P. Centers for head injury accused of earning millions for neglect. *New York Times.* March 16, 1992(sec)D4:1.

44. House Committee on Government Operations. *Fraud and Abuse in the Head Injury Rehabilitation Industry.* 102nd Congress, 2nd session; 1992. Report 102–1059.

45. Cowley RS et al. The role of rehabilitation in the intensive care unit. *Journal of Head Trauma Rehabilitation.* 1994;9:32–42.

46. Keith RA, Wilson DB, Gutierrez P. Acute and subacute rehabilitation for stroke: a comparison. *Archives of Physical Medicine and Rehabilitation.* 1995;76:495–500.

47. Evans RW, Preston BK. Day rehabilitation programming: a theoretical model. In Kreutzer JS, Wehman P (eds). *Community Integration Following Traumatic Brain Injury.* Baltimore, MD: Paul H Brookes Publishing; 1990:125–138.

48. Bistany DV. Overview of the economics of rehabilitation in the United States. In Christensen AL, Uzzell BP (eds). *Brain Injury and Neuropsychological Rehabilitation: International Perspectives.* NJ: Lawrence Erlbaum; 1994:244–255.

49. Evans RW, Ruff RM. Outcome and value: a perspective on rehabilitation outcomes achieved in acquired brain injury. *Journal Head Trauma Rehabilitation.* 1992;7:24–36.

3

Mechanisms of Traumatic Brain Injury and the Pathophysiologic Consequences

Rita J. Gillis and Jeffrey N. Pierce

Although the neuroanatomic and neurophysiologic aspects of brain injury are complex, and oftentimes presented with confusing terminology, it is essential that the rehabilitation clinician develop an understanding of the mechanisms underlying the neurobehavioral sequelae of traumatic brain injury. In most rehabilitation settings, the speech-language pathologist will be a member of a larger team of professionals, charged with the duty of developing and implementing an effective plan of care for the patient. A working knowledge of the underlying mechanisms of injury and the subsequent anatomic and physiologic changes to the brain will enable the speech-language pathologist to make informed decisions regarding both an expected course of recovery and the nature and timing of the treatment to be provided. This knowledge also will enhance an understanding of the factors outside of rehabilitative treatment that contribute to, and often determine, rehabilitation outcomes.

Most speech-language pathologists have a thorough understanding of the neuroanatomical correlates to speech and language functions, from their academic and clinical training. There are a number of texts that deal specifically with lesion analysis and localization theories of cognitive, linguistic, and motor functions. In this chapter, the authors assume that the readers have a basic understanding of the neuroanatomical correlates to these functions. This chapter deals largely with the anatomic and physiologic aspects of traumatic brain injury, with specific emphasis on nonmissile head injuries.

MECHANISMS OF INJURY

Our current understanding of the biomechanics of head injury comes largely from experimental animal studies, in which models of injury have been developed to reproduce the events of a traumatic injury to the head in man. The early, now landmark, experimental studies of Denny-Brown and Russell[1] heralded the more recent work of Gennarelli and colleagues,[2,3,4,5] who have contributed much toward the current thinking on the biomechanics of head injury . Denny-Brown and Russell were interested in determining the mechanisms of brain injury underlying concussion* (temporary neuronal disruption with loss of consciousness) in civilians, in part because they noted the relative absence of concussion secondary to missile head injuries in war time.[6] These early investigators used a pendulum to produce concussion in animals and determined that when the head was free to move, concussion resulted at a much lower velocity of force than when the head was supported and remained stationary. The authors referred to the former as "acceleration concussion" and the latter as "compression concussion" resulting from "crushing injury."*

Gennarelli and colleagues[7] have studied similar injuries using what is termed either a Penn I or Penn II device, in which inertially controlled, angular acceleration injuries to the head have been produced without direct impact to the skull. Through these experiments, and postmortem pathological studies of human brain tissue, they have refined our understanding of the mechanisms underlying brain injury resulting from trauma produced by mechanical forces. The principal forces that result in brain injury are impact, acceleration, and deceleration, as explained below.

Impact, Acceleration, and Deceleration Forces

Impact occurs when a moving object strikes the head, or the moving head strikes a slower moving or stationary object. The point at which the object hits the head is the *point of impact*. Impact or contact also occurs when portions of the brain strike rigid, immovable structures within the cranium. *Acceleration* occurs when an object increases in its rate of speed. This may occur when the head is suddenly propelled by an external force, such as a bat. Acceleration of the brain can occur without direct impact to the skull, as when the chest hits the steering wheel during an automobile accident, before the head comes into contact with the windshield, or as is commonly the case in football injuries. *Deceleration* occurs when an object in motion (such as the head) decreases in its speed or is forced to an abrupt stop when it hits a nonmoving object (such as the ground or the windshield of an automobile). Deceleration of the brain also occurs when the moving brain is "slowed" by the hard cranium.

Two types of acceleration have been presented in the literature, *translational* (linear) and *rotational* (angular). In translational acceleration, the head

*Note: *Concussion* is a widely disputed and poorly agreed upon term. A brief definition is provided here relative to the work of Denny-Brown. Concussion is addressed in greater detail under the classification of brain injury in Chapter Four.

abruptly moves in a linear direction. The brain's inertia causes it to remain stationary momentarily, until it is impacted by the moving skull and propelled forward. A blow or *coup* is delivered to this initial point of contact and generates a wave of force that spreads through the brain and causes it to strike the skull on the opposite side. This second blow is referred to as a *contrecoup* injury.[8,9] Some have suggested the contrecoup injury results in more severe impact damage than the initial blow,[9] although neuro-pathological studies have not supported this view.[7] Translational or linear forces are also present in deceleration of the brain, which may cause coup and contrecoup lesions.[8]

Rotational acceleration occurs with angular or rotational movements of the head. This may result in torsion or twisting of the relatively fixed brain stem by the more freely movable cerebrum. In both rotational and transla-tional acceleration, the soft tissues of the brain are forced against the irregu-lar and rigid contours of the cranial vault. The frontal and temporal lobes are particularly vulnerable to injury from the angular surface of the skull's base and the temporal and frontal bones.[10,11]

Because many studies that examine the effects of acceleration forces take place in the laboratory, the distinction between these two experimentally-controlled forces is of greater academic than clinical relevance. In the nonexperimental conditions of actual human head injuries, both directional forces are assumed to be present. The rotational forces, however, are thought to make the greatest contribution to the diffuse axonal injuries (discussed later in the chapter), now commonly accepted as the primary pathological alteration seen in nonmissile traumatic brain injuries.[12] Addi-tionally, in the laboratory setting, the magnitude of the forces of impact—velocity, direction, and duration of acceleration—can be individually manipulated and the effects of each examined. It is well accepted that the severity and type of brain injury encountered are dependent upon the configuration of these variables (for example, varying speeds of motor vehicle accidents), which are not controlled in common events. In non-experimental human brain injuries, both acceleration and deceleration of the brain occur; therefore, these injuries are sometimes referred to as *acceleration-deceleration injuries.*

Nonaccelerating injuries, in which the head is not in movement and is fixed (not free to move), are rare[8] but may be seen. These are the "crushing injuries" produced experimentally by Denny-Brown and Russell. Pang[8] pro-vides an example of the auto mechanic who is working under an automobile that falls and compresses the skull, yet little to no neurologic impairment is suffered. These laboratory and clinical findings emphasize the devastating effects of acceleration and deceleration forces, which may leave the skull virtually intact yet cause severe brain injury.

In defining mechanisms of injury, the distinction must again be made between injuries that compromise the integrity, and hence the sterility, of the cranial vault, and those that do not. By definition, open head injury requires that the meninges be exposed to bacterial contamination, and hence risk infection. This may occur after a scalp laceration alone, but usually occurs following a depressed skull fracture or as the result of penetrating trauma, such as a gunshot wound.[13] Gunshot wounds (missile injuries) are unique in that shock waves are generated by the penetrating bullet. The size or caliber of the projectile and the velocity of penetration are the primary variables that determine the forces generated. The pathophysiology presented in the next section largely addresses nonmissile traumatic brain injuries.

PATHOPHYSIOLOGY

Focal Versus Diffuse Damage

Many authors discuss the consequences of brain injury in terms of *focal* and *diffuse* damage.[10,14] Gennarelli[12] defines focal brain injuries as those "in which a lesion large enough to be visualized with the naked eye has occurred." Focal injury includes cerebral contusions, intracranial hematomas, hemorrhages, brain shift, and other mass lesions, discussed below. Diffuse injuries are characterized by widespread or global disruption of neuronal structures and function. Diffuse damage includes hypoxic and ischemic brain damage, diffuse axonal injury, and small, punctate hemorrhages. These injuries are discussed in the following sections.

The consequences of brain injury also are often classified as *focal deficits* or *diffuse deficits*. Focal deficits are associated with specific anatomic lesions; diffuse deficits reflect and are attributable to the widespread disruption of cortical and subcortical functions. These distinctions are useful in the acute medical setting, where course of treatment is based on the pattern of neurologic deficits. It is particularly important for the speech-language pathologist to understand such distinctions because traditional training places much emphasis on lesion analysis and localization of language functions. In the rehabilitation setting, where traumatic brain injury is common, it is not unusual to observe mixed patterns of brain damage. In such cases, the decisions for treatment should be based on the predominant patterns of impairment[10] (that is, cognitive, linguistic, speech, and/or behavioral).

Although the focal/diffuse dichotomy is useful, it is also important to understand the pathophysiology of traumatic brain injury in regard to its chronology. The pathological events of traumatic brain injury are discussed most frequently in terms of *primary* and *secondary* injuries. Primary injuries are those that occur immediately upon impact of the head; secondary injuries are the complications resulting from, and subsequent to, the initial injury. *Injury, damage, trauma,* and *insult* are frequently used interchangeably in the literature, in terms such as primary injury and secondary insult, or primary trauma and secondary damage. *Epiphenomena* is a term also used to refer to the secondary events of head injury.[8] The choice of terminology is one that is based largely on an author's perspective rather than on unique and specific meanings of the terms. The usefulness of the distinction between "primary" and "secondary" is that secondary injuries have a delay in onset and are the focus of many of the critical early medical and surgical interventions that attempt to prevent and ameliorate the delayed effects of the initial injury. Identification of these as potentially preventable or reversible secondary effects has served to reduce mortality and morbidity through aggressive treatment.

Primary Injury

Lacerations, Contusions, and Skull Fractures

As previously stated, primary injuries are those sustained immediately upon impact (at the moment of impact) and may yield both focal and diffuse brain damage. They sometimes are referred to as impact injuries and are rarely affected by treatment.[15] The types of injuries sustained immediately include *lacerations, contusions, skull fractures,* and *diffuse axonal injury.* Hematomas (an accumulation of blood) are in some instances discussed as primary injuries because of the instantaneous nature with which they can occur, but they are considered here as secondary because they occur only following disruption of the blood vessels. They are discussed thoroughly in the following section. Management of hematomas is a critical early intervention and, in that sense, they are of primary concern. The classification of injuries as strictly primary or secondary is somewhat arbitrary, but is a commonly used system.

Lacerations are cuts that may occur to the scalp, meninges, brain, or vascular structures. They are differentiated from *tears,* which are the result of opposing forces pulling upon tissues or vessels. Lacerations to the scalp are significant in that rapid blood loss may occur. Lacerations to the bridging veins of the subarachnoid space and meningeal vessels are significant for their ability to produce hematomas that may expand and compress the brain. Lacerations to the brain produce focal hemorrhagic lesions.

Contusions (bruises) are defined as a "structural alteration of the brain usually involving the surface characterized by extravasation [leakage from the vessel] of blood cells and tissue death."[16] Contusions are heterogeneous in their makeup (as compared to hematomas) and consist of necrotic brain tissue, hemorrhage, and in the acute stages, edema. Contusions begin as areas of hemorrhage and resolve over time to become encapsulated areas of hemorrhagic infarction (tissue death),[17] also observed as "shrunken brown scars."[7]

Contusions and lacerations occur in patterns of some predictability because of the structure of the cranium. The regions of the brain most susceptible to these injuries are the frontal and temporal poles (tips) and the undersurfaces of these lobes, because of their proximity to bony structures of the cranium. The frontal damage following traumatic brain injury has come to have great clinical significance as researchers have learned more about the role of the frontal lobes in cognitive functions. This point is expanded further, later in the text. Although contusions are found predominantly in these regions, they may extend into the white matter of the subcortical regions.[13,14] Focal damage may occur at the point of primary contact (coup injuries) or at the point where the cortex is contused or lacerated by the bony prominences and rigid structures of the skull, falx cerebri, and tentorium. Typically, contusions are found at the site of injury only when there is a depressed skull fracture.[15]

Skull fractures are significant diagnostically for the implications they bring to the emergency setting. Fractures of the skull are more common in patients who have sustained a severe head injury.[13] Depressed skull fractures increase the potential for infection and are likely to produce focal damage and swelling at the site. Fractures that allow communication between the intracranial cavity and the sinuses also present an increased risk of infection. Skull fractures are associated with a higher incidence of intracranial hematomas, and are almost always found in the presence of extradural hematomas. (See discussion of hematomas below.) Contusions are more severe when there has been a fracture of the skull.[14] However, fractures to the skull, in and of themselves, are not an indication of the severity of brain damage. Similarly, the absence of a skull fracture does not signify absence of brain damage.[18] A Left occipital bone fracture with contrecoup injury is shown in Figure 3.1. Figure 3.2 demonstrates the type of frontal lobe damage commonly observed in acceleration-deceleration injuries. Together these figures show the extensive nature of brain damage that may occur following a severe traumatic brain injury.

Diffuse Axonal Injury

Diffuse axonal injury (DAI) is now understood to be the principal type of injury in nonmissile traumatic brain injuries.[7,8,10,12,14,15,19] Much of our understanding of the pattern of diffuse axonal injury comes from pathology studies of brain tissue during autopsy, and from the study of experimentally produced injuries in animals.[15] Diffuse axonal injury was first identified as diffuse degeneration of white matter thought to be the result of the shearing of the axons during rotational acceleration of the brain.[20,21] Therefore, diffuse axonal injury has previously been referred to as *shearing injury* and *diffuse white matter shearing injury.*[22] The presence of diffuse axonal injury is diagnosed definitively by microscopic examination only. Indeed, it is now accepted that a normal (that is, negative) computerized tomography (CT) scan does not rule out brain injury.[23]

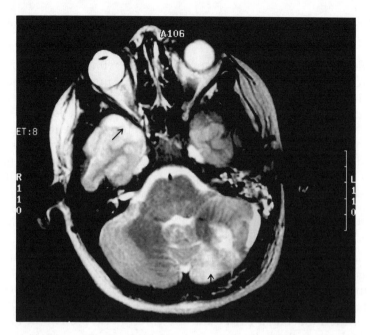

Figure 3.1 MRI of the head in a transverse plane showing a left occipital bone fracture and left cerebellar contusion with contrecoup edema in the anterior temporal lobes.

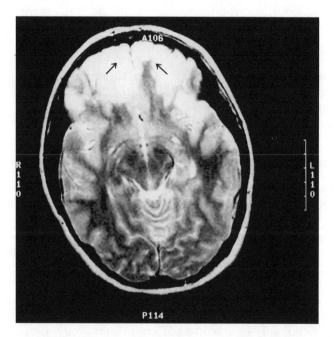

Figure 3.2 MRI of the head in a transverse plane showing anterior frontal lobe contusions in the same patient as Figure 3.1.

The distribution of axonal injury is neither symmetrical nor uniform, and axonal swellings may "occur particularly in the parasagittal white matter, in the corpus callosum, . . . in the internal capsule, in deep grey matter and in various tracts in the brain stem."[11] The histological findings vary over time such that, following survival of several months, evidence of myelin breakdown can be found in the white matter throughout the hemispheres, cerebellum, and brain stem fiber tracts.

In the clinical setting, the presence of diffuse axonal injury is assumed when small hemorrhagic lesions,[22] referred to as *tissue tear hemorrhages*,[24] are present. These have a characteristic pattern of diffuse distribution in the cortical and subcortical regions with propensity for the corpus callosum, the superior cerebellar peduncle, and the dorsolateral quadrant of the rostral brain stem,[12] although Wilberger et al.[24] noted a spectrum in location of tissue tear hemorrhages. Adams et al.[7] have observed that patients with multiple small hemorrhages die soon after injury. Therefore, individuals with diffuse injury of this nature would not be seen in rehabilitation settings. However, these patients are sometimes seen in the clinical setting.[24] Tissue tear hemorrhages predict a poor prognosis in terms of outcome, as they are indicative of severe diffuse axonal injury, but they represent a clinically challenging population to the rehabilitation clinician.

Coma of more than six hours is also clinical evidence of diffuse axonal injury.[12] Gennarelli[22] has classified diffuse axonal injury into three categories: mild, evidenced by coma of six to twenty-four hours; moderate, evidenced by prolonged coma of more than twenty-four hours with prominent signs of brain stem dysfunction; and severe, evidenced by coma of more than twenty-four hours, with clear brain stem dysfunction. The latter two categories indicate the presence of diffuse axonal injury in the brain stem as well as the cortex. Although damage to the axons is commonly accepted as a primary injury produced in movement trauma, the progression of axonal disruption is still under investigation. Microscopic investigations by Strich[20,21] and others[2,3,5,25] have since demonstrated that primary damage occurs to the axon as a result of stretching during rotational acceleration. With enough force, the axon is transected and severed from its connection with the cell body, and hence is said to be *deafferentated*. Following transection, the axon's severed ends pull away from each other and retract. The axon stump swells and forms a retraction ball or bulb, which is the hallmark microscopic finding of diffuse axonal damage. Whether the majority of axons suffer structural damage at the time of injury, as suggested by the early work of Strich, or suffer structural damage secondary to intracellular metabolic disruption, is a topic of current controversy and ongoing investigation. It is not surprising that new theories of the nature of axonal damage are being developed that challenge the structural view of axonal damage. In fact, Strich's work was challenged initially by those who thought that the widespread degeneration of the white matter was due largely to secondary factors such as hypoxia and edema, rather than to primary structural damage at the time of injury.[11] The experimental studies by Gennarelli and colleagues, over the last 20 years, may be credited for definitively demonstrating that primary structural axonal damage occurs that is not attributable to secondary insults.[14]

The more recent controversy over the nature of axonal injury has to do with the onset of the damage. Investigations within the last ten years suggest that axotomy (severing of the axon) may be the result of a more progressive, degenerative process in which trauma disrupts the axolemma (the membrane surrounding the axon) and subsequently impairs the transport of axoplasm.[17,19] The result is continued reactive swelling at the site of trauma which, if unarrested, leads to separation. The more distant segment of the detached axon eventually degenerates (referred to as Wallerian degeneration). The fact that pathologists are unable to identify axonal retraction balls (with light microscopy) for a period of twelve hours following the initial injury[22] suggests that the axonal changes are largely progressive and occur over time.

Diffuse axonal injury is the most important single factor that determines recovery and ultimate outcome in traumatic brain injury.[12,26] Consequently, the potential for this exciting area of study is apparent. If the nature of the axonal injury is more progressive than originally presumed, early intervention, designed to affect the neurochemical processes that lead to axonal loss, may ultimately reduce the severity of diffuse axonal damage.

Secondary Injury

Following a head injury, a number of complications may occur that adversely affect the patient's course of recovery and hence rehabilitation outcome. As stated previously, the early identification of these potential complications can reduce the morbidity of the initial injury. In part, it is the extent of the secondary complications, along with the severity of the diffuse axonal injury, that accounts for the significant differences observed within the heterogeneous population with traumatic brain injury. When traumatic brain injury is the result of an automobile accident, the brain is rarely the only injured structure. Injuries to other organs and systems (for example, lungs and heart) can compromise the functions of the already stressed brain, resulting in further insult.

Hematomas

Hematomas are collections of extravasated blood, and are therefore *space occupying lesions* (also called *expanding lesions*). Several classification systems of hematomas are found in the literature and include: *extradural* and *intradural* (including *subdural* and *intracerebral*) or *extracerebral* and *intracerebral*. Alternately, they have been grouped as *epidural* (extradural), *subdural*, and *intracerebral* or *intracranial*. Hematomas should be detected and managed immediately because of their potential to produce further brain damage by expansion.

Extradural hematomas (EDH), also epidural hematomas, occur as a result of direct trauma to the skull with concomitant tearing of meningeal vessels.[27] These occur mostly in the temporoparietal region in the location of the middle meningeal artery and vein.[13] With the inbending of the skull, the vessels are torn, and arterial blood pressure forces blood into the "potential" space between the dura and the skull. The dura and underlying brain are compressed within the confines of the cranial vault by arterial bleeding. Although fractures are frequently associated with extradural hematomas, the meningeal arteries may be torn in the absence of a fracture and produce a hematoma.[27]

Subdural hematomas (SDH) occur between the inner surface of the dura and the brain. Like contusions, they are somewhat predictable in their location, occurring most frequently in the frontal or temporal lobes. Subdural hematomas are common in traumatic brain injury, especially in injuries involving deceleration forces traveling in an anterior-posterior path. These forces tend to shear the veins that bridge the brain and dural sinuses. Since the dura is adherent to the brain, the veins may be torn as the brain moves within the cranium. Small unilateral injuries are more frequent and usually clot quickly, since the venous blood is under relatively low pressure. Massive injuries may be bilateral and result in large subdural hematomas that lead to herniation.[28]

Temporal lobe hematomas are associated with increased risk of brain stem compression.[29] The so-called "temporal lobe burst" or exploded temporal lobe, which is poorly defined but frequently cited in the literature, occurs when a subdural hematoma develops over a contusion (or intracerebral hematoma) at the temporal pole.[30] These may also occur at the frontal poles. Figure 3.3 shows a contusion with hemorrhage and edema in the left temporal lobe of an individual who sustained a traumatic brain injury.

Intracerebral hematomas probably develop from the tearing of the cerebral vessels during acceleration-deceleration of the brain, and may occur deep within the hemispheres. The difference between hemorrhagic contusions and hematomas, as provided by Cooper,[27] is that "intracerebral hematomas are well-defined, homogeneous collections of blood [and] hemorrhagic contusions are mixtures of blood and contused and edematous cerebral parenchyma." Like contusions, intracerebral hematomas occur principally in the temporal and frontal lobes and are rare in the posterior cranium.[27] These areas are, of course, important to the speech-language pathologist because of the location of speech and language functions.

Cortical contusions and hematomas result in neurological dysfunction both by causing local brain damage and by causing masses within the cranium. If not carefully managed, these masses can lead to secondary brain shift, herniation, and ultimately brain stem compression and death. *Brain distortion, midline shift, and herniation* often occur with hematomas, edema, or

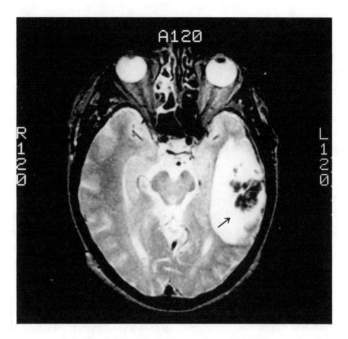

Figure 3.3 MRI of the head in a transverse plane showing a left temporal lobe contusion with hemorrhage and edema.

any lesion that occupies space. *Brain distortion* is the impingement upon the brain from any mass-producing lesion. *Midline shift* refers to the radiographic appearance of midline intracranial structures that are displaced laterally by pressure-producing masses. If sufficient force has been generated on one side of the brain to displace a midline structure, midline shift is said to be present. *Herniation* occurs when the brain, under pressure, is squeezed through the boundaries of the tentorium and falx. Compression of the underlying brain stem causes fatal complications when respiratory and cardiac functioning are compromised. Even if not fatal, the compression usually results in severe impairment because of the extensive brain damage. Figure 3.4 below provides an excellent example of a subdural hematoma with a mass effect resulting in midline shift.

Hypoxemia and Hypoxia

The brain's requirement for energy is great. As much as fifteen percent of all blood flow is directed to the brain, which is responsible for more than 50 percent of all glucose consumption. Nourishment for the brain comes from the oxidative metabolism of glucose.[13] Because the brain does not store energy, the demand is continuous, and so must be the supply. Consequently, any disruption in the brain's energy supply can cause neuronal

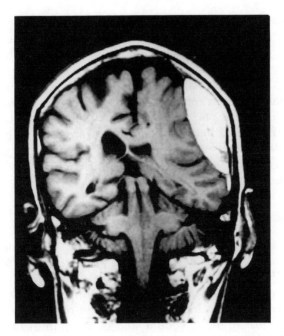

Figure 3.4 MRI of the head in the coronal plane showing a left subdural hematoma with midline shift to the right.

dysfunction in a matter of seconds, and permanent, irreversible damage can ensue in minutes.[11,18] In view of the brain's high demand for energy, systemic events have a dramatic effect on the maintenance of adequate oxygen supply to the brain.

One of the most common and impairing secondary injuries in traumatic brain injury is hypoxemia. *Hypoxemia* is a decrease in the oxygen content of the blood, and is diagnosed when the partial pressure of oxygen in the blood falls below 50 millimeters of mercury (PO_2 below 55 mmHg). The brain is extremely sensitive to changes in oxygen supply. Any number of events may happen in an accident that compromise oxygen supply and lead to hypoxemia. The upper airway may be obstructed by the back of the tongue (tongue prolapse), by tracheal fracture and edema, by edema of the soft tissues surrounding the neck, or by a foreign object. The gastric contents may be regurgitated and aspirated. Pulmonary injuries are common in trauma cases and may be the direct cause of decreased oxygenation. Depending upon the severity of the injury, there may be diminished respiratory drive.[31] Hypoxemia, therefore, may be the result of some systemic injury that compromises the supply of oxygen, or it may be due to the brain injury itself. Acute respiratory distress and the effects of alcohol or drugs on pulmonary effort may also contribute to hypoxemia. Direct injury to the lungs and chest wall can be a cause of impaired respiration. If unchecked, hypoxemia leads to *hypoxia* (insufficient oxygen supply, which can result in cell death). The importance of airway maintenance and ventilation is evident.

Because oxygen is carried via the cardiovascular system, obstructions in blood flow to the brain can also result in a loss of oxygen to neurons. This type of hypoxia has been referred to as *hypoxic-ischemic injury*[32] or *ischemic (hypoxic) encephalopathy*.[33] *Ischemia* (insufficient blood flow) is discussed below. The terms *hypoxic* and *anoxic brain damage* are commonly used to refer to neuronal damage resulting from a loss of oxygen, regardless of the etiology (that is, decreased oxygen supply, or decreased blood supply subsequently resulting in decreased oxygen).

Hypotension and Ischemia

Hypotension also is a frequent secondary event in traumatic brain injury. *Hypotension* is defined as a systolic blood pressure below 90 millimeters of mercury (<90 mmHg). Although there are a number of possible causes for hypotension following traumatic brain injury, the principal causes are hypovolemic, neuropathic, cardiogenic, and obstructive. Hypovolemic shock is due to loss of blood volume and is common in cases of multiple trauma.[34] Damage to the brain stem's autoregulatory mechanisms can affect respiration and circulation, resulting in neuropathic shock. Cardiac causes include trauma to the heart as well as other causes of contusion and infarction. Obstructive causes are uncommon, but serious. They include pulmonary embolus, pneumothorax, cardiac tamponade (obstruction of the inflow of blood to the heart as a result of fluid accumulation in the pericardial sac or other expanding masses in the chest), and dissecting aortic aneurysm.

Blood normally flows through the cerebral structures at a rate of 50 to 55 milliliters to 100 grams per minute (50 to 55 ml/100 g/min). Normal brain activity is maintained until flow falls below 18 to 20 ml/100 g/min. *Ischemia* or tissue damage occurs below this rate as a result of an insufficient supply of glucose and oxygen.[35,36] Ischemic neurons are capable of recovery, but only if flow is reestablished within a maximum time of two hours. Although the brain can tolerate hypoxia in varying degrees, ischemia is tolerated poorly.[33] Decreased blood flow results in an ineffective delivery of the nutrients needed to sustain the brain. The cellular reserve of energy, stored in the form of adenosine triphosphate (ATP), is exhausted within four minutes following a loss of blood supply. Waste products, such as lactic acid, quickly accumulate and alter the cellular pH. These initial changes lead to a complex cascade of events, including a disruption of the integrity of the cell membranes.[37] Disruption of the cell membrane permits an accumulation of intercellular calcium and of excitatory amino acids known as excitotoxins.[38,39] Further tissue destruction occurs as oxidative molecules, known as free radicals, are generated. If cerebral blood flow is not restored to functional levels and the ischemic process reversed, cell death or infarction will ensue. Although ischemia may exist as a relative state, infarction is absolute and irreversible. The brain's ability to tolerate ischemia is dependent upon the degree and duration of decreased blood flow, and upon the subpopulation of neurons that is affected. Cells with a high metabolic rate, such as those in the hippocampus, tolerate ischemia poorly and hence are highly susceptible to ischemic damage.[33,40] Within the cerebral hemispheres, ischemia occurs largely along the major cerebral artery territories, particularly between the anterior and middle cerebral arteries, or "watershed regions."[7,11,33]

Adams and colleagues[7] have found hypoxic brain damage to be common following severe traumatic brain injury, and indicate that it is a "further cause of traumatic coma in the absence of an intracranial mass lesion." It is associated with severe disability. In some studies of traumatic brain injury, hypoxic brain damage has been found to be more common in the hippocampus and basal ganglia than in the cortical regions.[11] Damage to the hippocampus has been suspected as a cause of memory impairment in a variety of amnesic syndromes for several years,[41] and has been implicated as a source of severe memory impairment in traumatic brain injury with hypoxia.[42]

Brain Swelling and Edema

The terms *brain swelling* and *edema* are used commonly in reference to the same process, although they are distinct phenomena from a medical perspective.[13,43] *Brain swelling* refers to an increase in cerebral blood volume or engorgement,[13] also referred to as *cerebral hyperemia*.[44] This is in contrast to *edema*, which, in strict usage, refers to an excessive accumulation of cellular fluid in the tissues of the brain. A number of types of brain edema are described in the literature. Edema may be focal (at the site of a lesion) or diffuse. From a rehabilitation perspective, understanding these as different processes is important only as it contributes to a better understanding of the dynamic nature of the pathophysiologic processes in general. Functionally, brain swelling and edema result in an increase of fluid volume within a limited space, raising intracranial pressure, and threatening compression of the brain stem. The following discussion of forms of edema is provided solely to assist the clinician in reading and understanding medical texts and medical records.

The cause of *vasogenic edema* is thought to be a disruption in the blood-brain barrier due to increased permeability of the cerebral capillaries. (The term blood-brain barrier refers to the selectively permeable membrane that restricts passage of some blood-borne molecules into the brain.) Following trauma, the epithelial lining of the blood vessels may become more permeable than in normal conditions, resulting in leakage of protein-rich fluids into the interstitial or extracellular space. The edema is often localized to the area of contusion or hemorrhage, and is sometimes referred to as perifocal edema.

Hydrostatic edema is also the result of extracellular fluid accumulation, but the fluid is considered protein poor.[43] Hydrostatic edema occurs when there are abrupt changes in cerebral perfusion pressure or intracranial pressure (an abrupt increase in the hydrostatic pressure gradient). This form of edema may occur with the sudden decompression of a mass lesion and may also occur when the brain's autoregulation of blood pressure is impaired, resulting in a rapid increase in arterial pressure without a simultaneous rise in intracranial pressure. The higher intravascular pressure pushes fluid into the extracellular space.

Cytotoxic edema is differentiated from vasogenic edema partially on the basis of intracellular rather than interstitial accumulation of fluid. This form of edema occurs when there has been a disruption in the energy supply to the cells, usually as the result of decreased cerebral blood flow.[43] There is a disruption in the functioning of the cell membrane pump (sodium-potassium pump), which becomes ineffective in the dying cell, resulting in an accumulation of fluids within the cells; potassium accumulates outside of the cells (the extracellular space) and calcium enters the cells. Intracellular equilibrium is disrupted, and the electrical excitability of the neurons may be affected.

Osmotic edema, alternately *hypo-osmotic edema*, occurs subsequent to a drop in serum osmolality, usually caused by low levels of serum sodium or hyponatremia. *Osmolality* is a term used to describe the concentration of a solute (for example, sodium) in a solution. The resulting imbalance between a high intracellular osmolality and low serum osmolality causes water to move into the cell in an attempt to reach an equilibrium in solute concentration. This may occur as a result of fluid loss replacement and dilution of electrolytes (see hyponatremia). *Congestive brain swelling*, or *cerebral hyperemia*, is the result of increased cerebral blood volume and is visualized by computerized tomography scan quite acutely. Increases in cerebral blood volume may be due to dilation of the arteries, to impairment in the autoregulation of cerebral blood pressure, or to a venous obstruction.[43] An increase in intracranial pressure, with its associated complications, may result.

Intracranial Pressure

Intracranial pressure (ICP) is a measurement of cerebrospinal fluid pressure. Like arterial pressure, it is compared to a range of normative values. In normal adults the mean intracranial pressure is between 0 and 10 millimeters of mercury (0–10 mmHg). It is a cause for concern when elevated to 20 mmHg or higher, and at levels of 40 mmHg there is neurologic dysfunction. Highly elevated intracranial pressure restricts cerebral blood flow, and at severely elevated levels (60 mmHg) it leads to death.[18] Elevated intracranial pressure may occur secondary to brain edema or as an immediate result of obstruction of the flow of cerebrospinal fluid though the cerebral aqueduct.

Hyponatremia

Hyponatremia results when the serum sodium levels in the bloodstream fall below critical levels (120 milliequivalents per liter; 120mEq/l). In severe trauma involving a number of injuries, fluid loss may be significant. With fluid loss and subsequent replacement, there is increased likelihood of electrolyte loss. Fluid replacement, which is often accomplished with dextrose solutions, may not include an adequate mixture for electrolyte replacement.[18] A loss of sodium in the blood can result in a reduction of serum osmolality that leads to brain cell edema (discussed above under osmotic edema). Hyponatremia may occur when there is damage to the hypothalamus, which regulates sodium metabolism by controlling the secretion of antidiuretic hormone (ADH).

Seizures

A *seizure* may be described as a "temporary physiologic dysfunction of the brain" characterized by the abnormal electrical discharge (excessive and hypersynchronous) of cortical neurons.[45] Seizures following traumatic brain injury occur with an incidence of up to 7 percent;[45] thus, they present a frequent complication. Seizures are generally divided into early (occurring within twenty-four hours of injury) or late. Early seizures may be a transient phenomenon that does not require treatment. Prolonged or recurrent seizures, especially during the acute phases of recovery, may cause further damage by increasing cerebral energy consumption and promoting hypoxia and hypercapnia (increased carbon dioxide in the blood). Seizures are discussed in greater detail in Chapter Four.

MECHANISMS OF COMA

Since antiquity, the literature has made reference to loss of consciousness associated with injuries to the head.[46] Coma can only be considered relative to consciousness, which is a concept or state without clear definition. As a point of reference, consciousness, as defined by Miller and Pentland,[47] "represents a state of arousal and awareness of the external environment linked to the capacity to react to changes in that environment."

The *reticular formation* is a collection of nuclei in the brain stem with far-reaching connections (via axons and dendrites) throughout the central nervous system. Anterior connections to the hypothalamus, thalamus, and locus ceruleus make up the *ascending reticular activating system (ARAS)*. This neural network is credited with the establishment and maintenance of arousal. With its global connections, the reticular formation receives input from the entire nervous system and relays information in a widespread manner as well. It functions as an integrative and regulatory system that integrates information from both sensory and motor systems, regulates sleep, and establishes and maintains arousal.[48] Angevine and Cotman[48] have proposed that the neurons of the reticular system probably respond to the intensity or volume of information received, and hence relay information reflecting the degree of activity, not its specific details. For the purpose of alerting other parts of the nervous system, such as the cortex, information regarding stimulus intensity is of primary importance. The reticular formation activates the cerebral cortex by way of the thalamocortical connections. Perhaps because of its widespread connections, if the reticular formation is disrupted in trauma to the head, the result is impairment of consciousness. (The evaluation of coma is discussed in detail in Chapter Four.) The reticular system and the cerebral hemispheres form a complex feedback loop, each utilizing information from the other. Consequently, severe bilateral cortical damage may also disrupt consciousness, resulting in an inability either to receive information via the ascending reticular activating system or to provide information to the reticular system and other parts of the brain. Typically, loss of consciousness is not seen in focal brain lesions because there has not been damage to the reticular activating system.[47] Early investigations of traumatic brain injury tended to attribute coma to neuronal lesions in the brain stem because of the location of the nuclei of the reticular formation.[49] Contemporary views hold that coma is a result of diffuse axonal injury present in the cortex and brain stem, but not in the brain stem alone.[7,11,49] Interestingly, this view is not new; it was expressed by Russell in 1968.[50] It is often assumed that injury to certain areas of the brain stem causes the unconsciousness in concussion, but it is just as likely that the widespread damage to large areas of the cerebral hemispheres will lead to generalized suppression of brain mechanisms, not only in the cerebral hemispheres but also in the brain stem.

The mechanisms by which the reticular system serves to alert and arouse are not well understood. Its precise role in maintaining consciousness is poorly understood as well. Nonetheless, it is well accepted that the reticular activating system, with its long projecting axons, is highly vulnerable to the stretching and shearing that occur in acceleration-deceleration injuries.

SUMMARY

Although the terminology is complex, it is imperative that the rehabilitation clinician have a basic understanding of the nature of the injury process that occurs in traumatic brain injury. Unlike stroke- and tumor-related brain damage, which result most often in focal deficits, this process is extremely dynamic with a less predictable course. The nature of injury is diffuse and results in widespread disruption of the neuronal structures supporting cognitive and communicative functions. Injury to the brain is most often classified into primary insults (that which occurs immediately upon impact of the brain) and secondary insults (those occurring at a later point in time, but during the critical medical recovery period). Primary injuries include contusions, lacerations, skull fractures, tissue tear hemorrhages, and diffuse axonal injury, the latter being the hallmark of traumatic brain injury. The secondary insults can be numerous, and are the focus of early medical intervention, which offers the most promise for improving outcome, other than preventive measures. The practicing clinician is concerned with both, since their severity affects the recovery rate of cognitive and communication abilities.

REFERENCES

1. Denny-Brown D, Russell WR. Experimental cerebral concussion. *Brain.* 1941;69:93–164.
2. Ommaya AK, Gennarelli TA. Cerebral concussion and traumatic unconsciousness: correlation of experimental and clinical observations on blunt head injuries. *Brain.* 1974;97:633–654.
3. Adams JH, Graham DI, Gennarelli TA. Acceleration induced head injury in the monkey. *Acta Neuropathologica.* 1981(suppl)7:26–28.
4. Adams JH, Gennarelli TA, Graham, DI. Brain damage in nonmissile head injury: observations in man and in subhuman primates. In Smith WT, Cavanagh J (eds). *Recent Advances in Neuropathology.* Edinburgh, Scotland: Churchill-Livingstone; 1982:165–190.
5. Gennarelli TA et al. Diffuse axonal injury in the primate. In Dacey RG (ed). *Trauma of the Central Nervous System.* New York, NY: Raven Press; 1985:169–194.
6. Denny-Brown D. Sequelae of war head injuries. *New England Journal of Medicine.* 1942;227:771–780.
7. Adams JH, Graham DI, Gennarelli TA. Contemporary neuropathological considerations regarding brain damage in head injury. In Becker DP, Povlishock JT (eds). *Central Nervous System Trauma Status Report.* Bethesda, MD: National Institute of Neurological and Communicative Disorders and Stroke; 1985: 65–77.
8. Pang D. Pathophysiologic correlates of neurobehavioral syndromes following closed head injury. In Ylvisaker M (ed). *Head Injury Rehabilitation: Children and Adolescents.* San-Diego, CA: College-Hill Press; 1985:3–70.
9. Gurdjian ES. Acute head injuries. *Surgery, Gynecology and Obstetrics.* 1978;146:805–820.
10. Auerbach SH. The pathophysiology of traumatic brain injury. In Horn LJ, Cope DN (eds). *Physical Medicine and Rehabilitation: State of the Art Reviews.* Philadelphia, PA: Hanely and Belfus; 1989:1–11.
11. Graham DI. Trauma. In Weller RO (ed). *Nervous System, Muscle and Eyes, Vol 4.* New York, NY: Churchill Livingstone; 1990:125–149.

12. Gennarelli TA. Cerebral concussion and diffuse brain injuries. In Cooper PR (ed). *Head Injury, 3rd ed.* Baltimore, MD: Williams and Wilkens; 1993:137–158.
13. Jennett B, Teasdale GM. *Management of Head Injuries.* Philadelphia, PA: F.A. Davis; 1981.
14. Graham DI, Adams JH, Gennarelli TA. Pathology of brain damage in head injury. In Cooper PR (ed). *Head Injury, 3rd ed.* Baltimore, MD: Williams and Wilkins; 1993:91–113.
15. Mendelow AD, Teasdale GM. Pathophysiology of head injuries. *British Journal of Surgery.* 1983;70: 641–650.
16. Cook AW et al. Report of ad hoc committee to study head injury nomenclature. *Clinical Neurosurgical Journal.* 1966;12:386–394.
17. Povlishock JT, Valadka AB. Pathobiology of traumatic brain injury. In Finlayson MAJ, Garner SH (eds). *Brain Injury Rehabilitation: Clinical Considerations.* Baltimore, MD: Williams and Wilkins; 1994:11–3.
18. Miller JD, Pentland B, Berrol S. Early evaluation and management. In Rosenthal M, Griffith ER, Bond MR, Miller JD (eds). *Rehabilitation of the Adult and Child with Traumatic Brain Injury.* Philadelphia, PA: FA Davis; 1990:21–51.
19. Povlishock JT. Traumatically induced axonal damage without concomitant change in focally related neuronal somata and dendrites. *Acta Neuropathologica.* 1986;70:53–59.
20. Strich SJ. Diffuse degeneration of the cerebral white matter in severe dementia following head injury. *Journal of Neurology, Neurosurgery, and Psychiatry.* 1956; 19:163–185.
21. Strich SJ. The pathology of brain damage due to blunt head injuries. In Walker AE, Caveness WF, Critchley, M (eds). *The Late Effects of Head Injury.* Springfield, IL: Charles C Thomas; 1969:501–524.
22. Gennarelli TA. Cerebral concussion and diffuse brain injuries. In Cooper PR (ed). *Head Injury, 2nd ed.* Baltimore, MD: Williams and Wilkins; 1987:108–124.
23. Cope DN. The rehabilitation of traumatic brain injury. In Kottke FJ, Lehman JF (eds). *Krusen's Handbook of Physical Medicine and Rehabilitation, 4th ed.* Philadelphia, PA: WB Saunders; 1990:1217–1251.
24. Wilberger JE et al. Acute tissue tear hemorrhages of the brain: computed tomography and clinicopathological correlations. *Neurosurgery.* 1990;27:208–213.
25. Oppenheimer DR. Microscopic lesions in the brain following head injury. *Journal of Neurology, Neurosurgery, and Psychiatry.* 1968;3:299–306.
26. Levin HS. Pathophysiologic mechanisms. In Levin HS, Benton AL, Grossman RG (eds). *Neurobehavioral Consequences of Closed Head Injury.* New York, NY: Oxford University Press; 1982:3–48.
27. Cooper PR. Post-traumatic intracranial mass lesions. In Cooper PR (ed). *Head Injury, 3rd ed.* Baltimore, MD: Williams and Wilkins; 1993:275–329.
28. Vogel FS, Bouldin TW. The nervous system. In Rubin E, Farber JL (eds). *Pathology.* Philadelphia, PA: Lippincott; 1988:1416–1499.
29. Soloniuk DS, Aldrich EF, Eisenberg HM. Traumatic intracerebral hematomas. In Pitts LH, Wagner FC (eds). *Craniospinal Trauma.* New York, NY: Thieme Medical Publishers: 1990:49–58.
30. Gennarelli TA. Initial assessment and management of head injury. In Pitts LH, Wagner FC (eds).*Craniospinal Trauma.* New York, NY: Thieme Medical Publishers; 1990:11–24.

31. Wilberger JE. Emergency care and initial evaluation. In Cooper PR (ed). *Head Injury, 3rd ed.* Baltimore, MD: Williams and Wilkins; 1993:27–41.
32. Goldbaum ML, Zasler N. Hypoxic-ischemic brain injury: neurorehabilitative issues. Presented at National Head Injury Foundation 11th Annual Symposium; December 1992; Boston, MA.
33. Morris JH. The nervous system. In Cotran RS, Kumar V, Robbins SL (eds). *Robbins Pathologic Basis of Disease, 4th ed.* Philadelphia, PA: WB Saunders; 1989:1385–1449.
34. Braunwald E, Williams GH. Alteration in arterial pressure and the shock syndrome. In Petersdorf RG et al (eds). *Principles of Internal Medicine, 10th ed.* New York, NY: McGraw-Hill Book; 1985:171–176.
35. Astrup J, Siesjo BK, Symon L. Thresholds in cerebral ischemia: the ischemic penumbra. *Stroke.* 1981;112:723–725.
36. Heiss W-D, Graf R. The ischemic penumbra. *Current Opinion in Neurology.* 1994;7:11–19.
37. Beneviste H et al. Elevation of extracellular concentration of glutamate and aspartate in rat hippocampus during transient ischemia monitored by intracerebral microdialysis. *Journal of Neurochemistry.* 1984;43:1364–1374.
38. Meyer FB. Calcium, neuronal hyperexcitability and ischemic injury. *Brain Research Reviews.* 1989;14:227–243.
39. Faden AI et al. The role of excitatory amino acids, and NMDA receptors in traumatic head injury. *Science.* 1989;244:798–800.
40. Adams RD, Victor M. *Principles of Neurology, 5th ed.* New York, NY: McGraw-Hill; 1993:879–880.
41. Squire, L. *Memory and Brain.* New York, NY: Oxford University Press; 1987:175–201.
42. Prigatano GP et al. *Neuropsychological Rehabilitation after Brain Injury.* Baltimore, MD: Johns Hopkins University Press;1986:2–17.
43. Miller JD. Traumatic brain swelling and edema. In Cooper PR (ed). *Head Injury, 3rd ed.* Baltimore, MD: Williams and Wilkins; 1993:331–354.
44. Cooper PR. Delayed brain injury: secondary insults. In Becker DP, Povlishock JT (eds). *Central Nervous System Trauma Status Report.* Bethesda, MD: National Institute of Neurological and Communicative Disorders and Stroke; 1985:217–228.
45. Yablon SA. Posttraumatic seizures. *Archives of Physical Medicine and Rehabilitation.* 1993;74:983–1001.
46. Gurdjian ES. *Head Injury from Antiquity to the Present with Special Reference to Penetrating Head Wounds.* Springfield, IL: Charles C Thomas; 1973.
47. Miller JD, Pentland B. The neurologic evaluation. In Rosenthal M, Griffith ER, Bond MR, Miller JD (eds). *Rehabilitation of the Adult and Child with Traumatic Brain Injury.* Philadelphia, PA: FA Davis; 1990:52–58.
48. Angevine JB, Cotman CW. *Principles of Neuroanatomy.* New York, NY: Oxford University Press; 1981:230–252.
49. Povlishock JT, Becker DP, Miller JD, et al. The morphopathologic substrates of concussion? *Acta Neuropathologica.* 1979;47:1–11.
50. Russell WR. The traumatic amnesias. *International Journal of Neurology.* 1968;7:55–59.

4

Medical Management

Jeffrey N. Pierce

In approaching the subject of medical management of patients with traumatic brain injury, one is confronted with a confusing literature filled with obscure acronyms, and a clinical environment that is a chaotic blend of the exceptional and the mundane. The author's task is to assist clinicians in making some sense of this unusual mixture and, in so doing, to help prepare them to make meaningful contributions to the treatment team. An entire textbook could be devoted to the medical evaluation and treatment of patients with traumatic brain injury and similar conditions. Out of necessity, the author will limit this treatment of the subject to areas that are clinically most important to speech-language pathologists and other rehabilitation clinicians.

This chapter is designed to help the clinician understand the evaluation of brain injuries and the conditions that frequently develop as complications. Complications are subdivided by the various organ systems that may be affected. Under each organ system, evaluation and treatment techniques that impact directly upon the delivery of speech-language pathology services or clinical rehabilitative services are discussed. Special attention is given to pharmacological therapy and its side effects. Finally, a review of studies that have attempted to define prognostic variables is provided.

ACUTE NEUROLOGIC EVALUATION

Speech-language pathologists are frequently consulted to evaluate the cognitive status of patients in acute hospital settings. Before attempting to diagnose and classify the patient's level of consciousness, it is imperative the clinician consider the difficulty of this task. Short of seeing an open wound that involves the brain, or an image of a damaged brain on a diagnostic study such as a computerized tomography scan, one makes the diagnosis of brain injury based on a clinical examination that can at times be quite subjective. The dichotomy between the brain and the mind leads to further uncertainty, especially when one is confronted with patients whose deficits are disproportionate to their apparent degree of injury. Deficits may improve or worsen over relatively short periods of time, necessitating frequent, comprehensive evaluations. The task is complicated further by the frequent use of alcohol or other mind-altering drugs by patients who are involved in trauma. Finally, the clinician's task is made even more difficult by the emotionally charged state of the patient's family and treatment team, who depend upon the clinician's recommendations regarding further treatment and eventual placement.

The definition and mechanisms of coma were discussed in Chapter Three. In describing consciousness, it is useful to distinguish between *arousal* and *content*. *Arousal* is considered to be relative and occurs on a continuum from states of total unresponsiveness or obtundation, through states of partial responsiveness or lethargy, up to states in which the individual is fully alert. Likewise, *content* of consciousness is quantitative in nature and can be described in terms of intellectual capacity. Although content also may be defined in qualitative terms, these aspects are not particularly relevant to the evaluation of coma. At this point, the reader may surmise that there are multiple levels of consciousness, and hence of coma.

Glasgow Coma Scale

One of the most widely used assessment tools to evaluate coma is the *Glasgow Coma Scale*,[1] shown in Table 4.1. This rapid, reliable test is used nationally and internationally. Although its validity has been questioned, and its use has been controversial at times, clinicians should be familiar with its relative strengths and weaknesses, and with its appropriate use as an assessment tool. Three different behaviors are evaluated in the Glasgow Coma Scale. They are *eye opening, verbal response,* and *best motor response.* The absence of a response gives the patient a score of one on each of the

Table 4.1
The Glasgow Coma Scale.

Eye Opening	Verbal Response	Motor Response
Spontaneous 4	Oriented 5	Obey Command 6
To Voice 3	Confused 4	Localized Response 5
To Pain 2	Inappropriate 3	Withdrawal 4
None 1	Incomprehensible 2	Flexion 3
None 1	Extension 2	None 1

Adapted from Teasdale G, Jennett B. Assessment of coma and impaired consciousness—a practical scale. *Lancet.* 1974;13:81–84.

behaviors listed, with higher-level responses receiving a greater score, as depicted in Table 4.1. Eye opening is mediated through the *oculomotor,* or third cranial, nerve. Since patients with traumatic brain injury occasionally will have damage to this nerve, scores may be decreased even in the absence of coma. More commonly, however, the inability to open the eyes is due to dysfunction of the oculomotor nucleus, which is situated in the midbrain at the level of the superior colliculus and is near the midline just ventral to the cerebral aqueduct.

Reflexive eye opening occurs as a response to pain in most patients with moderate brain damage, and even in some who have severe brain damage if midbrain structures are relatively preserved. Likewise, individuals who are intoxicated or who attempt to feign unconsciousness will usually open their eyes in response to pain. Clinicians must be cautious in interpreting the lack of responsiveness to speech, since this ability to respond is contingent upon normal auditory and language functions. Although spontaneous eye opening is a fairly reliable indicator of level of consciousness in the acute post-traumatic phase, it becomes unreliable after approximately two weeks. Spontaneous eye opening will sometimes resume as a reflexive behavior in comatose patients, and has been widely described as a component of the persistent vegetative state, which is discussed later in the chapter.

When interpreting a patient's motor response, it must be remembered that one is testing fairly long neural segments that connect the brain and spinal cord to the peripheral nerves and muscles. Motor responses become an unreliable indicator of level of consciousness in the presence of suspected injury to the spinal cord or to the descending pyramidal tracks of the brain stem. Patients with lesions of these two areas, as well as any lesion inferior to the medulla, initially exhibit flaccid muscle tone and complete paralysis. Patients with lesions that occur superior to the medulla assume a posture of exaggerated extension of the extremities and also of the neck. This stereotypic posture is termed *decerebrate* and was first demonstrated in animal models by Sherrington[2], who transected the brain between the pons and the medulla. This posture is due to the extensor tone generated by the vestibular nuclei.

Normally, extensor tone is regulated by facilitory and inhibitory neurons from the reticular substance that extend from the medulla to the midbrain. In the absence of inhibitory neurons, extensor tone predominates. In patients with lesions that occur above the midbrain, specifically above the red nucleus and tectum, the predominant best motor response is that of flexion of the upper extremities. This posture is termed *decorticate* indicating that there has been loss of the inhibitory neurons from the cortex to the midbrain. Patients with lesions of the midbrain and brain stem frequently lie motionless when undisturbed and display stereotypic postures only as a response to noxious stimuli. Likewise, the next level of motor responsiveness on the Glasgow Coma Scale, *withdrawal,* cannot be tested unless a painful stimulus is administered to the patient. Although various techniques have been employed, the following three maneuvers are used most commonly in clinical practice: applying pressure to the superior orbital rim near the exit of the supraorbital nerve; applying pressure to the nail bed with a dull, rigid object such as a pencil; or, applying pressure to the chest over the sternum with one's knuckles. Of these three, the author recommends the first for its superior reliability, because the sensory nerve being tested is the ophthalmic division of the fifth cranial nerve and, as such, is a shorter neural segment.

In assessing the verbal response of an unconscious patient, one initially assumes that a substrate of intact hearing and language is present, just as in the assessment of motor response and eye opening. A normal verbal response is also contingent upon the patient's ability to speak, which is problematic in cases of trauma to the neck or oral cavity. Likewise, the presence of a tracheostomy or impaired respiratory function limits the assessment of verbal responses. The responses of patients with dysarthria may be incorrectly assessed as confused or inappropriate by some emergency personnel, and the expertise of the speech-language pathologist may be of great value in these cases.

In assessing the reliability of the Glasgow Coma Scale, some authors[3] have recommended that the three subscores be separately recorded and not summed. Retrospective studies[4] that have correlated improvement with Glasgow Coma Scale subscores have found the best motor response score to be the most accurate of the three subtests in predicting recovery.

Gross Examination of the Head

Although the Glasgow Coma Scale is a useful tool in coma assessment, it is by no means comprehensive. We will now consider some of the other elements of neurological exams that are useful in evaluating patients with suspected traumatic brain injury. In a general examination of the head, it is important to note the presence of *ecchymosis*, or bruising. Ecchymosis of the posterior auricular region or mastoid region is referred to as *Battle's sign*. Periorbital ecchymosis is commonly referred to as *raccoon eyes* or *the raccoon sign*. Both of these findings can be seen in patients with basilar skull fractures. It is also important to note the presence of any drainage of fluid from the ears or nose, since this may be *cerebrospinal fluid (CSF)*. Cerebrospinal fluid drainage from these locations is referred to as a *craniocerebral fluid fistula* and is discussed later, under complications.

Cranial Nerves

Cranial nerve evaluation can be helpful both in assessing a patient's level of consciousness and in determining the anatomical location of neural trauma. A brief discussion of the functional anatomy of the cranial nerves follows as a review. Cranial nerves are so named because they originate from the motor nuclei within the cranium, rather than from those in the spinal cord. They are diverse in their function and in some cases possess both motor (efferent) branches and sensory (afferent) branches. Cranial nerves I, II, and VIII contain only sensory fibers, and cranial nerves III, IV, VI, XI, and XII contain only motor fibers. The remaining cranial nerves (V, VII, IX, X) have both sensory and motor functions. Motor pathways are made up of two motor neurons: the upper motor neuron, whose cell body is usually located in the cerebral cortex, and the lower motor neuron, whose cell body is located in the brain stem. Sensory pathways are composed of three major neurons: a primary neuron, whose cell body is located outside of the central nervous system in a sensory ganglion; a secondary neuron, whose cell body is located in the dorsal gray matter of the brain stem; and a tertiary neuron, whose cell body is in the thalamus.

Cranial nerve synapses within the brain stem form anatomically distinct structures referred to as *nuclei*. The brain stem was thought to resemble a "bulb" by early neuroanatomists. Damage to these nuclei, therefore, may result in nuclear or *bulbar* palsy. Since the brain stem is frequently damaged in patients with traumatic brain injury, cranial nerve impairment (palsy) is a relatively common finding.

Cranial nerve impairment may be seen with any lesion along the course of the neural pathway. Some motor nuclei receive dual innervation, with connections from both cerebral hemispheres, and therefore have relative preservation of function in cases of unilateral cortical damage. Many cases of cranial nerve impairment are due to lesions of either the lower motor neuron or the primary sensory neuron, secondary to fractures of the facial bones or the skull. Facial fractures occur with approximately a 38 percent incidence in patients with traumatic intracranial injury.[5] Conversely, up to 58 percent of patients with facial fractures have associated traumatic intracranial injuries. Therefore, it is often difficult, if not impossible, to determine whether the cranial nerve palsy is due to a peripheral or central lesion.

Cranial Nerve I

The *olfactory*, or first cranial, nerve is the most frequently injured cranial nerve and may be damaged in cases of relatively mild brain injury.[6] Although the incidence of injury is reported as 7 percent,[7] it is impossible to test the sensory nerves in an unconscious patient. Testing is further complicated when one considers that some tastes and aromas are carried by the sensory division of the fifth nerve rather than the first. Strong odors, such as camphor and ammonia, irritate the nasal and pharyngeal mucosa, causing fifth cranial nerve stimulation. When testing the first cranial nerve, the examiner should use more subtle stimuli such as coffee, tobacco, or peanut butter.

The primary sensory olfactory neuron is a bipolar cell that connects structures in the olfactory bulb with olfactory receptors in the nasal mucosa. These neurons pass through the cribriform plate of the cranium and are vulnerable to shearing and compression forces. If these neurons are transected, the loss of smell, or *anosmia*, is usually permanent, but a recovery of olfaction has been reported in approximately 25 percent of patients with traumatic brain injury.[8]

The olfactory nerve is unique in that it is the only cranial nerve that does not synapse in the brain stem. Most of the tertiary neurons pass through the lateral olfactory stria to the primary olfactory area, which consists of the cortex of the uncus, limen insula, and part of the amygdaloid body. Lesions in this area of the brain may cause patients to experience olfactory hallucinations, and may be seen in temporal lobe epilepsy.

Cranial Nerve II

The *optic*, or second cranial, nerve carries the special sensation of light and must be intact for vision to occur. Light impulses stimulate special photoreceptor cells in the retina called *rods* and *cones*, which in turn stimulate the primary and secondary sensory neurons whose cell bodies are located in the retina. Neural impulses are then transmitted through the optic nerve to the lateral geniculate nuclei located in the thalamus. Tertiary sensory neurons transmit these impulses to the occipital lobes, where input is coordinated and integrated. Following traumatic brain injury, damage to the optic nerve chiasma can occur, but the incidence has been reported at approximately 0.7 percent in survivors.[5] The majority of lesions involving the optic nerve occur in cases of trauma to the eye or the bones that form the optic canal where the optic nerve passes from the eyeball to form the chiasma. An incidence of 5.2 percent has been reported for these injuries.[5]

Transection of the optic nerve anterior to the optic chiasma results in monocular blindness. Partial lesions of the optic nerve in this location, or lesions distal to this location, result in the loss of part of the visual field of one or both eyes. Lesions to the occipital lobe may result in an impairment of vision termed *cortical blindness*.[8] Clinical evaluation of the optic nerve is difficult in an unconscious patient, but may be partially assessed by the evaluation of the *pupillary light reflex*, which involves the optic as well as the oculomotor, or third cranial, nerve. Some of the optic nerve fibers do not terminate at the lateral geniculate body, but rather progress posteriorly to another region named the *pretectal nucleus*. Interneurons from the pretectal nucleus connect with two midline nuclear bodies called the *Edinger-Westphal nuclei*. Efferent motor fibers that originate in the Edinger-Westphal nuclei accompany the oculomotor, or third cranial, nerve to the ciliary ganglia found posterior to the eyeball. These ganglia synapse with lower motor neurons that innervate the sphincter muscle of the iris and cause pupillary constriction. Light shone in either eye causes constriction of the pupil in the same eye (the *direct light reflex)* and also in the other eye (the *consensual light reflex*). For example, if light is shone into the right eye and no pupillary reflex is observed in either eye, but a pupillary reflex is observed in both eyes when light is shone in the left eye, one may deduce that the optic nerve of the right eye is damaged.[9]

Cranial Nerves III, IV, and VI

The *oculomotor,* or third cranial, nerve; the *abducens,* or fourth cranial, nerve; and the *trochlear,* or sixth cranial, nerve are usually examined together, since they all control extraocular movements. The third cranial nerve not only functions in controlling most of the extraocular muscles, but it also controls the dilatation and constriction of the pupils. The upper motor neurons that control pupillary dilatation are located in the spinal cord from the cervical segment C8 down to the thoracic segment T2. These neurons ascend to the superior cervical ganglia where they synapse with lower motor neurons that travel with the internal carotid artery and through the ciliary ganglia to the iris. Stimulation of these nerve fibers results in pupillary dilatation. The upper motor neurons located in the spinal cord receive impulses from the brain stem and higher centers in the brain, but these connections are poorly understood.

It is important to note that the diameter of the pupil is not controlled solely by the relative presence or absence of light, but also is affected by neurotransmitters. It is generally believed that sympathetic neurotransmitters, such as epinephrine, result in pupillary dilatation, and the presence of parasympathetic neurotransmitters, such as acetylcholine, result in pupillary constriction.

In the absence of cranial nerve deficits, the size of the pupils may indicate the presence of lesions within the brain or brain stem. Lesions in the diencephalon result in small pupils that are reactive to light. Lesions in the tectal region result in large pupils that are poorly reactive to light. Lesions in the midbrain result in pupils that are fixed in a midposition and are unreactive to light. Lesions in the pons result in pupils that are pinpoint in size and unreactive.[10] Pupillary size may be influenced further by the presence of exogenous drugs such as cocaine and amphetamines, which result in large pupils, or by the presence of narcotics, such as morphine, which result in small pupils.

Injuries to the nerves controlling extraocular movement occur with an incidence of less than 3 percent in patients surviving traumatic brain injury[5] but are difficult to document in the acute setting, since patients are usually unable to move their eyes voluntarily or participate in a careful examination. The third and sixth cranial nerves are involved most frequently, but the fourth nerve has been reported to be involved in injuries of the dorsolateral midbrain that are associated with severe frontal blows to the accelerating head.[5]

The upper motor neurons of the third cranial nerve originate in the motor cortex and synapse in the midbrain at the level of the superior colliculus at the motor nucleus of the third cranial nerve. The third cranial nerve travels anteriorly through the red nucleus to exit through the anterior surface of the pons. It then joins the fourth and sixth nerves at as they pass together through the cavernous sinus and enter the orbital fossa or *orbit*. At this point, the nerve bifurcates, with the upper division innervating the levator muscle of the eyelid and the superior rectus muscle. The lower branch innervates the medial and inferior rectus muscle and the inferior oblique muscle. The motor nucleus of the fourth cranial nerve is located at the level of the inferior colliculus, in front of the cerebral aqueduct and inferior to the nuclei of the oculomotor nerves. This nerve follows a circuitous path and crosses the midline before exiting the dorsal aspect of the brain stem. It then winds around the brain stem just inferior to the midbrain, where it joins the third cranial nerve in the cavernous sinus. Upon entering the orbit, the trochlear nerve supplies only the superior oblique muscle.[1]

The motor nucleus of the sixth cranial nerve is located inferior to that of the third and fourth cranial nerves, and is found anterior to the cerebral aqueduct in the lower pons. It travels anteriorly and inferiorly before exiting through the pontomedullary junction just above the pyramids of the medulla. It then travels superiorly between the pons and the portion of the petrous temporal bone known as the clivus before joining the third and fourth nerves in the cavernous sinus, where it enters the orbit to supply a single muscle, the lateral rectus. The directions of gaze determined by the extraocular muscles are represented in a schematic drawing shown in Figure 4.1.

Although damage to the preceding three nerves frequently may occur as a group, in cases of orbital trauma, several syndromes of isolated cranial nerve dysfunction are known to occur. In complete oculomotor nerve paralysis, there are three findings: ptosis of the eyelid, fixed position of the eye with the pupil directed downward and laterally, and a dilated pupil nonreactive to light. Complete paralysis of the trochlear nerve is subtle and often missed, even by trained clinicians, unless the patient complains of diplopia. When the patient looks straight ahead, the axis of the diseased eye is higher than that of the other eye. When the patient looks downward and inward, the eye rotates. Paralysis of the abducens nerve causes the diseased eye to rotate inward, and it cannot gaze laterally. If all three motor nerves of one eye are interrupted, the eye looks straight ahead and cannot be moved in any direction, and its pupil is wide and nonreactive to light. Bilateral paralysis of the eye muscles is usually the result of nuclear damage secondary to infection, hemorrhage, or degenerative neurological conditions such as multiple sclerosis, rather than from trauma.[9]

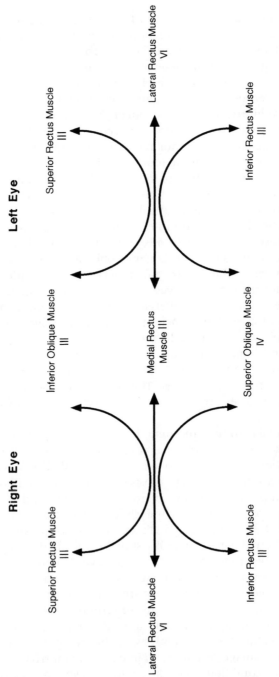

Figure 4.1 A schematic representation of the directions of eye gaze.

Eye movements may occur because of voluntary impulses from the cortex, but the majority of eye movements take place reflexively. In either case, eye movements are normally conjugate and are coordinated by inter-connections between the cranial nerve nuclei that control eye movements. These interconnections are provided by neurons located in the medial lon-gitudinal fasciculus, which runs parallel to the midline from the tegmentum of the midbrain down to the cervical cord. Further interconnections join the medial longitudinal fasciculus from the vestibular nerves, the reticular for-mation, the cerebral cortex, and from postural receptors in the cervical spinal cord.[9] These cranial nerve interconnections can be assessed in the acute neurological examination, and are helpful in the localization of sus-pected central nervous system lesions.

The integrity of these interconnections may be assessed grossly with a bedside examination to test the *oculocephalic reflex* or *doll's head eye phenom-enon*. Patients with an intact reflex are referred to in the vernacular as having "doll's eyes." During this examination, the patient may be assessed either in a supine or sitting position. The eyelids are held open, and the head is rotated from one side to the other. If the reflex loop is intact, the patient will appear to maintain a forward gaze. This reflex may be preserved even if the patient is unresponsive to other stimuli.[9,10] These maneuvers should never be performed on patients who are suspected of having cervical fractures or dislocation until appropriate x-rays of the neck have been obtained.

The integrity of the interconnections between eye movements and the vestibular apparatus can be tested by evaluating the *oculovestibular reflex*. This test requires the installation of cool and warm water into the auditory canal, and it should never be done unless the tympanic membranes have been thoroughly evaluated and found to be intact. However, since this procedure poses some potential risk for patients, it will be mentioned only in passing. The procedure is described in detail, along with several extensive evaluation techniques, in the well-known text of Plum and Posner,[10] *The Diagnosis of Stupor and Coma.*

Cranial Nerve V

The *trigeminal,* or fifth cranial, nerve is a mixed nerve with both sensory and motor function. Lower motor neurons originate from a motor nucleus well localized in the pontine tegmentum and travel anteriorly to the fora-men ovale where the trigeminal nerve descends to innervate the masseter muscle; the temporal, lateral, and medial pterygoid; the mylohyoid and the anterior digastric; and the tensor veli palatini muscles.[11]

The principal sensory nucleus of the fifth cranial nerve is lateral to the motor nucleus in the dorsolateral tegmentum of the pons. Sensory input is transmitted to this region via secondary neurons that originate in a peripheral sensory ganglion named the *trigeminal* or *gasserian ganglion*. This structure sits in a depression in the floor of the middle cranial fossa, where it is relatively protected except in cases of basilar skull fracture or in penetrating missile injuries to the maxillary region. The trigeminal ganglion receives primary sensory neurons from three separate branches, and so acquires its name. The most superior branch is the ophthalmic nerve (V^1), which is composed of the *lacrimal, frontal, nasociliary*, and *meningeal* branches. These neurons carry sensory impulses from the anterior scalp, forehead, bridge of the nose, and the skin surrounding the eye, including the cornea. These branches join and pass through the orbital fissure before synapsing with secondary sensory neurons in the trigeminal ganglion.

The maxillary branch of the trigeminal nerve (V^2) innervates the skin of the upper lip and cheek, but covers a relatively small area compared to the ophthalmic division. It also innervates the mucus membranes within the nasal cavity, palate, nasopharynx, and the meninges of the anterior and middle cranial fossa. Its branches are the *zygomatic, infraorbital, pterygopalatine*, and *meningeal*. These branches join and pass through the foramen rotundum prior to synapsing with secondary sensory neurons in the trigeminal ganglion.

The mandibular division (V^3) innervates the skin of the lower lip, chin, and anterior portions of the mandible, and extends posteriorly and superiorly to innervate the skin of the preauricular region. It also carries sensory input from the mouth and gums, the anterior portion of the auditory canal, portions of the tympanic membrane, and the meningeal region in the middle cranial fossa. Its branches, named the *buccal, auriculotemporal, lingual, inferior alveolar*, and *meningeal* branches, join to pass through the foramen ovale with the aforementioned motor branch of the trigeminal nerve before synapsing at the trigeminal ganglion.

Although injuries to the ganglion itself are uncommon, injuries to the primary sensory neurons are frequent in cases of trauma to the face, especially when there have been fractures of the frontal and ethmoidal bones. The incidence of injury to a branch of the trigeminal nerve is estimated to be as high as 4.5 percent in some series.[12] Patients with damage to a primary sensory neuron complain of loss of sensitivity to the corresponding area of supply, but do not usually complain of pain. Damage to the trigeminal nucleus, however, often results in excruciating pain, but, fortunately, this is extremely rare in patients with traumatic brain injury. The integrity of the ophthalmic branch of the fifth cranial nerve may be tested by eliciting the *corneal reflex* as follows. A sterile cotton swab is used to touch the cornea of the eye. With an intact reflex arc, the patient immediately attempts to shut the eye. The motor portion of this reflex is mediated by the seventh cranial nerve. Absence of this reflex may indicate an impairment of either the fifth or seventh cranial nerve. In either case, special care should be taken to provide adequate lubrication to the patient's eyes to prevent corneal abrasion.

As was previously mentioned in the description of the first cranial nerve, some stimuli that are commonly considered to be "smells" are actually conducted by the maxillary division of the fifth cranial nerve. Ammonia, or "smelling salts," occasionally used to assess arousal, stimulates this nerve.

Cranial Nerve VII

The *facial,* or seventh cranial, nerve also contains motor and sensory divisions. It is further divided by two separate motor divisions and two separate sensory divisions: The *branchial motor division* supplies the "muscles of expression" in the face; the *visceral motor division* supplies stimulation to the lacrimal, submandibular, sublingual, and nasal glands. The *general sensory division* supplies sensation to the portion of the external auditory canal and tympanic membrane not supplied by the fifth cranial nerve, and to a small patch of skin behind the ear; the *special sensory division* provides taste to the anterior two-thirds of the tongue and to the hard and soft palates. The *motor nucleus* lies immediately superior to the sensory nucleus in the ventrolateral portion of the lower pontine tegmentum near the medulla oblongata. All branches of the seventh cranial nerve exit through the internal auditory meatus. The *branchial motor division* exits through the stylomastoid foramen where it branches to supply the stapedius and stylohyoid muscles, the posterior belly of the digastric muscle, and the muscles of facial expression, including the buccinator, platysma, and occipitalis muscles.[11]

The temporal branches of this nerve receive innervation from the right and left cerebral motor cortex. This is important clinically because lesions of the motor cortex, if unilateral, result in paralysis only of the muscles supplied by the more inferior zygomatic, buccal, and mandibular branches of the facial nerve.[9] This is evidenced clinically by an asymmetrical smile but symmetrical wrinkling of the forehead, and in the vernacular is referred to as "paralysis of the facial nerve in a central pattern." Lesions of the facial nerve that occur distal to the motor nucleus result in paralysis of all muscles on either side of the face and commonly occur in temporal bone fractures. Evidence of injury may be immediate or may have a delayed onset. A delayed presentation may occur from one day to two weeks after the initial injury, and is generally thought to be due to swelling of the nerve within its fibrous sheath, or secondary to damage of the surrounding vasculature. The branchial motor branch of the seventh cranial nerve is the most superficial branch and, hence, the most commonly injured in cases of traumatic brain injury. The incidence of injury has been poorly studied in patients with traumatic brain injury.[5]

The visceral motor branch of the seventh cranial nerve separates into a superior division that innervates the lacrimal glands and the glands of the nasal mucosa, and an inferior branch that innervates the sublingual and submandibular salivary glands. The general sensory division of the seventh cranial nerve accompanies the branchial motor division through the stylomastoid foramen and is of little clinical importance. The special sensory branch accompanies the inferior portion of the visceral motor division through the pterotympanic fissure, and together they form the *chordae tympani nerve*. The special sensory branch splits away from the chordae tympani to supply taste to the anterior two-thirds of the tongue. Tastes supplied by this nerve primarily are those of sweet, salt, and sour.

Cranial Nerve VIII

The *vestibulocochlear*, or eighth cranial, nerve is a purely sensory nerve with two important functions. It receives auditory information from the cochlea and also postural information from the semicircular canals. The primary sensory neurons from both of these divisions make their first synapse at the vestibular, or Scarpa's, ganglion located in the internal auditory meatus. Secondary sensory neurons then make a series of multiple and complex interconnections within the vestibular nuclei located near the floor of the fourth ventricle. A thorough description of the multiple connections made between the vestibular nuclei and the centers that control posture and eye movements is beyond the scope of this chapter. The reader interested in a more thorough description of this subject is referred to other sources.[8,9] Injuries to the eighth cranial nerve occur most commonly in temporal bone fractures, but the incidence of these injuries is unknown in patients with traumatic brain injury. Patients who have received blows to the head occasionally will have transient high frequency hearing loss and tinnitus because of hair cell damage in the cochlea, which is distinguished from true eighth cranial nerve damage. Some degree of hearing loss occurs in approximately 50 percent of patients with severe head injuries and is usually of a sensorineural type. Conductive hearing loss occurs in approximately 3 percent of cases and is usually due to a hemotympanum (accumulation of blood behind the eardrum), which resolves when the hematoma is absorbed.[5] Additional information regarding hearing is contained in Chapter Seven.

Cranial Nerves IX, X, XI, and XII

In patients with traumatic brain injury, it is uncommon to find injuries to the peripheral branches of the *glossopharyngeal*, or ninth cranial, nerve; to the *vagus*, or tenth cranial, nerve; to the *spinal accessory*, or eleventh cranial, nerve; or to the *hypoglossal*, or twelfth cranial, nerve. They do occur, however, in patients who have penetrating wounds to the neck, or in patients who have severe basilar skull fractures or damage to the brain stem and medulla.[5]

Dysfunction also is seen in cortical injuries that affect the upper motor neurons of these nerves. Unilateral damage to all four of these nerves is a recognized clinical syndrome referred to as the *Collet-Sicard Syndrome*. Symptoms of this syndrome consist of cardiac irregularities, excessive salivation, loss of sensation and gag of ipsilateral palate, loss of taste sensation of the posterior one-third of the tongue, and hoarse voice with paralysis of the ipsilateral vocal fold, dysphagia, and hemiatrophy of the tongue.[5,8] Patients who have any of the above-named symptoms are at increased risk of aspiration and should receive a thorough dysphagia evaluation. Lesions of the brain stem and medulla also may present clinically with increased yawning, vomiting, or with hiccups, but the clinician should be mindful that these symptoms are nonspecific and may be representative of many other disease processes.

GENERAL NEUROLOGIC EXAMINATION

The patient's acute neurological assessment also should include observations of the respiratory rate and rhythm. Bilateral dysfunction of the diencephalon or deep regions of the cerebral hemispheres may produce a stereotypic pattern of respiration referred to as *Cheyne-Stokes respiration*. In this pattern of breathing, the depth of inspiration increases in a smooth crescendo with a subsequent smooth decrescendo interspersed with relative periods of apnea (no respiration). The presence of this breathing pattern is nonspecific and may occur in a variety of neurological conditions, but if it develops abruptly in a patient with a recent traumatic brain injury, it may herald an early transtentorial herniation.[10]

If a patient is suspected of having an expanding intracranial lesion or a gradual increase in cerebrospinal fluid pressure, it is imperative that the neurological exam be repeated at frequent intervals. With such lesions, progressive cerebral dysfunction often can be detected by the bedside clinical exam. Such dysfunction usually progresses in a rostral to caudal direction. In the early stages of a transtentorial herniation, a patient may exhibit the previously mentioned Cheyne-Stokes respirations, have small pupils, have doll's eyes, and may have some preservation of an appropriate motor response. As cerebral edema increases, the motor response may change to that of a stereotypic decorticate posture. Once the cerebral dysfunction progresses to the midbrain and upper pons, the pupils become fixed and in midposition, and the doll's eyes reflex is no longer present. Patients also may exhibit a decerebrate posture when noxious stimuli are administered. With advanced transtentorial herniation, the Cheyne-Stokes pattern of respiration will cease, and the patient will develop a shallow or irregular respiratory pattern.[10]

In cases of unilateral cerebral edema, herniation of the medial temporal lobe, or uncus, will sometimes occur, resulting in ipsilateral compression of the third cranial nerve. In the early stages of this syndrome, the ipsilateral pupil will be larger than the left contralateral, but will initially maintain its reactivity to light. Frequently, there also will be evidence of contralateral motor abnormalities such as decorticate or decerebrate posturing. As the syndrome progresses, a total third nerve palsy develops, as is evidenced by ipsilateral ptosis (partial closure of the eyelid), a nonreactive dilated pupil, and loss of the doll's eyes reflex in the affected eye.[9,10]

In evaluating patients who appear to be in coma, clinicians must be aware of a rare and unusual phenomenon referred to as the *locked-in syndrome*.[13,14] In this state, patients have paralysis of all four extremities, and loss of lower cranial nerve function, but have no alteration of consciousness. Subjects are unable to communicate verbally or through body movements, but retain extraocular movements and the capacity to blink. Although this condition may occur as a result of lesions in the ventral midbrain, or any lesion distal to the motor nuclei of the lower cranial nerves, in patients with traumatic injury it is usually due to a lesion in the pons. Since the abducens nerve exits the brain stem in this region, lateral eye movements frequently will be absent. The third cranial nerve, however, is usually intact, and the patient can be assessed by using eye blinks to represent "yes" and "no" responses. Patients with this syndrome may have intact cortical functioning with awareness of their surroundings, but they are "locked-in" in that they are unable to communicate except by eye movements.

CLASSIFICATION OF SEVERITY

Although many variables may be used to classify the severity of traumatic brain injury, classification is primarily determined on the basis of the length and depth of coma. The previously mentioned Glasgow Coma Scale is the most widely used measure to quantify coma, and therefore has formed the basis for classification. An initial Glasgow Coma Scale of 13 to 15 equates with a "mild" brain injury and may or may not involve a loss of consciousness. Patients with a "moderate" brain injury will have an initial Glasgow Coma Scale of 9 to 12, and will usually have a loss of consciousness lasting less than 24 hours. "Moderate" brain injuries are alternatively termed "moderately severe" injuries by some clinicians. Patients with "severe" injuries have an initial Glasgow Coma Scale score of 8 or less, and usually have a loss of consciousness for longer than 24 hours.[15]

An additional factor useful in determining the severity of brain injury is the persistence of *post-traumatic amnesia (PTA)*, which is the loss of memory for events occurring subsequent to the injury.[16] This implies that during the period of post-traumatic amnesia, the patient is unable to retain newly acquired information. Patients with moderate degrees of injury usually have periods of post-traumatic amnesia of less than 24 hours, whereas patients with severe injuries will have post-traumatic amnesia for periods greater than 24 hours.[17] Post-traumatic amnesia is discussed further in Chapters Five and Seven.

Mild traumatic brain injuries may be subdivided further into different grades of mild injury.[18] These gradations are based on the presence of amnesia and loss of consciousness. In the mildest forms of traumatic brain injury, there may be no amnesia or loss of consciousness, but merely confusion. Transient confusion, which occurs immediately following a traumatic brain injury, has been termed *concussion*. This term is widely used by clinicians as well as lay people, but it has no exact definition. Gennarelli[19] describes a spectrum of concussion-type syndromes, the least severe of which includes only transient visual disturbance, focal dysesthesia (painful or unusual tactile sensation), and motor dysfunction, implying a localized disruption of the cortex. Gennarelli defines the most severe level of concussion as the "classic concussion," in which the individual may have a period of coma lasting up to six hours. It is useful to classify the severity of brain injuries, since the prediction of outcome is based, to a large extent, on the severity of the injury and the duration of coma and post-traumatic amnesia.[20,21]

A widely used scale, the *Levels of Cognitive Function*,[22] was developed at Rancho Los Amigos Hospital in the 1970s and consists of eight levels of cognitive function. These levels are described briefly as follows: Level I, no response to external stimuli; Level II, generalized response; Level III, localized but purposeful response; Level IV, confused and agitated; Level V, confused but nonagitated; Level VI, confused but appropriate; Level VII, automatic but appropriate; and Level VIII, purposeful and appropriate. Patients typically progress from the lower levels of functioning to the higher levels as they recover from a traumatic brain injury. Some patients, however, may progress rapidly and appear to skip some levels. Other patients may reach a plateau and then fail to progress until weeks or even months have passed. The utility of the Rancho levels is in providing a common vocabulary for members of the treatment team. Familiarity with these different levels of functioning may help the team in providing therapy that is at an appropriate level for the patient's capacity to participate.

The Rancho classification system is relatively insensitive in detecting changes in the early stages of coma recovery. An alternative evaluation tool, the *Coma/Near-Coma Scale*[23], was designed to detect early signs of improvement in severely impaired individuals, and has shown promise in predicting recovery from coma. This assessment scale places patients in one of five levels of coma, according to their response to eleven separate modes of stimulation. Clinicians are referred to the original article for details regarding administration and scoring of this test.[23]

Patients who remain unresponsive for two weeks or longer frequently are described as being in a *persistent vegetative state*. This term was proposed initially by Jennett and Plum[24] to describe patients who develop reflexive eye opening, but have no response to commands and apparently lack all cognitive functioning. Although some authors have defended the term "vegetative state" as possessing greater dignity than many other terms, the use of this term is controversial and has led to many attempts at renaming this syndrome.[10] Synonyms include "prolonged post-traumatic unconsciousness" and "post-comatose unawareness."[25,26] Patients in a persistent vegetative state are characterized as having intact sleep-wake cycles, preservation of spontaneous eye opening and extraocular movements, and preservation of primitive brain stem reflexes including yawning, sucking, and chewing.

Although some authors consider the development of the persistent vegetative state to be a negative prognostic sign, other authors[25] claim its presence has no predictive value with regard to further improvement. Approximately 60 percent of patients with this diagnosis show some evidence of improvement during the first year. In the study by Bricolo and associates[25], who followed the recovery of 135 comatose patients, 52 percent of patients began to follow commands in the first three months, 13 percent did so between three and six months, and 1.5 percent only after the sixth month.

COMPLICATIONS AND TREATMENT

Seizures

The word *seizure* may be used loosely in medicine to refer to any type of sudden or catastrophic event. The root of the Greek word *epilepsy* literally means "to seize" and is commonly used to describe the condition or state of patients who are prone to have uncontrollable behaviors that are due to abnormal spontaneous activity of the neurons in the cerebral cortex. Although the term *epileptic seizure* is somewhat redundant, its use is advocated by some authors to avoid confusion.[27] Terminology regarding seizures is even more confused among the general public. "Fits," "convulsions," "attacks," and "spells" are terms commonly used to describe these events by patients and their families.

The classification of seizures is multifactorial in nature. The term *posttraumatic seizure* is descriptive with regard to the time of onset but it is demographic only; it does not describe the severity of the seizure or imply the specific anatomic focus of abnormal activity in the brain. Seizures may be described in terms of severity as well as in terms of time of onset following a traumatic brain injury. Seizures are subdivided with regard to severity according to the classification scheme developed by The International League Against Epilepsy.[28] Seizures that involve only a portion of the brain are termed *partial,* in contrast to *generalized* seizures, which involve both cerebral hemispheres.

Partial seizures that do not affect consciousness are termed *simple partial*, whereas those that alter consciousness or responsiveness are termed *complex partial*. Generalized seizures always affect consciousness. Post-traumatic epileptic seizures also may be classified as being either *early* or *late*. Early seizures occur within the first week following injury and have an incidence of approximately 5 percent.[29] Late post-traumatic seizures develop after the first week following injury. They occur with an approximate incidence of 4 to 7 percent in patients with closed head injuries,[30] but occur with a higher incidence in individuals who have received penetrating wounds to the brain, or in individuals who have severe focal contusions or hemorrhages.[31]

Treatment of post-traumatic epileptic seizure is controversial and is often determined by clinical custom and individual physician preference, rather than by a universally agreed upon protocol based on scientific study. It is well recognized that patients who develop early generalized recurrent seizures should be treated to prevent the destructive effects of hypoxia and increased metabolism. The prophylactic use of anticonvulsant medications to prevent seizures has been extensively debated in the literature. The case against using anticonvulsant prophylaxis was stated convincingly in the review article by Yablon,[32] who found little evidence to support this practice. Arguments against the use of anticonvulsants are based primarily on the avoidance of the central nervous system depressant effects.

Guidelines for treatment with specific anticonvulsant agents are beyond the scope of this chapter, but will be briefly reviewed to familiarize the clinician with the various agents. Phenobarbital, first introduced in 1912, was the only drug available for many years. Although it is an effective medication, it produces sedation and central nervous system depression even at small doses. Phenytoin (brand name Dilantin) was introduced in 1938 and has an advantage over phenobarbital in that it is less sedating within its therapeutic range. Carbamazepine (brand name Tegretol) was introduced in 1974 for the treatment of seizures. It is also recognized as a "membrane stabilizing" agent and has been used to treat a variety of other conditions, including behavior disturbances and pain syndromes. Carbamazepine causes less sedation in many patients and is the preferred anticonvulsant for the treatment of post-traumatic epileptic seizures, in the opinion of many authors.[32,33] Cognitive side effects of phenytoin and carbamazepine may be similar and idiosyncratic, necessitating individual evaluation of each patient.[34] Carbamazepine also has the disadvantage of a more frequent dosage interval and more frequent hematological monitoring when compared with phenytoin and phenobarbital. Although several other anticonvulsant agents have been used in the treatment of post-traumatic epileptic seizures, the above three agents are the most widely used.

Post-Traumatic Hydrocephalus

Cerebrospinal fluid is produced by the choroid plexus at a rate of 15 to 35 milliliters per hour (ml/hr). Fluid circulates through the lateral and third ventricles prior to passing through the cerebral aqueduct and fourth ventricle. It subsequently exits into the subarachnoid space, where it bathes the entire brain and spinal cord. Cerebrospinal fluid is absorbed from the arachnoid space through projections called arachnoid granulations, which project into the superior sagittal sinus and its tributaries.[8,9] Normally, an equal volume of cerebrospinal fluid is produced and absorbed, resulting in a steady state. If fluid is unable to exit the ventricular system because of an obstruction, it will accumulate within the ventricular system, causing the ventricles to expand under pressure. Expansion of the ventricles by an increased volume of cerebrospinal fluid is termed *hydrocephalus*. As cerebrospinal fluid pressure increases within the brain, the neural structures are compressed, resulting in dysfunction. If this condition is allowed to progress, the outcome is usually fatal.[8,9]

When hydrocephalus occurs as the result of a blockage in the outflow of cerebrospinal fluid, it is termed *obstructive hydrocephalus*. This condition may be seen in the acute setting in patients with traumatic brain injury, and may be due to a hematoma or cerebral edema that obstructs cerebrospinal fluid flow.[9]

Communicating hydrocephalus, also known as *normal pressure hydrocephalus*, is thought to develop as a result of impaired cerebrospinal fluid absorption from the arachnoid space. Patients with subarachnoid hemorrhage may develop scarring and fibrosis in the arachnoid space, predisposing them to communicating hydrocephalus. This condition usually develops over a period of several weeks and is accompanied by a reduction in cerebrospinal fluid production. Cerebrospinal fluid pressure subsequently returns to normal, hence the term normal pressure hydrocephalus.

Some patients recovering from traumatic brain injury will develop cerebral atrophy, as evidenced by dilated ventricles and shrinkage of the cortical gyri. Although these patients are sometimes referred to as having *hydrocephalus ex vacuo*, there is no increase in cerebrospinal fluid pressure, and the condition is not considered to be a true hydrocephalus by most authors.[35] Ventricular dilation due to either atrophy or hydrocephalus occurs in up to 86 percent of patients recovering from severe traumatic brain injury.[36] The true incidence of obstructive and communicating hydrocephalus is unknown.

Patients who develop communicating hydrocephalus usually do so within two weeks following injury, but its development may be delayed until as late as the second month after injury.[35] This is clinically important because the onset of symptoms may be subtle and go unnoticed by many members of the rehabilitation treatment team. This condition should be suspected in patients who develop a regression in cognitive function within the first two months following injury. The classic triad of progressive dementia, ataxia, and urinary incontinence is seen in patients with normal pressure hydrocephalus.[8,9]

Cerebrospinal Fluid Fistula

Normally, cerebrospinal fluid circulates through the ventricles and intracranial structures without making contact with the external environment. If the integrity of the cranial vault is broken by a skull fracture, a tract may form that allows cerebrospinal fluid to exit the cranial vault, usually through the auditory canal or structures in the posterior nasopharynx and sinuses. These tracts are referred to as *cerebrospinal fluid fistulas* and were briefly introduced earlier in this chapter.

Cerebrospinal fluid fistulas are not problematic because of the fluid loss that occurs, but rather because the tract that allows fluid to escape may also allow infectious organisms to enter into the cranial vault. If this leakage goes undetected for several days or weeks, the risk of meningitis or abscess increases dramatically. Among patients who develop a cerebrospinal fluid fistula, approximately 80 percent will develop fistulas during the first 48 hours following injury.[37] The remaining patients have a delayed presentation and may even develop their fistula several years after their original injury. The incidence of cerebrospinal fluid fistulas is reported to be as high as 11 percent in patients who sustain a basilar skull fracture.[38]

Speech-language pathologists are in a unique position to detect this uncommon complication. In the early stages of development, patients may complain only of a painless, watery discharge from the nose or ear, without other symptoms. This condition should be suspected in all patients with moderate to severe traumatic brain injuries, even if there is no clear history of a basilar skull fracture. If a fistula is suspected, the physician should be notified immediately and a sample of the discharge analyzed in a clinical laboratory for the presence of glucose. Glucose concentration is much higher in cerebrospinal fluid than in other discharges from the nose and ears. Initial treatment of a cerebrospinal fluid fistula is done with antibiotics, which prevent infection. If drainage persists for days to weeks, surgical repair of the tract is indicated.

Respiratory Complications

In the acute hospital setting, patients with traumatic brain injury who are suspected of having increased intracranial pressure are frequently treated with hyperventilation. This necessitates placement of an *endotracheal tube (ET)* that is usually introduced through the oral cavity. The rationale for this treatment is that hyperventilation causes a decrease in blood levels of carbon dioxide, which is known to cause cerebral vasodilation and, hence, increased intracranial pressure. Although endotracheal tubes may be well tolerated for several days, their prolonged use leads to vocal fold trauma.[39] Endotracheal tubes are also uncomfortable and may be poorly tolerated in patients emerging from coma, necessitating frequent sedation.

In patients with prolonged periods of coma, especially those with an impairment in spontaneous respiration, consideration is usually given to insertion of a *tracheostomy tube,* which is placed through the skin at a level below the vocal folds. Tracheostomy tubes avoid vocal fold trauma and decrease the noxious stimuli associated with an endotracheal tube. Patients with a tracheostomy have a reduced incidence of pneumonia and sinusitis when compared to patients with oral or nasal endotracheal tubes.[39,40] In addition, patients who have difficulty in clearing respiratory secretions are more easily suctioned through a tracheostomy tube. Disadvantages of tracheostomy include the necessity of a surgical procedure and a higher incidence of tracheal stenosis and stomal infection.[41]

Speech-language pathologists who treat patients with traumatic brain injuries may be expected to assist with tracheostomy management in some clinical settings. Clinicians who find themselves in this position should familiarize themselves with the various types of tracheostomy tubes, which are described in the following references.[41,42,43] Although academic knowledge of these devices is a prerequisite, the author recommends that the speech-language pathologist confer with the respiratory therapist and receive "hands on" instruction prior to suctioning or adjusting a tracheostomy.

Nutritional and Gastrointestinal Considerations

Patients who survive a traumatic brain injury frequently have impaired swallowing and gastrointestinal motility, limiting their ability to ingest and absorb nutrients. Paradoxically, these same patients have increased nutritional requirements, even though they may be perceived by the casual observer to be inactive.[44] In fact, patients with traumatic brain injury, as well as patients with stroke and other forms of cerebral injury, have increased energy expenditure ranging from 130 percent to 170 percent above the normal predicted basal metabolic rate.[45] This *hypermetabolic state* persists for several weeks after injury, but it may continue for as long as one year after injury in some cases. Patients in this state are prone to *catabolism,* which is defined as tissue destruction due to increased energy requirements. Tissues vulnerable to catabolism include muscle, fat, and circulating serum proteins, including the proteins that mediate immune responses. Such patients may experience muscle atrophy, lose the protection provided by subcutaneous fat, and have an increased risk of infection.

Total parenteral nutrition (TPN) refers to the intravenous administration of glucose, amino acids, fatty acids, vitamins, and minerals. During the 1980s, total parenteral nutrition was developed as an alternative to *enteral nutrition* (nutrition received through the alimentary tract) in individuals who had increased metabolic demands but who also had dysfunction of the gastrointestinal tract. Although total parenteral nutrition plays a role in the management of such patients, it is recognized that enteral feeding offers many advantages over total parenteral nutrition.[45] Patients who receive total parenteral nutrition must have a central venous catheter placed, usually in the subclavian vein, and may experience complications from this procedure. Patients receiving total parenteral nutrition also must be monitored carefully for evidence of metabolic abnormalities due to the intravenous administration of this concentrated solution. Patients receiving enteral feedings, in contrast, have a lower incidence of infection and other complications. Enteral feedings also are more convenient and less expensive.

In the first days following a traumatic brain injury, a conventional *nasogastric tube (NG tube)* may be used to provide adequate nutrition, but prolonged use is associated with an increased incidence of sinusitis and gastroesophageal reflux, and it may be a contributing factor to agitation due to patient discomfort.[46] These side effects may be lessened by using a small diameter tube such as the *Dobhoff tube*. This tube has a weighted tip that is propelled by peristalsis through the pyloric sphincter, and thus decreases the probability of regurgitation. The disadvantage of using a small diameter tube is that it may become clogged more frequently, especially if it is used to administer pulverized medications. It is most suited for continuous administration of a preformulated tube feeding.

The disadvantages of nasogastric tubes may be circumvented by the use of a *gastrostomy tube (G-tube)*, which enters the stomach through the skin of the anterior abdomen. This surgically created portal of entry is termed the *stoma*, literally translated from Greek as "mouth." Gastrostomy tubes come in many forms and are placed using a variety of surgical techniques. One very popular surgical technique is that of the *percutaneous endoscopic gastrostomy (PEG)*.[47] This technique has become so popular that all gastrostomy tubes are sometimes incorrectly referred to as "PEG tubes." Short tubes that terminate within the stomach are correctly termed to be gastrostomy tubes. Longer tubes that pass through the pyloric sphincter and duodenum into the jejunum are correctly termed *jejunostomy tubes*. Although gastrostomy and jejunostomy tubes offer several advantages over nasogastric tubes, it should be remembered that patients receiving these devices must undergo surgery and, therefore, face potential complications from this procedure. Other complications associated with gastrostomy tubes include bleeding and stomal infection. Occasionally, portions of the tube may erode the stomach lining, resulting in gastritis or even peritonitis.[48] It also should be remembered that aspiration may occur in patients with gastrostomy tubes if the stomach contents are regurgitated.

Pharmacotherapy

Patients recovering from traumatic brain injury often receive multiple medications for the treatment of complications, and, in some cases, to augment recovery. Although drug therapy may be directed toward treatment of a single problem, some medications have unintended side effects that may affect cognitive performance and behavior. The previous description of seizures and their treatment serves as a prime example of this phenomenon. In treating problems associated with the brain and nervous system, one may intuitively expect cognitive side effects, but similar effects may be observed from the treatment of conditions seemingly unrelated to mental function.

This section is presented to increase the clinician's awareness of medication side effects and the complex nature of pharmacologic treatment. Clinicians also are reminded that they may be called upon to evaluate drug effects if their patients are placed on a drug therapy trial. Since many of these drug effects occur idiosyncratically, it is often useful to study patients' responses to treatment by evaluating their behavior before, during, and after drug administration in a single case study design.[49,50]

At the risk of oversimplification, a review of neuropharmacology is provided before specific problems and their treatment are covered. This subject is extremely complex and does not lend itself easily to a brief review. The reader is referred to the referenced texts and the topic readings in Appendix B for a more thorough understanding of the topic.

The transmission of electrical signals from one neuron to another occurs at the synapse by way of chemical mediators. These molecules, termed *neurotransmitters*, act as chemical messengers that facilitate or inhibit neural activity. Neurotransmitters may originate at the synapse or may be carried to the synapse by way of the blood stream. Exogenous drugs (chemicals created outside of the body) may exert their effect by mimicking the action of endogenous neurotransmitters.

The chemical structure of neurotransmitters is diverse. Some are small molecules with ammonia derivatives on their side chain (amines), and others are large protein molecules (peptides), such as the endorphins. Four principal groups of neurotransmitters are recognized: monoamines, which include norepinephrine, dopamine, serotonin, and histamine; acetylcholine; amino acids; and peptides.[51]

Hypertension

Patients recovering from brain injury may have *hypertension* (elevated blood pressure) that requires medical treatment. Some antihypertensive drugs are associated with central nervous system depressant effects. These include clonidine, hydralazine, reserpine, and methyldopa.[52] Another class of antihypertensive drugs, the beta blockers, rarely affects cognition, with the exception of propranolol, which penetrates the central nervous system because of its unique solubility characteristics. Propranolol has, therefore, been advocated by some as a treatment for agitation, although others feel that its risks outweigh the benefits.[53,54]

Pain

Complaints of headache are common in patients with traumatic brain injury. Patients also may complain of pain in other regions of the body, especially following trauma involving multiple skeletal injuries. Narcotic analgesics are used commonly in the acute setting and are known to result in sedation and confusion.[55] Nonsteroidal anti-inflammatory drugs (NSAIDS), such as ibuprofen, also are used to treat pain. Although they have a much lower incidence of cognitive side effects, confusion has been reported in rare cases.

In patients with chronic headaches, some authors[53] recommend treatment with amitriptyline and related tricyclic antidepressants. Others[56] contend, however, that the sedating effects of these medications limit their usefulness in patients with traumatic brain injuries.

Spasticity

Patients may develop spasticity as a result of damage to the brain or spinal cord. Two medications commonly used to treat this condition, diazepam (brand name Valium) and baclofen (brand name Lioresal) are both known to cause sedation and confusion, especially at higher dosages. Baclofen also is associated with hallucinations if patients are abruptly withdrawn from this medication.[56]

Infection

Although cognitive side effects from antibiotics are rare, sensorineural hearing loss is associated with high doses of the aminoglycoside antibiotics gentamicin and tobramycin. Severe hearing loss may result in decreased responsiveness to auditory stimuli and may contribute to confusion.

Gastrointestinal Problems

An increased risk of gastric ulceration occurs in all patients recovering from the significant physical and emotional stress of a traumatic brain injury. Frequently, medications are prescribed to inhibit secretion of gastric acid. One class of drugs blocks the stimulant effects of histamine on the stomach mucosa. These drugs are named H^2 blocking agents and include cimetidine (brand name Tagamet), ranitidine (brand name Zantac), and famotidine (brand name Pepcid). These drugs, especially cimetidine, occasionally are associated with confusion and even hallucinations.[56]

Metoclopramide (brand name Reglan) may be used to facilitate gastric emptying and to inhibit emesis (vomiting). It is a dopamine antagonist and, as such, may cause the same side effects as the antipsychotic agents covered in the following section.[56]

Agitation and Insomnia

A variety of medications has been used to treat agitation associated with recovery from traumatic brain injury. Propanolol has been mentioned previously under the heading of hypertension. Antipsychotic agents, formerly known as "major tranquilizers," are used widely in the treatment of psychosis and its accompanying agitation and aggression. Theoretically, these medications work by antagonizing the effects of dopamine, which is necessary for the transmission of motor impulses. (Depletion of dopamine is present in Parkinsonism and is thought to be responsible for the impairment of motor planning and initiation seen in that disease). Although these drugs are effective as tranquilizers, studies[57] have demonstrated impaired recovery from brain injury in animals treated with them. These medications include haloperidol (brand name Haldol), chlorpromazine (brand name Thorazine), and prochlorperazine (brand name Compazine). Most authors discourage their use in patients recovering from traumatic brain injury, since dopamine depletion is thought to occur as a consequence of injury and should not be exacerbated by medication.[56]

Benzodiazepines, such as diazepam (brand name Valium), and lorazepam (brand name Ativan) also are effective in the treatment of post-traumatic agitation, but their sedating side effects impair cognitive function. In small doses, they may exert a paradoxical effect and increase aggressive behavior by decreasing impulse control. One benzodiazepine, triazolam (brand name Halcion), has been associated with transient global amnesia.[59] All drugs in this class are habit forming and their long-term use is associated with depression.[56]

Trazodone (brand name Desyrel) was originally marketed as an antidepressant, but is widely used as a hypnotic (sleep-inducing) medication. Its use in patients with traumatic brain injury is favored by many authors, since its sedating effects are relatively short lived, and its other side effects are few.[56]

Although their use is not advocated in the literature, antihistamines such as diphenhydramine (brand name Benadryl) are used widely in the treatment of insomnia and are available as nonprescription medications. These medications are relatively safe, but as with all drugs mentioned in this section, they may be associated with prolonged sedation in patients with central nervous system injury. Antihistamines also are known to dry the oral mucosa, potentially exacerbating dysphagia.[58]

Somnolence and Decreased Arousal

Stimulant drugs are used to improve alertness in selected patients who are excessively somnolent or lethargic. The most commonly used stimulant drug in patients with central nervous system disease is methylphenidate (brand name Ritalin). Amphetamines also may be tried but are used less frequently than methylphenidate because of their higher potential for abuse. Patients receiving high doses of stimulant medications may experience anxiety, resulting in an impairment rather than in an improvement in concentration.

Since patients with a traumatic brain injury theoretically have decreased levels of dopamine in the central nervous system, several drugs have been used to increase levels of dopamine and are termed *dopaminergic.* Although they are not stimulant drugs in the conventional sense, they may be used in a similar fashion to enhance recovery. The two most widely studied dopaminergic drugs used to treat patients with traumatic brain injury are amantadine (brand name Symmetrel) and bromocriptine (brand name Parlodel). The unwanted side effects of these drugs include nausea, anorexia, anxiety, and confusion.[56]

Depression

Antidepressant medications have the effect of increasing levels of neurotransmitters, especially norepinephrine and serotonin. Those that selectively increase norepinephrine are termed *noradrenergic,* and those increasing serotonin are termed *serotonergic.* Most antidepressants affect more than one neurotransmitter.

Tricyclic antidepressants such as amitriptyline (brand name Elavil) and desipramine (brand name Norpramin) also decrease acetylcholine and histamine, and may cause dryness of the mucous membranes, constipation, and urinary retention. They also may cause *orthostatic hypotension,* defined as a decreased flow of blood to the brain upon rising to a standing position. This can be a potentially disastrous side effect, since it may lead to falls and additional head trauma.

Serotonergic antidepressants are better tolerated by most patients with traumatic brain injury, but have not been studied as frequently as tricyclic antidepressants. These medications include fluoxetine (brand name Prozac), paroxetine (brand name Paxil), sertraline (brand name Zoloft), and venlafaxine (brand name Effexor). Fluoxetine may be useful in some lethargic patients since it tends to be stimulating. Sertraline, on the other hand, may cause sedation and may offer advantages to patients with insomnia if it is given as a bedtime medication.[60]

PROGNOSTIC FACTORS

Although the physician is the usual member of the health care team called upon to render the prognosis for recovery, all team members should be familiar with the variables that factor into making this "educated guess." Although there is no single approved method for determining prognosis, many studies have attempted to determine which factors are most important. These studies have been criticized, as have most clinical studies, as being poorly standardized and lacking consistent methods of data collection. An additional difficulty in determining significant prognostic variables is the lack of a uniform definition to indicate the factors that constitute a "good" outcome. Patients with understanding and supportive families, for example, often are able to return home or to work despite significant limitations.

Prognostic factors may be grouped into three broad areas: demographic descriptions, such as age, gender, and premorbid psychosocial background; clinical measures, such as the Glasgow Coma Scale, duration of coma, and duration of post-traumatic amnesia; and type and extent of injury, as defined by the presence of focal lesions on a computerized tomography scan, skull fractures, and medical complications. These variables have been evaluated carefully in a review article by Mack and Horn,[61] which has served as a basis for discussion since its publication in 1989. These authors concluded that there was no infallible system for determining prognosis "with even the best tools failing to categorize 10 percent of patients accurately."[61] Subsequent authors,[62,63] using retrospective and prospective methods, also have failed to demonstrate a reliable technique for determining prognosis. There are, however, two variables—duration of coma and age—which seem to correlate fairly well with outcome. They are discussed below to offer some guidance to the clinician.

Duration of Coma

Although there is no clear linear relationship between duration of coma and outcome, significant differences have been observed in individuals who experience a loss of consciousness of less than 24 hours, compared to those who have loss of consciousness of longer than 24 hours.[63,64] Stover[65] determined that coma duration of greater than four months is associated with loss of independence. His observation has been supported recently.[66]

Age

In general, an age greater than 20 years at the time of injury is associated with a relatively worse outcome than an age of less than 20 years at the time of injury. Significant declines in outcome also have been observed in those more than 60 years old and, in a recent study, in those more than 40 years old.[62] Other variables associated with the aging process itself (for example, general health) have not been examined for their potential contribution to outcome.

SUMMARY

The medical management of individuals with traumatic brain injuries is complex and difficult to present in a concise format. Because the acute stages of recovery can proceed with many complications, the recognition of early neurologic signs that indicate changes in the patient's status can be critical to the medical management of the patient's condition. To aid in this management, clinicians need to be aware of neurologic signs that indicate deterioration as well as progress, and of the many complications that often accompany a traumatic brain injury.

This chapter has provided a review of the acute neurological examination, with special attention given to the evaluation of coma and the general examination of the head and cranial nerves. Each cranial nerve has been discussed with regard to anatomy, function, and techniques for evaluation. The classification of brain injury severity as mild, moderate, or severe was discussed with a review of the criteria for each severity level. Additional attention was given to the *persistent vegetative state* as a controversial term and condition.

The medical complications of traumatic brain injury were discussed with particular regard for those conditions that may impact directly upon the delivery of services by the speech-language pathologist. These topics include seizures, hydrocephalus, cerebrospinal fluid fistulas, respiratory complications, and nutritional considerations. Pharmacotherapy that may affect cognitive functioning was discussed. This chapter concluded with a brief presentation of prognostic indicators related to outcome in traumatic brain injury.

REFERENCES

1. Teasdale G, Jennett B. Assessment of coma and impaired consciousness—a practical scale. *Lancet.* 1974;13:81–84.
2. Sherrington CS. Decerebrate rigidity and reflex coordination of movements. *Journal of Physiology.* 1898;22:319.
3. Jagger J, Jane JA, Rimel R. The Glasgow coma scale: to sum or not to sum. *Lancet.* 1983;9:97.
4. Choi SS et al. Enhanced specificity of prognosis in severe head injury. *Journal of Neurosurgery.* 1988;69:381–385.
5. Murali R, Rovit RL. Injuries of the cranial nerves. In Barrow DL (ed). *Complications and Sequelae of Head Injury.* Park Ridge, IL: American Association of Neurological Surgeons; 1992:109–126.
6. Minderhoud JM et al. Treatment of minor head injuries. *Clinics in Neurology and Neurosurgery.* 1980;82:127–40.

7. Sumner D. On testing the sense of smell. *Lancet.* 1962;2:895–897.
8. Adams RD, Victor M. *Principles of Neurology.* New York, NY: McGraw-Hill; 1993.
9. Duus P. *Topical Diagnosis in Neurology.* New York, NY: Georg Thieme Verlag; 1983:104–183.
10. Plum F, Posner JB. *The Diagnosis of Stupor and Coma.* Philadelphia, PA: FA Davis; 1982:1–86.
11. Wilson-Pauwels L, Akesson EJ, Stewart PA. *Cranial Nerves—Anatomy and Clinical Comments.* Toronto, Ontario, Canada: BC Decker; 1988.
12. Russell WR. Injury to cranial nerves and optic chiasm. In Brocks (ed). *Injuries of the Brain and Spinal Cord and Their Coverings, 3rd ed.* Baltimore, MD: Williams and Wilkins; 1949:116–124.
13. Patterson JR, Grabois M. Locked-in syndrome: a review of 139 cases. *Stroke.* 1986;17:758–764.
14. Haig AJ, Katz RT, Sahgal V. Locked-in syndrome: a review. *Current Concepts in Rehabilitation Medicine.* 1986;3:12–15.
15. Andrews BT. Initial management of head injury. In Kraft GH, Berrol S (eds). *Traumatic Brain Injury: Physical Medicine and Rehabilitation Clinics of North America.* Philadelphia, PA: WB Saunders; 1992;3(2):249–258.
16. Levin HS, O'Donnell VM, Grossman RG. The Galveston Orientation and Amnesia Test: a practical scale to assess cognition after head injury. *Journal of Nervous and Mental Disorders.* 1979;167:675–683.
17. Katz DI, Alexander MP. Traumatic brain injury. In Good DC, Couch JR (eds). *Handbook of Neurorehabilitation.* New York, NY: Marcel Dekker; 1994:493–549.
18. Esselman PC, Uomoto JM. Classification of the spectrum of mild traumatic brain injury. *Brain Injury.* 1995;9:417–424.
19. Gennarelli TA. Mechanisms and pathophysiology of cerebral concussion. *Journal of Head Trauma Rehabilitation.* 1986;1:23–29.
20. Katz DI, Alexander MP. Traumatic brain injury: predicting course of recovery and outcome for patients admitted to rehabilitation. *Archives of Neurology.* 1994;51:661–670.
21. Ross BL et al. Neuropsychological outcome in relation to head injury severity: contributions of coma length and focal abnormalities. *American Journal of Physical Medicine and Rehabilitation.* 1994;73:341–347.
22. Hagen C, Malkmus D, Durham P. Levels of cognitive functioning. *Rehabilitation of the Head Injured Adult: Comprehensive Physical Management.* Downey, CA: Professional Staff Association of Rancho Los Amigos Hospital; 1979.
23. Rappaport M, Dougherty AM, Kelting DL. Evaluation of coma and vegetative states. *Archives of Physical Medicine Rehabilitation.* 1992;73:628–634.
24. Jennett WB, Plum F. The persistent vegetative state after brain damage: a syndrome in search of a name. *Lancet.* 1972;1:734–737.
25. Bricolo AB, Turazzi S, Feriotti G. Prolonged post traumatic unconsciousness: therapeutic assets and liabilities. *Journal of Neurosurgery.* 1980;52:625–634.
26. Sazbon L, Costeff H, Groswasser Z. Epidemiological findings in traumatic post-comatose unawareness. *Brain Injury.* 1992;6:359–362.
27. Engel J. *Seizures and Epilepsy.* Philadelphia, PA: FA Davis; 1989.
28. Commission on Classification and Terminology of the International League Against Epilepsy: proposal for revised clinical and electroencephalographic classification of epileptic seizures. *Epilepsia.* 1981;22:489–501.
29. Jennett B. *Epilepsy after Non-missile Head Injuries, 2nd ed.* Chicago, IL: William Heinemann; 1975.

30. Jennett B, Lewin W. Traumatic epilepsy after closed head injuries. *Journal of Neurology, Neurosurgery, and Psychiatry.* 1960;23:295–301.
31. Salazar AM et al. Epilepsy after penetrating head injury: I. clinical correlates. *Neurology.* 1985;35:1406–14.
32. Yablon SA. Posttraumatic seizures. *Archives of Physical Medicine and Rehabilitation.* 1993;74:983–1001.
33. Bontke CF, Baize CM, Boake C. Coma management and sensory stimulation. In Kraft GH, Berrol S (eds). *Traumatic Brain Injury: Physical Medicine and Rehabilitation Clinics of North America.* Philadelphia, PA: WB Saunders; 1992;3(2):259–272.
34. Smith KR et al. Neurobehavior effects of phenytoin and carbamazepine in patients recovering from brain trauma: a comparative study. *Archives of Neurology.* 1994;51:653–660.
35. Doherty D. Posttraumatic hydrocephalus. In Kraft GH, Berrol S (eds). *Traumatic Brain Injury: Physical Medicine and Rehabilitation Clinics of North America.* Philadelphia, PA: WB Saunders; 1992;3(2):389–405.
36. Van Dongen KJ, Broakman R. Late computed tomography in survivors of severe head injury. *Neurosurgery.* 1980;7:14.
37. Park J-I, Strelzow VV, Friedman WH. Current management of cerebrospinal fluid rhinorrhea. *Laryngoscope.* 1983;93:1294–1300.
38. Cooper PR. Cerebrospinal fluid fistulas and pneumocephalus. In Barrow DL (ed). *Complications and Sequelae of Head Injury.* Park Ridge, IL: American Association of Neurological Surgeons; 1992:1–12.
39. Astrachan DI et al. Prolonged intubation vs. tracheostomy: complications, practical and psychological considerations. *Laryngoscope.* 1988;98:1165–1169.
40. Marsh HM, Gillespie DJ, Baumgartner AE. Timing of tracheostomy in the critically ill patient. *Chest.* 1989;91:190–193.
41. Taya VS. Tracheostomies. In Morgan JA, Stack LB (eds). *Patients with Indwelling Devices: Emergency Medicine Clinics of North America.* Philadelphia, PA: WB Saunders; August 1994:707–727.
42. Weilitz PB, Dettenmeier PA. Test your knowledge of tracheostomy tubes. *American Journal of Nursing.* February 1994:46–50.
43. Hoit JD, Shea SS, Banzett RB. Speech production during mechanical ventilation in tracheostomized individuals. *Journal of Speech and Hearing Research.* 1994;37:53–63.
44. Glenn MR, Rosenthal M. Rehabilitation following severe traumatic brain injury. *Seminars in Neurology.* 1985;5:233–246.
45. Hadley MN. Hypermetabolism following head trauma: nutritional considerations. In Barrow DL (ed). *Complications and Sequelae of Head Injury.* Park Ridge, IL: American Association of Neurological Surgeons; 1992:161–168.
46. Desmond, Raman R, Idikula J. Effect of nasogastric tubes on the nose and maxillary sinus. *Critical Care Medicine.* 1991;19:509–511.
47. D'Amelio LF, Hammond JS, Spain DA, Sutyak JP. Tracheostomy and percutaneous endoscopic gastrostomy in the management of the head-injured trauma patient. *American Surgeon.* 1994;60(pt 3):180–185.
48. O'Keefe KP. Complications of percutaneous feeding tubes. In Morgan JA, Stack LB (eds). *Patients with Indwelling Devices: Emergency Medicine Clinics of North America.* Philadelphia, PA: WB Saunders; August 1994:815–826.
49. Pierce JN et al. The use of a double-blind, placebo, crossover design in the evaluation of psychostimulant drug therapy efficacy: a case study. Poster presen-

tation at American Academy of Physical Medicine and Rehabilitation 56th Annual Assembly. Anaheim, CA; October 1994.

50. Evans RW, Gualtieri CT, Patterson D. Treatment of chronic closed head injury with psychostimulant drugs: a controlled case study and an appropriate evaluation procedure. *The Journal of Nervous and Mental Disease.* 1987;175:106–110.

51. Zasler ND. Advances in neuropharmacological rehabilitation for brain dysfunction. *Brain Injury.* 1992;6:1–14.

52. O'Shanick GJ, Zasler ND. Neuropsychopharmacological approaches to traumatic brain injury. In Kreutzer JS, Wehman P (eds). *Community Integration Following Traumatic Brain Injury.* Baltimore, MD: Paul H Brookes; 1990:15–27.

53. Cardenas DD, McLean A. Psychopharmacologic management of traumatic brain injury. In Kraft GH, Berrol S (eds). *Traumatic Brain Injury: Physical Medicine and Rehabilitation Clinics of North America.* Philadelphia, PA: WB Saunders; 1992;3(2):273–290.

54. Haas JF, Cope DN. Neuropharmacologic management of behavioral sequelae in head injury: a case report. *Archives of Physical Medicine and Rehabilitation.* 1985;66:472–474.

55. Ross LK. The use of pharmacology in the treatment of head-injured patients. In Long CJ, Ross LK (eds). *Handbook of Head Trauma: Acute Care to Recovery.* New York, NY: Plenum Press; 1992:137–164.

56. Gaultieri CT. *Neuropsychiatry and Behavioral Pharmacology.* New York, NY: Springer-Verlag; 1991:37–88.

57. Feeney DM, Gonzalez A, Law WA. Amphetamine, haloperidol and experience interact to affect rate of recovery after motor cortex surgery. *Science.* 1982;217:855–857.

58. Douglas WW. Histamine and 5-hydroxytryptamine (serotonin) and their antagonists. In Gilman AG et al (eds). *Goodman and Gilman's The Pharmacological Basis of Therapeutics, 7th ed.* New York, NY: Macmillan Publishing; 1985:605–638.

59. Morris HH, Estes ML. Traveler's amnesia. Transient global amnesia secondary to triazolam. *Journal of the American Medical Association.* 1987;258:945–946.

60. The Medical Letter. Choice of an antidepressant. *The Medical Letter.* 1993;35:25–26.

61. Mack A, Horn LJ. Functional prognosis in traumatic brain injury. In Horn LJ, Cope DN (eds). *Traumatic Brain Injury: Physical Medicine and Rehabilitation State of the Art Reviews.* Philadelphia, PA: Hanley and Belfus; 1989;3(1):13–26.

62. Ross BL et al. Neuropsychological outcome in relation to head injury severity: contributions of coma length and focal abnormalities. *American Journal of Physical Medicine and Rehabilitation.* 1994;73:341–347.

63. Katz DI, Alexander MP. Traumatic brain injury: predicting course of recovery and outcome for patients admitted to rehabilitation. *Archives of Neurology.* 1994;51:661–670.

64. Levin HS, Eisenberg HM. Neuropsychological outcome of closed head injury in children and adolescents. *Child's Brain.* 1979;5:281–292.

65. Stover SL, Zeiger HE. Head injury in children and teenagers: functional recovery correlate with duration of coma. *Archives of Physical Medicine and Rehabilitation.* 1976;57:201–205.

66. Wisdom PJ. Correlation of disability rating scale with duration of unresponsiveness. Poster presentation at the American Society of Neurorehabilitation. Minneapolis, MN; June 1994.

5

The Nature of Cognitive and Communication Impairment: Theoretical and Clinical Considerations

In the early 1970s, traumatic brain injury piqued the interest of many health care professionals in the United States and Europe. As with any other condition of growing proportions, the initial concerns were centered around the evaluation of the problem, and then the delineation of its characteristics. In the neurosurgical field, the evaluation of coma was critical, as discussed by Pierce in Chapter Four. Numerous studies[1,2,3,4] during the seventies addressed coma and the severity of brain injury. Our knowledge of impaired consciousness and its underlying mechanisms owes much to these early works, although there is still much to be discovered.

At the same time, there was increased interest in the sequelae to traumatic brain injury, aside from coma and the severity of the injury itself. Countless articles and texts have addressed the findings of clinical evaluation and research studies. Their findings have been reviewed and summarized in numerous other works,[5,6,7,8,9,10,11,12,13,14,15] and are, therefore, not reviewed here. Much of this early work was directed toward the delineation of the cognitive, psychological, and social consequences of traumatic brain injury because of their overwhelming prevalence and long-term impact, in contrast to the physical consequences, which typically have been the focus of attention in other conditions, such as spinal cord injury and stroke. *Neurobehavioral consequences*[5] is a term frequently used to describe the primary sequelae of traumatic brain injury. Table 5.1 presents a summary of what have come to be known as the hallmarks of traumatic brain injury. Although a somewhat fixed constellation of deficits is presented in overviews of traumatic brain injury, our understanding of these is far from fixed. Nor do we have definite knowledge of if, and how, these impairments are affected by treatment.

This chapter largely addresses the cognitive and communication impairments commonly observed following traumatic brain injury, although other behavioral variables are considered. Again, terminology in the field is

Table 5.1
Commonly Reported Neurobehavioral Sequelae.

Cognitive-communicative	Behavioral
Impaired memory	Irritability and restlessness
Impaired attention and concentration	Childishness and egocentricity
Slowed information processing	Impulsivity
Decreased initiation, planning, and organization	Disinhibition
Inefficient word recall	Dependency
Tangentiality	Apathy
Diminished self-awareness/self-appraisal	Emotional lability
Talkativeness	Depression

unclear, and multiple terms are often used to refer to the same or related phenomena. Problems in terminology are addressed as they arise in context.

TERMINOLOGY CONFUSION IN SPEECH-LANGUAGE PATHOLOGY

One of the greatest problems in terminology within the field of speech-language pathology is the description of neurobehavioral sequelae, in particular the breakdown in communication skills. It is widely acknowledged that traditional terminology is inadequate,[16,17,18,19,20,21] if not inaccurate, for describing the communication problems following traumatic brain injury with diffuse damage. The reasons for the terminology shortcomings, however, are quite varied. One problem, not often discussed in the traumatic brain injury literature, rests in the fact that the term aphasia has been highly debated. Before one can decide whether or not aphasia is an appropriate term to use, one must first know what aphasia is. Whether the relationship between cognition and language is one of independence or interdependence is a question central to the issue of how to define aphasia. This controversy has not come about with the renewed interest in traumatic brain injury, even though the literature leads us to think otherwise. A simple review of developmental language studies will bear this out. The classic article of Wepman[22] in 1976, *Aphasia: Language Without Thought or Thought Without Language* demonstrates that the relationship between language and cognition has been intriguing and challenging clinicians for some time.

In 1982, at the Clinical Aphasiology Conference in Oshkosh, Wisconsin, the issue of terminology was addressed by a group of scholars in the field. Rosenbek[23] spoke on the topic of "When is aphasia aphasia?" In doing so, he discussed the opinions of at least a dozen other scholars who have contributed to our understanding of aphasia. In part, the view of aphasia (or any other disorder) depends upon the viewer. A neurologist will tend to view lesions, a psycholinguist will want to investigate cognitive-linguistic relationships, and a speech-language pathologist will analyze the impaired input and output aspects of language. Rosenbek did not offer another definition of aphasia, but rather presented the characteristics of the person who has aphasia. These are summarized as follows: The person who has aphasia has a verifiable lesion of the major hemisphere, specifically within the distribution of the middle cerebral artery or border zones. The aphasic has characteristics that reflect stability, motivation, reasonableness, and responsiveness. He or she is oriented. The aphasic is admirable and respect-worthy because of the nature of this disorder and his tolerance in the face of it. He or she remains as good a person as before the aphasia. Good long-term memory is retained, as are preinjury interests, if these are of a nonlinguistic nature. The aphasic recognizes communication success even if unable to achieve it, establishes eye contact, and, "says he is aphasic."[23] From this perspective, aphasia is obviously not the correct term to use in traumatic brain injury, which is characteristically accompanied by some degree of cognitive disruption, loss of previous self, and inadequate recognition of the problems experienced.

A number of alternate terms have been used in the traumatic brain injury literature to refer to the impairment of speech-language that pathologists might find themselves confronting. These have included *nonaphasic language impairment, subclinical aphasia, cognitive-linguistic impairment, cognitive-language disorders*, and *cognitive-communicative impairment/disorders*. Some authors[16,18,20] have indicated a preference for *cognitive-language* to reflect the relationship between cognition and language, and to eliminate the confusion with motor speech disorders, which may be implied by the term communication impairment. Others[21,24] have adopted the term *cognitive-communicative* to reflect the behavioral aspects of communication not necessarily indicated by the term *linguistic*. Cognitive-communicative is the term proposed by the American Speech, Language, and Hearing Association. This author uses cognitive-communicative, when indicated, in an attempt to improve consistency in terminology. Labeling is useful to the extent that it represents a definitive, predictable constellation of characteristics that may serve to guide a particular course of action. However, it is often best to describe the characteristics of the breakdown more fully, since these tend to be highly variable from individual to individual. At some level, these issues are merely philosophical. It is, however, vitally important to understand communication in relation to cognitive and linguistic skills, in order to develop effective treatment plans for persons with traumatic brain injury.

Speech-language pathologists are presumed to be knowledgeable of language theory and language constructs; therefore, these subject areas are not reviewed. Cognition is of interest to all clinicians working in the field of traumatic brain injury rehabilitation, and an understanding of terminology and concepts is essential. In the words of Ben-Yishay,[25] it is "preferable to have an imperfect or incomplete conceptual framework than to have none at all."

COGNITIVE FUNCTIONS

Four key aspects of cognition are discussed in the following sections: *attention and information processing, memory, reasoning and problem solving,* and *metacognition and executive functions.* Attention, learning, memory, and problem solving are processes that have interested clinicians and scientists for decades. Executive functions are of more recent clinical interest.

Experimental psychologists Hermann Ebbinghaus (1885) and later William James (1890) were among the first to conduct experimental laboratory studies of memory. Much of what has been done since has been in search of resolution to the controversy raised by these early works. The definitive answers to questions such as: "How do we process information? How do we learn? What happens when we forget?" are yet to come, but our knowledge has increased tremendously over the last century. Experimental psychology, with its many contributions, has not been the only source for this growth in knowledge. For the most part, cognitive processes have been examined in three different environments that are not entirely distinct, although they have used different techniques and subject matter for study. In the clinical arena, hypotheses about memory have been formulated on the basis of memory disorders, and on the localization of functions as determined by brain studies (much in the same manner aphasia research has been conducted). In the arena of experimental or cognitive psychology, studies designed to test various hypotheses have been conducted on normal subjects (remember those psychology experiments during college?), and also carried out through the use of computer models designed to simulate cognitive processes (artificial intelligence). A third major area of contribution has come from physiological psychology, or psychophysiology, in which animal studies provide the basis for models of cognitive processes. Electroconvulsant shock is one technique that has been used to study memory functions in animals. Additionally, some psychophysiologists are interested in the electrophysiology of cognitive processing, and employ *electroencephalography (EEG)* in their studies of humans. *Evoked potentials (EPs)* are considered to "reliably assess stimulus-dependent neural activity in sensory pathways and primary sensory cortex" and cognitive *event-related potentials (ERPs)* are thought to "index cognitive processes independent of sensory parameters."[26] Both have greatly aided in our understanding of brain functions. The field of neurobiology or the broader neurosciences also studies memory through biologic models.

Within the "cognitive sciences," individuals have been divided in their views, in part depending upon their orientation. Thus, it would be optimistic to approach the cognitive processes as if there were consensus and a clear understanding. Speech-language pathologists, and most other rehabilitation clinicians, typically do not take course work in information processing or learning and memory theory; yet, in the rehabilitation setting, they rely on these skills for the success of virtually all treatment. Although it is unrealistic for the clinician to have an exhaustive understanding of normal cognitive processes, particularly since a unified perspective cannot be offered, it is important to have a base of knowledge from which to view the cognitive skills of persons who have sustained brain injuries, in order to render effective treatment.

Attention and Information Processing

Theories of the mechanisms of attention are key to models of information processing. Our knowledge of attentional processes is based primarily on theoretical models, although imaging (for example, positron emission tomography) offers a promising future for improving our knowledge of cognitive processes. It is not necessary, however, to adhere to a single theory in order to understand certain aspects of attention that are pertinent to the clinical setting.

Arousal

Most models of attention have been developed within experimental settings, and there has been little concern for the neuroanatomical correlates to attention, or for the physiological state of the subject under investigation. Therefore, arousal is typically not discussed outside of the clinical literature, yet it is an important aspect to consider, particularly with regard to traumatic brain injury.

Arousal refers to a general state of readiness to process sensory input and/ or respond to environmental stimuli.[27,28] Some have referred to this readiness as *alertness*,[29,30,31] and it is considered the initial stage of attentional processing. The term alertness is sometimes used to indicate more of a cognitive than a physiologic process,[29] but it is here used to refer to the physiologic state. The reticular activating system, with its far-reaching connections, has a predominant role in the mediation of arousal. The reader is reminded of the two-way information relay between the reticular system and the cortex, and the influence each has on the other. Arousal is not a steady state but undergoes fluctuations. *Tonic arousal* refers to slow fluctuations in the readiness state that are influenced primarily by internal or physiological changes that occur with variables such as food and drug intake, circadian rhythm, and temperature. Van Zomeren and colleagues[30] refer to "'tonic alertness' as a continuing receptivity to stimulation." *Phasic arousal* refers to fluctuations that arise from the external environment and occur more rapidly.

Arousal response is related to the nature of tasks, although the relationship between arousal and task stimulation is quite complex.[28] We can often become "aroused" by challenging or particularly interesting activities, or "drift off" during monotonous tasks or tasks of low interest. Although it is apparent that adequate arousal is necessary for information processing to occur (for example, we do not process information in sleep states), extreme levels of arousal (for example, when in pain) can also interfere with attention and information processing.[32]

Perception

Numerous theories of perceptual processes exist and cannot be summarized adequately in a short section. Although perceptual processing occurs with all sensory input, visual and auditory perception have been examined most frequently. Most theories of perception are concerned with the way in which sensory input is matched to stored information so that recognition occurs. Perhaps the most widely held view is that sensory information is recognized on the basis of certain physical properties or distinctive features (for example, the frequency of sounds).[33]

The neurophysiologic correlates to perceptual experience are not well localized within the brain.[20,34] Rather, most perceptual experience requires the integration of numerous features, and this integration relies upon a distributed neural network. At a basic level, perception may be thought of as detection of certain features in sensory information. However, even at the level of simple features, detection is immediately influenced by memory, previous experience, and the environment in which the stimulus occurs. For example, shape recognition can be influenced by position or possibly by color, depending upon one's previous experience. Although many researchers examine perception as a distinct process, the need to attend to information that is not well perceived, and the reliance on representational stores, makes it difficult to separate perception from other aspects of cognition.[20]

Definitions and Theories of Attention

One is pressed to find a single, concise definition of attention, and this is perhaps an indication of the complexity of the process.[30,31,35,36] From a neurophysiologic framework, Whyte and Rosenthal[27] consider *attention* to be "the selective channeling of arousal." Although simplistic, this definition is appealing because it implies a level of activity (energy), or effort, from the organism. Treisman[37] has broadened the definition by including *response*, and considers attention to be the "selective aspect of perception and response." Sohlberg and Mateer[35] go a step further and define attention as "the capacity to focus on particular stimuli over time and to manipulate flexibly the information," which implies more than a simple stimulus-response process. Finally, Weber[38] focuses more on the nature of stimuli and considers attention as "the ability to be aware of stimuli, both internal stimuli such as thoughts and memories and external stimuli such as sights and sounds." This definition is somewhat encumbered by the term "aware."

At this point, some additional terminology is needed. *Capacity* is the term used to refer to the amount of information that can be attended to at any one instance,[38] or the amount of mental effort required by a task. *Information processing capacity* is used synonymously. Some tasks require relatively little effort, and others can exceed capacity. When attentional supply is less than the demands of a task, performance declines.[33] Simply put, the amount of information one can process cannot exceed attentional capacity. *Working memory* and *short-term memory* are used by some[38] to refer to this limited capacity for information, but they are more appropriately discussed under memory. *Control* refers to the process of guiding or directing one's attentional capacity where needed.[38] *Concentration* may be thought of as a product of control, and the term is typically used to refer to deliberate attentional effort.[38,39]

The meaning of *speed of information processing* is self-evident; however, it is almost always studied as *reaction* time. Reaction time is defined by the nature of the task. *Simple reaction time* is assessed when only one stimulus is presented and a single response is required, such as tapping the space bar on a computer keyboard when an object or letter appears on the screen. *Choice reaction time* is measured when one must choose a response from a number of options, in the presence of more than one stimulus; the response must match a particular stimulus. As an example, the letter F on the keyboard is to be depressed in response to a green square presented on the screen, the letter G in response to a red square, the letter H in response to a black square, and so on. The complexity in choice reaction time tests can vary considerably, and in many instances multiple skills are needed to complete the task. Information processing speed also can be examined by varying the rate of the presentation of information, such as with the *Paced Auditory Serial Addition Task* described by Gronwall.[40] This task is cited frequently in the literature, and is therefore described for the reader. It requires that the subject add a series of numbers presented auditorily (from a tape recording). The subject must add the first number to the second, state the answer, then add the second number to a third number, state the new total, and so on, for 61 digit presentations. There is a total of four trials with the interstimulus presentation time decreasing in each trial by .4 seconds, from 2.4 seconds in the first trial to a rate of 1.2 seconds in the last trial. The decreased time between stimulus items results in a faster presentation rate, thus requiring a faster rate of information processing in order to complete the same type of activity.

It is well agreed that attention is not a single process that can be localized to a particular area within the brain.[28,36] The controversy appears to be more concerned with the manner in which attention should be divided, and with the nature of attentional processes (discussed later in this section). Several definitions of attention have been presented to demonstrate some of the controversy. The definitions also reflect certain biases consistent with a researcher's theoretical framework.

Van Zomeren et al.[30] and Sohlberg and Mateer[34] have reviewed the theoretical models of attention that have held prominence in research studies. Briefly, the primary differences among models have centered around the selectivity of stimuli (information) in relation to the control and allocation of attentional capacity. Some theories have considered that the selection of information to be processed occurs at a perceptual level (physical characteristics).[37,41] According to these models not all information is perceived (that is, detected by the physical properties or features). The amount of sensory input to be processed is limited or filtered by the brain. Other theories[42] have considered a later stage of selectivity whereby all perceptual information is recognized, but only salient or pertinent information is processed. The discussion of selection theories is cursory, out of necessity, given that each view of selectivity has numerous "slants" or theoretical interpretations. In the literature, schematic models of information processing are often simplistic so as to account for simple feature analysis, but they are inadequate to explain complex task performance typical of daily human activity.

Attentional control is an area of more recent interest to researchers than stage of selection. Information processing can be considered to be either *automatic,* which requires little to no allocation of attention, or *controlled,* which requires directed attention.[43] Automatic processing occurs when overlearned, habitual activities are performed, such as reading familiar words. It accounts for our ability to perform multiple tasks simultaneously (for example, drive a car and have a conversation). It also accounts for our ability to recognize certain perceptual features (for example, lines, angles, curves, sounds) at a level of complete unawareness. Although the automatic processing of some perceptual features may be innate, other processes become automatic through practice.[33] Reading is perhaps the best example of a complex process that becomes automatic. The automaticity begins with the recognition of letters as single units, instead of as combinations of individual features; it then advances to the recognition of words as units, instead of combinations of individual letters. Table 5.2 provides a quick test for the reader that illustrates this point.

Controlled processing or *conscious processing* is required for novel information, and for complex information that has not yet been overlearned. Weber[38] refers to controlled processing as deliberate and effortful processing. Automatic processing would appear to be absolutely necessary for efficiency. If all activity required controlled processing (implying effort), we would be greatly slowed in our daily activities. Problems in attention arise in automatic processing when irrelevant or new information is attached to

Table 5.2
A test of letter recognition.

How many Fs are in the following sentence?

FINISHED FILES ARE THE RESULT OF YEARS OF SCIENTIFIC
STUDY COMBINED WITH THE EXPERIENCE OF MANY YEARS.

The answer is six Fs. Some may be overlooked because they are processed as part of a word instead of as letters.

(Adapted from Reed SK. *Cognition: Theory and Applications.* Monterey, CA: Brooks/Cole Publishing; 1982.)

something that has become automatic.[30] In experimental studies, automatic processing has been disrupted using the *Stroop Color Word Test*[44] In this test, the subject first reads color names (such as black, green, blue), then identifies the colors of blocks printed on a card. Finally, the subject identifies the color of the ink in which certain color names are printed. Because the color names in the latter subtest conflict with the color of the ink in which they are printed, the automatic processing of overlearned color words becomes effortful, and controlled processing is required to name the colors. An example using a more familiar experience is the case when one needs to take a different route home from work, but takes a wrong turn and ends up on the habitual route, because of interference from the automatic behavior. Whyte[28,45] refers to the prioritization of attention as "strategic control" and indicates that effective performance requires the ability to direct attention toward performance priorities and, at the same time, monitor the environment for unforeseen, critical information. "Ongoing monitoring" of the environment is not addressed by the previously discussed models, but would seem an important aspect to consider.

Related to the two-system model of automatic and controlled attentional processes is Norman and Shallice's concept of the *Supervisory Attentional System (SAS)*.[46] Their model is much more elaborate and includes higher and lower order mechanisms. Lower levels of the system involve the activation of well-learned routines or "action and thought schemas" analogous to computer programs. Once engaged, the program can run automatically. Mechanisms are included to account for competition between schemata through "contention scheduling," which prevents the selection of schemata that require the same resources. The Supervisory System is responsible for modulating the contention scheduling and has what might be thought of as oversight responsibilities. The Supervisory System must be involved in activities that require planning, decision making, error correction, troubleshooting, novel actions (or ones that are difficult or dangerous), and overriding strong habitual responses.[46] Given the range of responsibility of the Supervisory System, the Supervisory Attentional System model would appear to incorporate aspects of ongoing monitoring of the environment.

While some researchers have moved to a "higher level" of attentional processes, others have separated attention into components. These divisions or levels are not agreed upon, and again this is reflected by inconsistent use of terminology. Sohlberg and Mateer[34,35] assume the largest breakdown of attention and consider five levels: focused, sustained, selective, alternating, and divided. They define these as follows:

Focused Attention: The ability to respond discretely to specific visual, auditory, or tactile stimuli.

Sustained Attention: The ability to maintain a consistent behavioral response during continuous or repetitive activity.

Selective Attention: The ability to maintain a cognitive set that requires activation and inhibition of response dependent upon discrimination of stimuli.

Alternating Attention: The capacity for mental flexibility that allows for moving between tasks having different cognitive requirements.

Divided Attention: The ability to simultaneously respond to multiple tasks.

Others[30,31,38] do not consider selective attention and focused attention to be distinct properties of attention. When deficits in focused attention are considered, there appears to be considerable disagreement. Shiffrin and Schneider[43] and van Zomeren et al.[30] use *focused attention deficits (FADs)* to refer to the problems that arise when an automatic process interferes with the ability to process new information or perform nonhabitual tasks, as occurs during the Stroop Test. Mack[47] uses *focused attention* to refer to attention in the presence of background noise, which would include the *freedom from distractibility* concept. A number of the auditory perceptual batteries and activities used by the speech-language pathologist examine the ability to focus attention in the presence of background noise in order to identify an auditory target (for example, Goldman-Fristoe Tests of Auditory Discrimination).[48]

Divided attention is generally agreed upon as the term for the ability to move attention between several sources of input or activity. It is frequently assessed by tasks such as reciting digits backward, serial addition (for example, counting forward by multiples of three), or serial subtraction (for example, starting with 100, subtracting by seven). The *Paced Auditory Serial Addition Task (PASAT)* also is a task that divides attention, by requiring the manipulation of more than one piece of information at a time. Some[47] include *alternating attention* tasks as tests of divided attention, because capacity must be "divided" between tasks, but it appears more useful, particularly in the clinical setting, to view these two as distinct. Divided attentional tasks require the sharing of attentional capacity; alternating tasks require the shifting of attention from one activity to another, and hence require the disengagement of attention. Van Zomeren et al.[30] use the term *divided attention deficits (DADs)* for the failure of controlled processing when attentional capacity is divided over several cognitive operations.

Sustained attention is generally agreed upon to be attention maintained over time, but the term also encompasses consistency of performance over time. Sustained attention is frequently assessed by the so-called vigilance tasks in which an individual must select (respond to) stimuli that are presented infrequently against a background of nontarget stimuli. Visual cancellation tasks (for example, letters, numbers, or designs) also assess sustained attention.[39]

Weber[38] considers attention from a dual perspective of *capacity* and *control*. Problems in the performance of selective attention and sustained attention tasks are predominantly the result of problems in attentional control. Poor performance on divided attention tasks indicates an "attentional capacity deficit," and poor performance on alternating attention tasks may reflect problems in capacity and control.

It is important to remember that internal stimuli as well as external stimuli make demands on attentional capacity. Pain is an obvious instance of an internal stimulus that can occupy attentional capacity, but other, less obvious, internal demands, such as worry or preoccupation with some personal concern, demand capacity as well. The manner in which internal stimuli affect component aspects of attention has not been discussed in the literature, but must be considered in the clinical setting.

Memory Functions

Sensory Stores

Memory, like attention, is not a unitary construct, nor can it be considered truly distinct from attention, or vice versa. Some consider information processing from a memory perspective, and others place greater emphasis on attentional components. This, in part, accounts for some of the confusion one experiences when reading the literature. The first aspect of information processing that can be considered as a "store" is the sensory memories, also referred to as *sensory stores* and *sensory registers*. The two that have been examined in experimental studies most frequently are visual sensory store or *iconic memory* and acoustic sensory store or *echoic memory*. Although large in capacity, these sensory memories are quite brief in duration (measured in milliseconds). Because of the brevity, "register" may be the preferred term (as in "sensory register"). In attentional models, these stores or registers represent the same stage as *perceptual feature analysis*. Some consider feature analysis to be innate and part of automatic processing (low to no attentional demands).[33,49] Others view sensory stores as a brief holding tank for memories that must receive attention in order to be processed further, as in the case of early selection theories of attention discussed previously. Automatic processing still requires normal sensory processes and intact perceptual abilities. Whether processing is automatic or controlled, the management of sensory information is at the beginning of all information processing.

Encoding and Retrieval

When examining memory, one must make some important distinctions that have great bearing on the conclusions drawn from task performance. *Encoding* refers to the actual processing of information, that is, sensory registration and the extraction of some level of meaning from the information (for example, the word *star* may have *twinkling, sheriff, actor* and/or *Christmas* associated with it).[39] The meaning extracted or attached is influenced by each individual's unique associations and perceptions, although there are certain associations we all share. Encoding is a term used similarly in both experimental and clinical settings. Numerous theories regarding the manner in which information is encoded or processed have been proffered. One theoretical framework that has received much attention has been the *levels-of-processing* approach introduced by Craik and Lockhart in 1972.[50] These authors proposed that the likelihood information will be stored (and retrievable) depends upon the "depth" of processing that occurs. Initial sensory registration is the shallowest level of processing, consisting of the analysis of physical features only. The deepest level of processing occurs at a level of semantic analysis and includes "mental elaboration" that increases the likelihood of retention.[50]

Craig and Lockhart's information processing theory is contrasted with a *multistore* view of memory discussed under the next heading. (The reader is cautioned not to be overly concerned with the either/or theoretical dimensions [that is, theoretical alliance] that are discussed so frequently in the literature, but rather to use all the information presented to gain a better understanding of the complexity of information processing and retention.)

The organizational components of memory have a significant bearing on the way information is processed. The ability to categorize, or organize, information is an important aspect of encoding, storage, and ultimately retrieval. For example, familiar, concrete categories are accessed quickly, hence information that is familiar and concrete is processed quickly.

Retrieval is the act of accessing information from memory, but it can be accomplished in a number of ways. Recall is the term used to refer to the act of "remembering" or accessing a memory store without the assistance of cues or prompts. *Free recall* is a term used to refer to a test condition in which subjects or patients are not required to recall test information in the order of presentation. When cues are used to facilitate the recall act, it is referred to as *cued recall*. An example is the use by speech-language pathologists of a variety of cues (for example, semantic, phonemic, contextual) to facilitate word retrieval. Cuing (verbal or nonverbal) can be used to improve visual recall as well. *Recognition* is similar to cued recall, but a full representation of the test information is provided, among foils or in a multiple choice format. For example, a person is shown ten words printed on cards; then, following a delay, or perhaps after recall has failed, the subject is presented with a group of twenty cards and asked to indicate the words "recognized" from the first group of ten. The distinction between recall and recognition is important in order to determine if encoding has occurred. If recall is the only method of assessment used to determine if material has been learned, and recall fails, one should not conclude that learning has not taken place. The problem could be in retrieval or encoding. Recognition and cued recall assist in ruling out retrieval problems. *Relearning* is another way to examine what has been stored, but assessment must be performed properly (that is, comparisons must be made to new material as well as old). Material that is present in long-term memory (has been learned, but cannot be recalled) is relearned at a faster rate than novel, test control information.

Short-term and Long-term Memory Processes

A dual-process, or two-stage, view of memory has been recognized for many decades, although terminology has varied. The terms *primary memory* and *secondary memory* were first introduced by William James in 1890[51,52] and are terms still used by some.[47,51] Zechmeister and Nyberg[51] summarize the way James used *primary memory* as "the conscious experience that results from our attention to something." This is a useful conceptualization, as it brings together the role of attentional processes and memory at the point at which they are basically indistinguishable (that is, as a memory process or an attention process). For James, secondary memory referred to the reservoir of stored information that must be called back to consciousness to be used.[51]

Short-term memory and *long-term memory* are terms that have been used to differentiate between the time period when information is presented and the point when it is to be recalled.[51,52] In this context, the terms refer to tasks, not to memory processes. Despite this imprecision, nonetheless, the short-term/long-term dichotomy appears to be the terminology used most often, especially in the clinical literature, to refer to memory stores.

Short-term Memory

Short-term memory refers to the temporary and limited-capacity storage of information that, when processed in some effortful manner, can be learned and then retrieved at a later time. If not continuously acted upon (for example, rehearsed), information in short-term memory decays in thirty seconds to a few minutes;[39,51,52] the times stated in the literature vary.

Short-term memory is most often assessed using the *digit span format* with either numbers, words, sentences, or paragraphs. When information can be retrieved from short-term memory, sensory registration can be assumed.[53]

Working memory is a more recent term used by Baddeley and Hitch[54] to refer to the active processing that must occur if information is to be remembered. It implies effort as well as a holding place. Most experts accept short-term memory and working memory as the same entity or concept. Nissen[31] considers short-term memory as "working space" for active attentional processing. Parenté and colleagues,[55,56] however, make the distinction that short-term memory is "where information is stored," while working memory refers to the actual processing of information. According to these authors, working memory is limited in capacity, (which is defined as the classic seven plus or minus two digits), and it employs rehearsal to keep information activated for storage. This description, however, appears more accurate when applied to their view of short-term memory as a fixed and limited concept. Working memory, as the label implies, should encompass a variety of processing strategies other than rehearsal. In the context of effortful processing, a variety of strategies or "processes" may be employed including rehearsal, visual imagery, verbal elaboration, and chunking.[49] The distinction made by Parenté and others is intended to clarify that the stage of information processing immediately preceding long-term memory storage represents more than merely a holding ground or temporary storage; it also includes processing (attention), as has already been stated. The distinction between short-term and working memory appears frequently in the literature as a controversial issue. Since all tasks designed to examine short-term memory require either recognition or recall, and some type of response, it seems unlikely that one can separate "storage space" from "working space," (that is, the space from the process), except as a theoretical construct. With the understanding, then, that these terms are not always used synonymously, short-term memory appears to be an adequate term (at this time). Different processes, however, can be distinguished from each other, as discussed below.

Processing Strategies

Although they are rarely discussed in the literature, there are individual differences in the capacity of short-term memory that are dependent upon the efficiency of the processing strategies employed.[51] Numerous experiments have demonstrated not only that there are differences in memory span between individuals, but that some individuals can improve their memory span through practice (much practice).[51] *Rehearsal*, typically considered as auditory-verbal, is one strategy employed to maintain information in short-term memory. The *auditory-verbal rehearsal strategy* is the one most often reported, because it is the one that has been the most investigated. This alone is not sufficient reason to expect that other strategies are not employed, but for many years verbal rehearsal was the only processing strategy considered.[52]

Visual rehearsal is a strategy that could be employed for objects or pictures in which the visual replica (rather than a verbal code) is reviewed in short-term memory. *Visual imagery* might be employed to remember high-imagery words (for example, an apple is a high-imagery word, democracy is not), or to connect information together by a single visual representation. *Verbal elaboration* is yet another technique that can be used to facilitate processing and learning of verbal information. *Chunking*, whereby individual units are grouped together to form a larger unit, is another processing strategy. Table 5.3 presents an example of a chunking strategy that improved the recall of the experimenter, Nobel prize winner Herbert Simon.[51]

All of the processing strategies discussed above are internal and are sometimes referred to as *internal memory aids*. There are other internal memory aids that are used to facilitate recall but are not a part of initial processing, for example, retracing one's actions or conducting an alphabet search. These can be distinguished as retrieval strategies as opposed to processing strategies. An interesting, and clinically relevant, point must be made about the use of internal strategies. Processing strategies have been investigated the most frequently, but in natural contexts they are used the least. Further, external aids such as calendars, lists, and schedules appear to be used by normal subjects with greater frequency than any of the internal strategies.[57] Finally, when researchers use self-reporting techniques to determine subjects' use of strategies, there is an apparent underreporting of use,

Table 5.3
Chunking strategy used by Herbert Simon.

Test items presented one at a time:	Chunking strategy:
Lincoln	Lincoln's Gettysburg Address
milky	Milky Way
criminal	Criminal Lawyer
Gettysburg	Differential Calculus
differential	
way	
lawyer	
address	
calculus	

(Adapted from Zechmeister EG, Nyberg SE. *Human Memory: An Introduction to Research and Theory.* Monterey CA; Brooks/Cole Publishing Company, 1982.)

which improves when individuals are prompted and given examples of specific strategies.[57]

There is, no doubt, much to be learned from individual differences in approach that are often masked by group results. In the past, experimental studies have seldom examined these differences, nor have they extended beyond the laboratory setting. Studies in long-term memory, however, have begun to examine memory in natural contexts and have already greatly extended our knowledge beyond the "permanent holding space" perspective.

Long-term Memory

As with attention and short-term memory, different terms are often used to refer to the same aspect of long-term memory. The concept of long-term memory does not appear to cause great confusion at a basic level: it is the permanent storage of information and has no limits in capacity. How the information is stored and the type of information that is stored (that is, kinds of memories) do present areas of much debate. We do not yet know how information is stored, but it is an area being investigated with vigor. *Consolidation* is an important concept in relation to storage. It refers to the changes in memory structure that develop over time. It refers both to the concept that information is not immediately "consolidated" or permanently fixed, and to the idea that information storage is a neurophysiologic process.[58,59] Information is stored in neuronal networks that are both dynamic and susceptible to damage. That is to say if neuronal structures are changed with stimulation (sensory input), this occurs over and over as new information enters the system.[59] Neuronal networks (hypothetically, the memory traces) are believed to be strengthened over time when like information or information reoccurs (for example, one's name). Networks that are activated repeatedly are thought to be more permanently altered[60] and, hence, more resistant to damage. Forgetting may actually be the result of neuronal change or loss, and not simply an issue of retrieval failure, as was once thought.[52] This explanation is obviously limited. Additional readings regarding the neurobiology of memory are included in the recommended readings list in Appendix B.

Procedural and Declarative Memory

The term *procedural memory* refers to the acquisition and storage of information embedded in skills or behaviors that are rule-based and ordered. The ability to verbalize the sequence or procedure for a particular task is not the same as procedural memory. Procedural knowledge is implicit in a behavior and accessible only through performance.[52,59] Procedural memory is often associated with motor skills, such as riding a bicycle, but can involve other types of skill acquisition as well, such as learning to read words in a mirror.[52] Because the information stored is implicit in task performance, some authors use the term *implicit memory*.

Declarative memory is the term used to refer to stored information that is, directly accessible to retrieval. Squire[59] defines declarative memory as that which is "explicit and accessible to conscious awareness, and it includes the facts, episodes, lists, and routes of everyday life. It can be declared, that is, brought to mind verbally as a proposition or nonverbally as an image." Declarative memory has also been referred to as *explicit memory*[31] and *propositional memory.*[61]

There are more distinctions between these two memory systems than just the type of information stored. Squire[52] puts forth the position that procedural learning may be more phylogenetically older than is declarative learning. Procedural information may only be accessible through the information-processing systems involved in original learning, whereas declarative information may be more "modality-general" allowing greater accessibility. He argues that different processes (and neural structures) are involved in the acquisition of these two kinds of knowledge.

Semantic and Episodic Memory

Included under the rubric of declarative memory are semantic and episodic memory. The term *semantic memory* refers to the well-learned facts, word meanings, and abstract concepts that one generally thinks of as knowledge. It is decontextual, without spatial and temporal codes. *Episodic memory* is contextual. Information is stored along with temporal and spatial information, that is, with the time and place, or when and where, aspects. Episodic memory reflects personally relevant or autobiographical experiences[52] (for example, a sixteenth birthday, a parent's death, college graduation).

Although these two systems of memory are often viewed as distinct, they are probably not. Information in semantic memory is used in episodic memory during information processing. Similarly, at some point in time episodic memories, at least aspects of them, must be incorporated into our general knowledge.[62]

Material Specific Memory

The question of whether or not memories are stored in different regions of the brain, according to the nature of the information involved has not been answered. Visual information processing of nonverbal material has been investigated in normal subjects,[63,64,65,66] but not to the same extent as auditory-verbal information. Most studies have examined the differences between these two modalities at the level of sensory store, which holds information only long enough for specific features or patterns to be automatically detected. Sensory stores are not available to controlled processing, and a review of the differences found at this level is not within the scope of this chapter. Several researchers[65,67,68] have demonstrated that subjects have superior recall for pictures, which is considered to be the result of dual-coding (that is, visual and verbal).

A number of investigations have been conducted in the patient population exhibiting *Korsakoff's syndrome*. For the most part, the drive of these investigations has been to determine or to prove that the severe memory impairment characteristic of the disorder is limited to verbal-semantic information. A primary criticism of the research in this area has been that there is multifocal, bilateral brain pathology associated with the syndrome, and that one should therefore expect a range of results.[69] The studies conducted with this population, or with those suffering from other types of multifocal pathology, have produced mixed results. Some studies support a selective verbal memory impairment[70,71,72,73,74] and others support a multimodality, generalized memory impairment.[75]

Other authors[76,77,78] have put forth the view that site of lesion is a determining factor in the nature of memory impairment. According to this view, lesions in the dominant hemisphere result in verbal memory impairment and those in the nondominant hemisphere produce memory impairment for nonverbal information.[78] It would appear difficult to draw conclusions about memory impairment from a patient population with brain damage that may have perceptual problems and language problems.[34] Although memory may be impaired, it is, most likely, quite difficult to distinguish memory impairment from impairment of other aspects of processing.

Squire[52] has argued that memory stores cannot be easily separated from the processing systems that give rise to them. In other words, the modality employed in the initial processing of information determines the storage and, possibly, the subsequent retrieval. At the level of everyday experience, his perspective has strong value. Most people know individuals who have preferred processing modalities, at least for processing particular kinds of information. Consider the individual who states "if you draw a picture for me, I'll be able to understand," and then is able to reproduce a near replica weeks later.

More Aspects of Memory: Metamemory, Prospective Memory, Source Memory, and Schemata

Metamemory is a term that was introduced by Flavell,[79] specifically with regard to developmental aspects of memory. The prefix "meta" comes from the Greek and means "beyond" or "after."[51] Metamemory is used to refer to what one knows about one's own memory, both in terms of content and the way in which information is stored and retrieved. Prior to Flavell's coining of the term, aspects of metamemory were investigated under different names. The most familiar aspect is the *feeling-of-knowing* phenomenon. Hart[80,81,82] conducted a number of experiments in which he asked subjects to rate their feeling of knowing or not knowing answers to questions, and then compared these ratings to both recall and recognition responses. The conclusions drawn were that strong feelings of knowing related to generally high recognition levels, but there was not a perfect linear relation in terms of "memory monitoring."[51]

The feeling-of-knowing phenomenon also has been studied in patients with amnesia from various etiologies.[83] Not all patients with amnesia demonstrate impaired accuracy of memory judgments when compared to normal controls. Patients with Korsakoff's syndrome, typically characterized by a severe impairment in new learning, have been found to have an impairment of metamemory as well as semantic memory. The differences in patient populations suggest that the neural networks involved in metamemory functions are distinct from those involved in the consolidation of new memories. Additionally, impairment of metamemory may provide some indication of overall severity of memory impairment following brain injury.

Other aspects of metamemory that have been investigated include ease of learning and memory for remembered events. The term *ease-of-learning judgments* refers to the predictability that information will be learned. Experiments with college students have shown that there is a high correlation between the prediction of how easy an item will be to learn and actual learning.[51] *Memory for remembered events*, or memory for previous test outcomes, also has been studied in college students, and results have shown that subjects can remember previous test outcomes. In these studies, subjects have been given lists to learn and learning was first tested by recall, then by recognition tests that assessed the subjects' recognition of items remembered and not remembered.[51] An important theoretical premise in multitrial learning experiments is that knowing which information is remembered, or not remembered, aids in the distribution of memory processes for subsequent learning. This appears to be a fact and not merely a premise.[51] From a learning perspective, this may be thought of as an efficiency function of metamemory.

Prospective memory refers to the ability to remember to perform future actions. It is distinguished from retrospective memory, which solely involves information about the past.[84] In a strict sense, prospective memory is neither long-term memory nor metamemory, but requires both. For example, when asked to deliver a message to someone at a future time, the messenger must do more than remember the information and the person to whom the message is to be delivered. To be successful, he or she must also devise a plan for remembering, based on personal knowledge of previously used strategies. Shimamura et al.[83] have suggested that prospective memory is analogous to a prospector searching for gold, in that it concerns "self-initiated searches and retrieval of information in memory." Prospective memory is no doubt related to planned behavior. Additionally, the ability to remember to perform future actions may be influenced by and certainly influences, "one's self-concept as an efficient, reliable, or well-organized individual."[84] The person who forgets to go to the grocery store on the way home from work may be considered unreliable. The person who always remembers appointments and birthdays, and reminds others of their future activities, is considered to be "highly efficient," "very productive," even "indispensable." Prospective memory, in and of itself, has been investigated little. It has been studied in most cases by examining the use of external aids to facilitate remembering.

Source memory is an aspect of metamemory that specifically addresses the "where and when" of information learning. Where did you learn to swim? When did you learn to speak French? Reportedly, normal subjects record and can recall learning episodes,[52] particularly when strong emotion or shock is associated with them. Where were you when you learned that President Kennedy had been assassinated? Highly charged memories of this nature have been referred to as *flashbulb memories*, to indicate that the memory is established at the moment and is vivid, like a photograph.[85] However, this concept has been challenged,[86] perhaps the notion of source memory as well. Frequently, investigations of flashbulb memories, and other aspects of memory, have accepted subjects' reports as truth, without verification of the information. Further, in the case of emotional or shocking events, it is difficult to ascertain what is part of one's original memory and what has been encoded from conversations, newspapers, television reports, or radio.

Schemata, scripts, and frames are newer concepts to memory theory, although the use of schemata was first introduced by Bartlett in 1932.[51] The definitions of these terms and the distinctions between them are not clear. A general perspective is provided. The term *schemata* refers to large clusters of stored information or concepts, and the many associations that are part of them. The term is used broadly. *Scripts* and *frames* may be thought of as generalized examples such as cocktail parties, restaurants, libraries, and so on, and the linking together of these examples (for instance, a restaurant in the suburbs). Schema theory has been used to explain the complex process of text comprehension and the interrelationship between new information and knowledge.

These last areas of memory discussed reflect the move in psychology to examine memory more in natural contexts and less in the laboratory. Although the utility of these broader views of memory may seem obscure for the clinical setting, an introduction to this area serves to provide the clinician with some knowledge of how information is stored and accessed, beyond the over-reviewed, verbal-semantic trail. It thus offers an additional perspective on why some memories may be preserved and why generalized information can be recalled when specific details cannot.

Reasoning and Problem Solving

There are hundreds of articles from the fields of cognitive and educational psychology and business that discuss human reasoning and problem solving.[34,87] Although numerous concepts are borrowed from these fields, it would be impractical to review the research in this area. Readings from these fields are recommended in Appendix B.

Reasoning is usually discussed in terms of the information one must consider and the type of conclusion that follows the evaluation of the information. In short, it is the process of evaluating information in order to reach a conclusion. In the clinical literature, the two types of reasoning most often discussed are deductive and inductive reasoning. *Deductive reasoning* results in a conclusion being drawn about a particular (individual fact, circumstance, or detail) from premises offered or known. Deductive reasoning involves formal relationships between the premises and the conclusion (for example, if A is true, then B must follow).[88] A practical example of deductive reasoning is: Payday is every Friday. I was not paid today. Therefore, today is not Friday. In this example, one can understand the importance of the truthfulness of the "payday is every Friday" statement to the drawing of correct conclusions.

Inductive reasoning results in a conclusion that is a generalization (from one instance to a broad interpretation, or from one person to a general concept about people) drawn from particulars. In inductive reasoning there is not a formal relationship between the premise(s) and the conclusion, therefore, true premises can lead to false conclusions, and often do. For example, Jane knows the following to be true: Some of her friends like ice cream. Sally is her friend. Therefore, Sally likes ice cream. Based on the particular that some of Jane's friends like ice cream, she erroneously generalizes that Sally does too. Ylvisaker et al.[88] have stated that, in inductive reasoning, conclusions are drawn from experience. It is inductive reasoning that we most often apply in our everyday lives.[88,89] In common everyday situations, conclusions also are reached indirectly from experience, based on analogies. This is referred to as *analogical reasoning* and is a type of inductive reasoning.[88]

Problem solving and reasoning frequently are considered together. From a practical perspective, they are quite difficult to separate. Problem solving involves the evaluation of a situation (information) in order to find an answer (reach a conclusion). Many times tasks that involve reasoning are called problems. Before delving into a discussion of some of the types of problems and skills needed to solve them, let us consider a common problem (using hypothetical Jane as a subject). Jane *always* drinks a cup of coffee in the morning, but the timer failed and none has been made. The magnitude of the problem depends on a number of variables, including previous experience. Jane has never made coffee. Bill always made it, and he left early. Solutions to the immediate problem of NO COFFEE! would include trying to make the coffee, drinking tea instead, stopping by a fast food vendor, visiting a neighbor, or waiting until arriving at work, to list a few. The person who is unable to "see" the possibilities and is intent on having a cup before leaving the house could have major difficulty if: she is already late for work, has never observed coffee being made, cannot find an instruction book, and so on. Sometimes people are considered to be "rigid" or "inflexible" when they do not consider or act upon alternative solutions because they are unfamiliar.

Problem solving and reasoning are required by a variety of situations (problems). It is the nature of the problem that defines the skills needed. Problems can quickly cut across many modalities, requiring an integration of skills. Consider the task of learning to drive a car as a problem, and the importance of skill integration becomes apparent (to both the driver and teacher). Because a variety of skills frequently is required in problem-solving tasks, the tasks themselves should be analyzed carefully to determine skill demands before conclusions are drawn about performance.

The following are examples of some of the problems often seen on tests or used in experiments.

Analogy Problems: simple verbal analogy problems
    hammer:nail saw: _____
    dentist:teeth mechanic: _____
Arrangement Problems: rearrangement of an anagram
    LLJEO JELLO
Series Completion: numerical sequence problem
    1 3 5 2 4 6 3 5 _____

The ability to identify relationships among the components of the problem is essential to solving analogy and series completion problems. Although the anagram problem seems simple, it requires a number of skills, if the answer is not immediately apparent. A skill that is required by virtually all problems is the ability to generate multiple possibilities that can lead to the correct solution, a skill sometimes referred to as fluency.[33] The anagram problem also requires retrieval of information from memory (in particular words), and knowledge of how sounds (letters) occur in the English language (for example, J and L rarely occur adjacent to one another). Although the knowledge of letter relationships is not essential to solving the problem (that is, one could compare whole words until the solution was reached), it is a more efficient strategy. Often, efficiency is the aspect that is evaluated and rated in problem solving.

Another type of problem is the *transformation problem*. These involve a goal state (the desired solution), an initial state (the current status of a situation), and some series of operations needed to transform the initial state into the goal state.[33] Transformation problems are different from anagrams and analogies in that the "answer" or solution is known. The "how to get there" is the unknown. These types of problems might be seen as the "heart" of industry and invention. For example, Ford Motor Company wants to produce a more fuel efficient car with a goal state of 45 miles per gallon. The current status is a car that can achieve 35 miles per gallon. The individual who defines the operations that will "transform" the initial state to the goal state will most likely be quite valuable to the company—particularly if the process is efficient.

Although efficiency and effectiveness share the meaning of producing a desired result or "effect," efficiency has the additional aspect of "with a minimum of effort, expense, or waste."[90] With regard to problem solving, *effectiveness* is used to refer to a solution that works, the one that solves the problem. When multiple solutions are available, the best solution is often referred to as the most effective one. *Efficiency*, on the other hand, has come to refer not only to a correct solution, but to one that can be accomplished in a timely manner and/or with the fewest resources. These distinctions become quite important in the "real world" where time and money are being evaluated constantly. Sometimes, the solution that is perceived to be the most efficient actually may not be, if "short cuts" are taken, and the solution is not effective. Then, additional time and resources may be required to prepare alternate solutions. People who choose solutions based on perceived efficiency or effectiveness alone are sometimes referred to as being "short-sighted." As one can surmise, like prospective memory, problem solving abilities produce a variety of labels that can affect self-esteem.

METACOGNITION AND EXECUTIVE FUNCTIONS

The term *metacognition* refers to knowledge about all cognitive processes, their products, and anything related to them. It is involved in the monitoring of cognitive processes (input and output). This monitoring includes knowing how and when to attend to and organize information; knowing how, when and what to remember; knowing when a problem exists and which solutions have worked or failed; and knowing the individual strengths and weaknesses of different processes and strategies. These skills have a developmental curve and largely have been examined in normal children[79] and in children with special education needs.[91] Metamemory, a subcategory of metacognition, was reviewed earlier in the chapter.

Unlike attention and memory, executive functioning has not occasioned a rich body of information from experimental psychology. This, no doubt, is due in part to the fact that psychological experiments, by design, are well-organized and highly structured, frequently require little interaction with other people, are conducted in a low distraction environment, and require little initiation or planning. It is under conditions in which there is little control for these variables that a breakdown in executive functioning is observed. Much of the information concerning executive functions has come from studies on individuals with brain injuries.

The term *executive functions* comes from the verb to execute,[92] to carry out. An analogy often is made to the functions performed by a business executive, especially a "chief executive officer." These functions or skills include anticipation, goal direction, planning, internal and external monitoring, and the interpretation and application of feedback.[39,93,94] Behaviorally these may be observed as inhibition, deliberation, coordination, and self-regulation. The executive system is employed in the control of nonroutine processes. In order to plan and monitor behaviors, the executive system must "activate the appropriate memory information [necessary] to carry out those plans."[95] The Norman and Shallice model previously discussed may also be thought of as a model of executive functioning, with regard to the allocation of attentional resources and information processing. The label "Supervisory" implies an executive function. As will be recalled, the model draws upon schema theory, where schemas (or schemata) are analogous to programs or sets of operations. The *Supervisory System* is responsible for "modulating the activation level of schemas." The Supervisory System is "called to action" when nonroutine (effortful) processes are required.

Executive skills are thought to be mediated by the frontal lobes. Therefore, literature regarding frontal lobe functions will lead one to information about the hypothetical executive system. Although a detailed review of the frontal lobe functions cannot be provided, a synopsis is offered, for many of these functions are thought to be impaired following traumatic brain injury.[96]

The frontal lobes are thought to be central in the integration of many forms of information, because of their numerous direct and indirect connections to virtually all other parts of the brain. A great deal is known about the functions of the motor and premotor areas of the frontal lobes, as the result of the study of stroke patients (for example, hemiplegia, Broca's aphasia, apraxia). The functions of other areas of the frontal lobes, in particular the prefrontal regions, are less well-known and have been the focus of much recent attention. Mesulam[97] discusses the prefrontal lobes as heteromodal association areas. *Heteromodal* association areas are differentiated from *unimodal* regions that deal with a single sensory modality, such as the primary auditory cortex. The interrelation of sensory information (and motor output in the prefrontal area) occurs in heteromodal areas. The prefrontal heteromodal association area receives paralimbic input, input from all unimodal regions, and input from all other heteromodal association areas (for example, tempoparietal heteromodal area).[97] Immediately, one can envision the complexity of functions based on the amount of input alone.

The frontal lobes and their many connections are involved in the regulation of both cognitive and psychosocial functions. Emotional control and tone are probably mediated by frontal lobe-limbic connections, and arousal and selectivity functions are supported through frontal lobe-reticular and frontal lobe-thalamic connections.[93] The prefrontal cortex is thought to be associated with the highest function in humans: self-awareness and the ability to be self-reflective.[94,96,98]

Newcombe[99] has reviewed some of the research on patients with known frontal lobe dysfunction and delineated supporting evidence for a variety of impairments. Studies were categorized based on locus of lesions (as opposed to etiology): anterior/posterior, left/right frontal, and specific verified focal lesions. Collectively, the studies indicated disorders of attention, planning and organization, anticipation or search, fluency, and switching sets.

Gualtieri[15] has identified two major types of frontal lobe dysfunction that correlate to the *prefrontal* and the *orbitofrontal* (inferior-medial surface) neuroanatomical areas. The complex functions of the prefrontal regions are best presented by a description of behaviors that arise following prefrontal lesions. Gualtieri[15] has described the plight of patients with prefrontal lesions with a most vivid presentation:

> Patients with lesions in this area tend to have little spontaneous behavior or initiative, they do not initiate interaction, although they are perfectly pleasant if someone else does. If you watch them sitting in the waiting room, you may be struck by their quiet, passive demeanor . . . [they] may deny their disability (anosagnosia); they may be compliant to a fault, or, alternatively, as stubborn as mules. They are not flexible people, or as thinkers, and they prefer to deal with simple, agreeable issues. They have difficulty when the rules are changed, when there is the requirement for readjustment to a new set of demands. They tend to get stuck in a rut; a personal rut, or a cognitive rut. In extreme cases this may be so dramatic that they perseverate or engage in stereotyped behavior. They tend to be socially inappropriate, but in an innocent kind of way, like a bumpkin. They are not very good in complex or ambiguous situations, they prefer structure and predictability in their environment, they are not good planners, and they have real difficulty with complex tasks. They are easily distracted, they can be absentminded, they can stare off for long periods without a thought in their head.

In contrast, patients who exhibit predominantly orbitofrontal lesions are described as being impulsive, disinhibited, excitable and restless, sometimes childlike, and emotionally labile. The condition of these individuals can be worsened by stress, lack of structure, and intoxicants.[15]

Phylogenetically, the frontal lobes are the most recently developed cortical regions. The behaviors that are thought to distinguish humans from other species are regulated by the frontal lobes. As we have come to have a better understanding of some of the frontal lobe functions, so have we come to better understand the impairment following traumatic brain injury, since this region of the brain and/or its many connections are frequently injured.[96,100]

DELINEATION OF AREAS OF IMPAIRMENT

The delineation of impairment following traumatic brain injury is much easier when one understands the complexity of cognitive skills. The range of impairment is diverse, often within the individuals as well as across the population. One should not conclude, however, that the impairment can be neatly compartmentalized, any more than one should conclude that cognitive functions are neatly compartmentalized. The above discussion of cognitive functions was intended to elucidate the complexity of, rather than to oversimplify, the skills. Often in rehabilitation, especially when therapists are overwhelmed with numerous patients to treat, there is a tendency to overgeneralize impairments and not investigate thoroughly the aspects of the impairment that might be most amenable to treatment. It is much more important that clinicians be able to think critically about the nature of impairment and understand the type of skills an evaluation tool measures, than it is to administer batteries of tests in order to derive a label.

Because of the diversity of impairment observed following traumatic brain injury, it does not seem fruitful to attempt to list all possibilities. An overview of commonly observed impairment is provided at this point. It is of particular importance to understand that one of the most predictable aspects of traumatic brain injury is change. Cognitive and communication impairment, and behavioral and emotional control, all change over time as recovery occurs. Memory impairment observed within the first month of injury is not necessarily predictive of memory impairment in twelve months. Linguistic abilities vary considerably over time, as do attentional abilities. A more detailed discussion of the types of impairment common to the different stages of rehabilitation is presented in Chapters Seven and Eight.

Perceptual Impairment

There has been little documented evidence of specific perceptual deficits following traumatic brain injury, yet perceptual disturbances often are listed as an area of concern in the clinical literature.[20,29] Sohlberg and Mateer[34] have presented a model for the physiological bases of visual processing and have described the nature of visual impairment accompanying lesions in these areas. The extent to which specific problems have been observed following traumatic brain injury was not presented; however, their discussion is informative. Levin[5,8] reviewed some of the research on perceptual disorders secondary to closed head injury. In his review, select cases of prosopagnosia (impaired recognition of familiar faces) were documented, although the condition is rare. Other cases of impaired recognition for unfamiliar faces (photographs) have been documented with an incidence as high as 25 percent of the subjects studied. Another study found patients with closed head injury to have impaired perception of facial affect. This finding is of particular interest in view of the social inappropriateness often cited as a problem following traumatic brain injury. One study of auditory perception was reviewed in which impairment in sentence comprehension during a dichotic listening task was found in the presence of a unilateral temporal lobe lesion.

It is not a great surprise that perceptual deficits are "believed" to be present following traumatic brain injury, nevertheless they have not been well documented. They are difficult for the clinician to delineate and for the patient to describe. It is not within the scope of this text to review the types of visual impairment that may accompany traumatic brain injury and that contribute to problems in visual perception. Pierce's review of the cranial nerves in Chapter Four provides an indication of the complexity of the visual system. Determining the cause of visual perceptual impairment (that is, at what point within the visual system a deficit occurs) requires a great deal of skill and knowledge. Most speech-language pathologists would not begin to treat what they believed to be an auditory perceptual impairment without first obtaining audiological and otological consultations. The same should be true for visual perceptual impairments. A referral to a neuro-opthalmologist or similar specialist frequently is indicated. Clinicians should suspect perceptual deficits when evaluating patients and should determine their potential effects on test performance and daily activities, but this should not take the place of formal assessment by the most appropriate professional.

Attentional Impairment

From a neurophysiologic perspective, unconsciousness must be viewed as an attentional impairment. Tonic arousal is disrupted initially following traumatic brain injury as evidenced by loss of consciousness. In the initial stages of recovery following the regaining of consciousness, problems in virtually all aspects of attention are evidenced. The confusion and disorientation that are hallmarks in early recovery are indices of disrupted attention. The nature of more permanent attentional problems is less clear. Many researchers[34,35,60] now think that impairment of attentional processes underlies many of the other cognitive problems experienced by individuals with traumatic brain injury.

A few researchers have attempted to investigate particular aspects of attention, effortful versus automatic processing, divided attention, sustained attention or vigilance, and speed information processing. These studies have been reviewed by several authors.[30,40] With the exception of information processing speed, specific deficits have not been delineated with any confidence. With regard to the speed of controlled information processing, several researchers[28,30,36,60] have concluded that it is reduced following traumatic brain injury in an overwhelming majority of cases. As would be expected, speed of processing has been shown to be greatly affected by complexity of information.[14,47,30] When attention must be divided over several tasks, or a novel response is required, information processing speed is slowed.[20] It is not entirely clear, however, that other aspects of attention, such as the ability to inhibit interfering information, do not contribute to problems in speed of processing.[47] Whyte[28] has noted that in the clinical setting, it may be difficult to separate problems in arousal from processing speed.

Memory Impairment

Amnesia is the inability to remember. It is a term used to refer to memory impairment in a variety of medical conditions. Three types of amnesia are identified in traumatic brain injury rehabilitation. *Anterograde amnesia* refers to the inability to acquire and retrieve new information, and to recall day-to-day events since an injury or illness.[53] *Retrograde amnesia* refers to the inability to remember information preceding an injury or illness. In traumatic brain injury, retrograde amnesia typically affects the most recently acquired information. Patients can often remember their names and can access semantic memory (word knowledge, general concepts, et cetera), but they may have difficulty recalling events preceding the injury, from a few minutes to several months before the injury, sometimes longer. These memories usually improve over time. The length of retrograde amnesia is measured from the time of the earliest event that can be recalled to the injury date. Ritchie[101] noted that the extent of retrograde amnesia can only be assessed accurately if the patient was awake at the time of the injury. Therefore, the ingestion of alcohol or other drugs prior to the time of injury could adversely affect the degree of retrograde amnesia. Additionally, it may be difficult for patients to differentiate what they actually remember from what information they have been told by friends and family.

It is the post-traumatic amnesia of traumatic brain injury that has been of most interest to clinicians and researchers and accordingly it presents another bit of confusing terminology. The term *post-traumatic amnesia (PTA)* refers both to the inability of patients to remember events preceding the injury and to their inability to remember information on a day-to-day basis since the injury. The confusion in terminology is not so much with the concept, as with the criteria used to determine the termination point of post-traumatic amnesia.[102] The restoration of memory for day-to-day events (referred to as ongoing memory) is not an all-or-none phenomenon. The popular term "islands of memory" refers to recall for only some events, or recall on a sporadic basis. For this reason, many clinicians think that the establishment of continuous memory is an important aspect to the determination of the end of post-traumatic amnesia.[102] Within the clinical setting, it is certainly preferable that all clinicians use the same reference point, particularly in regard to assessment and prediction. Post-traumatic amnesia is highly variable from individual to individual and can range in duration from minutes to months.[11] It is considered to be related to the severity of the injury, and for many years was thought to be highly predictive of cognitive outcome. As duration of post-traumatic amnesia increases, it becomes more predictive of outcome, but the relationship should not be considered linear.[14]

Before ending a discussion of the amnesias, it is important to make a distinction between those observed following traumatic brain injury and the "classic" amnesic syndrome. The *"classic" amnesic syndrome* refers to a profound impairment in the ability to acquire and store new information in the presence of relative preservation of other cognitive abilities and in the absence of confusion.[53] It is well documented[27,52] that damage to the medial temporal lobes and to the hippocampus results in this type of memory impairment.[27,52] Although hippocampal structures have been implicated in memory impairment following traumatic brain injury,[10,14] severe or profound damage to these structures caused by traumatic brain injury is considered uncommon by some.[27,103] Accordingly, the pure amnesic syndrome with profound anterograde amnesia is relatively uncommon following traumatic brain injury. The definition of amnesia as a profoud memory impairment coupled with a sparing of other cognitive faculties explains why the term (although perhaps technically correct) is generally not used to refer to the type of memory impairment following traumatic brain injury, unless these criteria fit. This is not to say that hippocampal structures are not impaired to some extent following traumatic brain injury, particularly when hypoxic-ischemic injury is known to be present, but rather that the injury and amnesia are a matter of degree.

The nature of long-term memory impairment cannot be determined until the patient is no longer experiencing post-traumatic amnesia. Predictions about other cognitive functions also should not be made. Although attentional problems may be paramount, and frequently underlie problems in learning and memory, in the clinical setting a number of persistent memory impairments may be observed. Short-term memory impairment, following the initial stages of recovery, is most often found to be spared, except in cases of severe injuries.[14] Semantic memory may be impaired, but rarely is there a complete loss of previously acquired information. More typical is loss of memory for particular facts or an apparent reduction in knowledge that cannot always be attributed to a problem in retrieval. This is sometimes referred to as a loss in "fund of general knowledge." Again, the most recently acquired memories appear to be the most vulnerable, a phenomenon that is evidenced frequently in clinical settings where students are found. It is not unusual for students to have difficulty recalling the coursework in which they were involved for weeks and sometimes even months prior to the injury.

Brooks[14] has reviewed many of the studies that have attempted to delineate particular aspects of memory that may be selectively impaired following traumatic brain injury. He concluded that "the exact nature of memory disturbances has proved difficult to unravel." Shimamura et al.[83] have indicated that prospective memory is impaired following frontal lobe damage (not necessarily attributable to a traumatic brain injury). Indeed, this is an area of significant interest to traumatic brain injury rehabilitation clinicians. Although there are few documented studies of prospective memory impairment following traumatic brain injury, clinicians in the field know that it is a critical aspect with respect to successful community and work re-entry.

In the clinical setting, memory is often divided into three stages or types based on temporal aspects of recall testing.[39,52,104] *Immediate memory* is often used synonymously with working memory or short-term memory and is assessed with digit-span-type activities. A second type, *recent memory*, is also thought to be a short-term memory, because the recall being assessed is within a few hours to a few days. The third stage or type is *remote memory*, which refers to long-term storage and older memories. The distinction between immediate and recent memory has some utility in the clinical setting, where short-term memory is frequently used to refer to both, without a clear point of reference. In the author's experience, clinicians unfamiliar with experimental psychology often use *short-term memory* to refer to memory for recent events or recently presented information. As an example, clinicians often refer to a patient's failure to recall the items eaten for breakfast as a short-term memory impairment. Sometimes, patients are still in post-traumatic amnesia and may, in fact, have a short-term memory impairment, but more often it is incorrect terminology usage. Generally, errors of this nature are harmless, but sometimes they can lead to confusion, such as in a team or family conference. Consider the family's level of confusion when, in a family conference, one clinician announces that "Short-term memory is intact, and that's a good sign." Then, another clinician states "I found short-term memory to be severely impaired. Mary can't remember what she ate for breakfast this morning or if she came to therapy" (four hours earlier). Because clinicians and researchers are often confused among themselves, description and examples should be preferred to labels.

Impairment of Problem Solving, Reasoning, Executive Functions, and Metacognition

There is great inconsistency in the literature regarding what to call the "higher order functions" in humans that seem to become so terribly dysfunctional following traumatic brain injury. Are executive system problems and problems in metacogntion the same, or are they separate? Are breakdowns in problem solving unique to a "problem solving skill" per se, or are they the result of problems in planning and monitoring, or due to the inability to draw conclusions? Are motivational problems psychosocial or cognitive? For many years there has been a tendency to compartmentalize these skills,[105] but by their very nature they are multiprocesses. The author has chosen to group these central nervous system functions together because, in reality, they are not distinctive processes, but overlapping ones that require the integration of numerous skills. Aspects of each, as they have been presented in the literature, are discussed.

Impairment in reasoning and problem solving is frequently listed among the cognitive sequelae to traumatic brain injury. However, following a review of numerous texts[7,10,11,20,24,29,34,88,106] in which impaired reasoning and problem solving were cited as sequelae, no studies were identified that specifically addressed the frequency with which these problems occur, the characteristics of the problems, or the characteristics of the patients. Typically, the particular components or subskills of problem solving are listed with suggestions that any or all aspects may be impaired. These have included organization, convergent and divergent thinking, ordering and sequencing, deductive and inductive reasoning, and abstract concept formation. Regarding problem solving ability, Adamovich et al.[29] noted that patients with traumatic brain injury frequently do not know how to approach problems and tend to perform concrete analysis of problem situations, often failing to think problems through. They have difficulty generating hypotheses, recognizing when information is incomplete, and employing alternate strategies to develop solutions. Descriptions such as this are common in the clinical literature. Clinicians in the field, in fact, will immediately recognize that these often are areas of breakdown.

Definitions of metacognition typically address the awareness of one's knowledge of personal cognitive abilities (refer to preceding sections), but do not necessarily encompass knowledge of one's feelings and emotional state; yet, no one would deny that knowledge of these is critical to self-awareness. With increasing frequency, it is the term *self-awareness* that appears in discussions of metacognition and executive functions.

Ylvisaker and Szekers[91] have discussed metacognition in terms of *static* (knowledge based) and *dynamic* (anticipatory and regulatory) aspects of self-knowledge. They have suggested that problems in the area of "executive system function" include self-awareness, goal setting and planning, flexible problem solving, self-initiation and direction, self-monitoring and inhibition, and self-evaluation.

Lezak[107] has proposed four broad areas of the executive system that may be impaired following brain damage:

(1) *volition*, including capacities for awareness of one's self and surroundings and motivational state;

(2) *planning*, including abilities to conceptualize change (look ahead), be objective, conceive of alternatives and make choices, develop a plan conceptually, and sustain attention;

(3) *purposive action*, including productivity and self-regulation; and

(4) *performance effectiveness*, or quality control.

She has included self-awareness as an executive function, with knowledge or awareness of motivation as a subcomponent. Stuss and colleagues[94,98] have presented a model of the "self" that places self-reflectiveness and metacognition at a higher level than executive control, which they describe as being regulatory in nature and including sub-functions such as anticipation, plan formulation, and goal articulation. Disruptions of executive control may yield fragmentary behavior that can be reflected as errors in sequencing or timing of actions,[94] or as an inability to inhibit familiar actions (routine schemata) in the presence of novel tasks.[108] Problems of this nature are referred to as "errors of action."

One way clinicians can conceptualize these differences is to think of executive functions from an action perspective, and metacognitive functions (including knowledge of emotional states) from an analytical one. Collectively, they can be conceptualized as a feedback loop capable of fine adjustments. In reality, it may be quite difficult to separate motivation from planning or initiation. Can self-awareness be separated from self-monitoring or use of feedback? Can attempts to improve self-awareness improve monitoring? Or, can self-awareness be developed gradually if an individual is taught to recognize concrete feedback? It is not as imperative that clinicians learn to separate these states, as it is that they understand the interrelatedness.

Many authors[96,98,100,109] have begun to refer more specifically to frontal lobe function(s) and dysfunction(s) because of the importance of the frontal lobes in integration of basic cognitive skills with regulatory functions and emotional states. This view tends to focus on the anatomy of the injury, but is perhaps preferable to labels with arbitrary boundaries.

Frontal lobe dysfunction increasingly is recognized as a common feature of traumatic brain injury,[96,98,100] although Levin et al.[109] have cautioned that "a potential problem in evaluating the neurobehavioral consequences of traumatic frontal lesions is the frequent presence of concomitant extrafrontal lesions." Nonetheless, there is a pattern of impairment that clinicians have come to consider "frontal lobe dysfuntion." The two distinct types of frontal lobe dysfunction, as previously reviewed in this chapter, do not necessarily differ with the etiology of traumatic brain injury. The difference between select focal frontal lesions and frontal lesions following traumatic brain injury is that the latter frequently are seen in the presence of temporal lobe damage and diffuse axonal injury while the former are not. For this reason, as Levin and colleagues have suggested, frontal lobe dysfunction pattern may not be completely accurate.

It must be stated, however, that the specific consideration of frontal lobe function, and the high risk for impairment following traumatic brain injury, have yielded a great deal of relevant information for rehabilitation. For example, problems in executive control have been overlooked in neuropsychological studies, in large part, because test instruments traditionally employed to evaluate cognitive functions are not sensitive to executive functions.[94,107] Problems in self-awareness and motivation have been reported in the literature for many years, but have been viewed as distinct psychosocial phenomena, with only marginal incorporation into rehabilitation frameworks. (Exceptions of course can be found, such as Ben-Yishay's[25] program and the work of Prigatano.[10]) Understanding the importance of the prefrontal regions to self-awareness has helped clinicians recognize that self-awareness itself can be impaired, and that poor self-awareness is not merely the byproduct of impaired cognitive functioning or psychosocial maladjustment. These relatively new insights have great bearing on the approach taken in rehabilitation. Altered awareness, often referred to as poor or limited awareness of deficits, denial of deficits, or *anosognosia*, frequently is seen as one of the greatest obstacles to successful rehabilitation and outcome, whether this is a valid view or not.[96]

Motivation, observed as a lack of drive in the negative state, also has been considered to be important to rehabilitation outcome. Prigatano[96] has suggested, however, that in the presence of frontal lobe damage it may not be a motivational state that affects performance and behavior, but rather the inability to integrate a feeling state into a plan of action.

Understanding the vulnerability of frontal lobe functions following traumatic brain injury can guide clinicians in their evaluation and treatment planning, beyond the knowledge of basic skills acquisition. In particular, these functions have great bearing on communication, as discussed below.

Cognitive-Communicative Impairment

The aspects of cognition that must be considered in relation to communicative functioning have been reviewed thoroughly at this point. A breakdown in any one of these cognitive skill areas can impact evaluation performance and daily living. When administering standardized, formal test procedures, it is important that clinicians analyze the skill requirements of each instrument in order that accurate conclusions can be drawn. Most test instruments require the application of more than one skill, even though they are designed to measure a single skill. (Reading paragraphs is a good example.) It is important to recognize specific problems in attention, memory, and organizational skills. These are best evaluated through both structured and unstructured assessment. Several authors[20,24,29,110,111,112] have reviewed standardized procedures commonly used in the field of speech-language pathology and have discussed their relevance to various cognitive and linguistic domains. These resources are listed in Appendix B, as well as in the reference list at the end of the chapter.

Comments on Aphasia

In studies that have included large sample sizes (over 600 patients) of persons with traumatic brain injury, the incidence of aphasia must be considered low (less than 2.5 percent).[113] The type of aphasia most frequently reported in the literature is anomia or amnesic aphasia. Severe anomia, disproportionate to other memory impairment, however, has not been carefully investigated or at least reported as such. The literature regarding aphasic disturbances has been reviewed by several authors,[18,19,21,100,113] and, given current consensus that aphasia is not a predominant feature of traumatic brain injury, these studies are not reviewed here. Some points regarding investigations into aphasia syndromes, however, should be discussed.

Aphasic symptoms of almost every type can be seen in the acute stages of injury, when the patient is disoriented and confused, and has low arousal. Depending upon one's definition, transient symptoms do not typically constitute aphasic syndromes. In the author's opinion, a definitive picture of a patient's language impairment following traumatic brain injury cannot be ascertained until attentional abilities and responsiveness have improved.

The issues concerning the presence or absence of focal lesions were mentioned in Chapter One. Some studies[114] have documented the presence of focal lesions, but then examined the results of a mixed group. The results of studies are typically the points referenced in other studies or reviews, so findings may continue to be grouped into still larger groups (that is, the population with traumatic brain injury).

Problems in terminology were introduced at the beginning of this chapter. It is important to note, however, that problems in the definitions of aphasia and language disorders will affect the outcome of studies. The perspective taken by the evaluator regarding the nature of language disorders will necessarily influence the manner in which data are collected and the conclusions drawn. As an example, Sarno[115] noted in her study that "in a few instances there was disagreement among speech-pathology staff members as to whether a patient was indeed aphasic." In another study[116] she clarified that the "designation 'aphasia' was limited to patients whose use of speech for expression and/or reception was impaired." Few would argue that individuals who are unable to "keep up" in a conversation do not have problems in the reception of speech, for whatever reasons (for example, attention or auditory comprehension problems). *Subclinical aphasia* is a term used by Sarno[115,116] to refer to "evidence of linguistic processing deficits on testing in the absence of clinical manifestations of linguistic impairment." Those familiar with traumatic brain injury know what this definition is attempting to describe, but one must ask: How can a linguistic processing deficit *not* be a clinical manifestation of language impairment? These examples elucidate the degree of confusion that arises when one is attempting to operate within the confines of traditional labels. Hart and Hayden[117] have suggested that in neuropsychological assessment, clinicians tend to evaluate only what tests "test." As an example, if one is "looking for patients" who fit into a fluent/nonfluent aphasia classification scheme, and if one employs an evaluation tool designed to classify patients in this way, one is apt to find some of those patients. It is, therefore, perhaps best not to use an abundance of labels, but rather to describe characteristics.

Specific Aspects of Communication Impairment

When individuals are confused, they say confusing things. Bizarre comments, perseveration of responses to questions or expression of ideas, confabulation, tangential and irrelevant comments may all be observed at various stages following traumatic brain injury. Problems in auditory comprehension may be observed, particularly as length and complexity of information increase. This is also true for reading comprehension.

Nelson and Schwentor[118] have reviewed the literature that has addressed reading and writing disorders following traumatic brain injury, and the literature is scant of studies that have investigated reading and writing specifically. Most of the studies in which reading and writing impairments have been noted, have investigated overall intellectual skills or memory and language skills and utilized tests of intelligence (for example, the Wechsler Adult Intelligence Scale) or aphasia test batteris (for example, the Boston Diagnostic Aphasia Examination). The reader can conclude that reading comprehension for lengthy and complex information and written language expression beyond the level of sentence construction have not been well investigated.

Nelson and Schwentor reported on the results of a survey they conducted with clinicians responsible for the assessment of reading and writing abilities in rehabilitation facilities that support this conclusion. The *Reading Comprehension Battery for Aphasia*[119] was utilized by the largest number of respondents, followed by the informal testing. Writing skills were most commonly assessed through informal testing followed by the *Boston Diagnostic Aphasia Examination.*[120]

Severe impairment of reading and writing skills, as seen in patients with aphasia and/or alexia and agraphia, can be addressed as they would be with the stroke population, with the exception that other cognitive deficits, such as attentional deficits, must be considered simultaneously. Often, severe cognitive deficits must be addressed at a basic level before the treatment of reading and writing impairments can be initiated. In patients who do not exhibit severe reading and writing impairment, reading and writing activities frequently are used to address other problems (for example, sequencing and organization). When working with patients who evidence moderate or mild impairments, it immediately becomes apparent that reading and writing cannot be separated from other cognitive skills. Reading and writing, both, are complex cognitive activities and should be approached as such.

Regarding language, complexity must be evaluated in terms of the abstractness of the message as well as the complexity of linguistic structure, because both can significantly affect comprehension (for example, metaphors and figures of speech may be missed). Specific impairments in word retrieval and verbal fluency may be observed and, as noted above, are the most commonly reported linguistic deficits in investigations of aphasia following traumatic brain injury. In the presence of focal lesions, isolated areas of language impairment may be observed. This appears to be the exception, rather than the rule.

Structured language (aphasia) batteries, like numerous other neuropsychological batteries, have not proven to be highly sensitive to the communication impairment of traumatic brain injury.[121,122] Figure 5.1 demonstrates how communication exists at the interface of cognitive, linguistic, and psychosocial/emotional abilities. It is at this interface that traumatic brain injury seems to have the greatest impact on daily functioning. Therefore, clinicians have turned their investigations more toward discourse assessment[100,123,124] and the assessment of pragmatic skills.[118]

Discourse assessments have included measurements taken during narrative, procedural, and conversational discourse production. Structured discourse assessment typically includes tasks such as picture description, story re-telling (narrative), or describing a procedure (procedural). Measures of productivity (for example, words per minute), content (for example, number of propositions), and cohesion (for example, number of units used to tie a story together) are usually taken. Although there is a growing body of

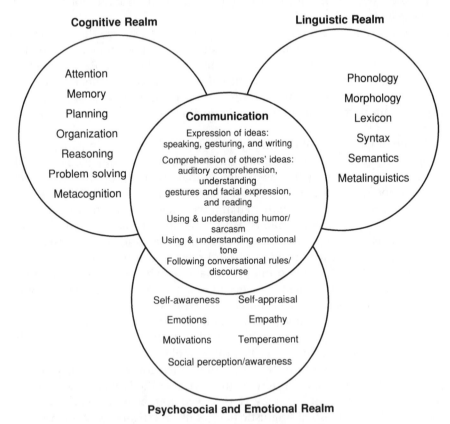

Figure 5.1 Communication depicted as the interface of cognitive, linguistic, and psychosocial abilities.

discourse research in various clinical populations (for example, stroke, Alzheimer's disease), very little research has been conducted in the field of traumatic brain injury. Those who have conducted research in the area[118,123,125,126] have found that persons with traumatic brain injury often verbally produce less and/or produce less efficiently. Hartley and Jensen[127] examined the discourse of speakers with traumatic brain injury and then classified the discourse into one of three profiles: *confused discourse, impoverished discourse,* or *inefficient discourse* (the latter being a case of overproduction compared to controls). They did note that the cases of confused discourse were closer in time to the injury than were the other cases. Coelho and colleagues[126] have also noted evidence of subtypes of discourse production following traumatic brain injury.

Structured discourse procedures offer the advantage of providing the clinician with some controls over the nature of the test condition. However, these procedures still lack the interactional nature of conversation, and it is only at this level that all aspects of oral communication can be assessed. Again, the research is quite limited, but clinical reports abound with comments such as "socially inappropriate," "interrupts others," "uses inappropriate language," "doesn't say anything," "stands too close," "talks too loudly," and the list could continue.

In conversational discourse, topic maintenance is often observed to be a problem.[121] Failure to observe turn-taking rules (in terms of initiation, interruption of others, and termination), recognition of speaker's intention or authority, and floor dominance (often in the form of rambling) may all be observed. As should be surmised, many of these problems are subsequent to a breakdown of cognitive and executive abilities. Attentional problems, as pointed out, can result in numerous subsequent difficulties such as the inability to maintain the topic of conversation or to observe turns. Patients with problems in generalized initiation of activity, to no one's surprise, often display poor or limited initiation of conversational exchange and lack of initiation during conversation. In conversation, perseveration may be observed as reiteration of the same comment or theme. Individuals who have difficulty making cognitive shifts also have difficulty shifting from one topic to another. Limited awareness and perceptual difficulties can result in poor observance of the personal space of others during conversational exchange, failure to recognize speaker position, poor recognition of facial expression and gestural cues, as well as poor monitoring of output. Individuals who have slowed information processing may miss information during conversation, particularly when the rate of exchange and linguistic complexity are variable.

These are the problems that have come to be the hallmarks of communication impairment following traumatic brain injury. The highly structured, formal testing environment does not assess this aspect of communication. Very often, the testing situation itself allows for adequate comprehension and expression by providing needed structure. This is true for information processing and responding in general.

Some Evaluation Guidelines

As stated above, a number of texts have reviewed test instruments that can be used in the evaluation of cognitive-communication impairment following traumatic brain injury. Evaluation is a process, however, and must go beyond the confines of a particular instrument. Some general concepts regarding the evaluation and delineation of impairment following traumatic brain injury should be considered:

- A thorough history inclusive of premorbid personality traits, learning style and academic performance, use of alcohol and drugs, current medications, communication style, employment, family history and relationships, and medical findings is essential to the accurate interpretation of evaluative findings and to treatment planning.
- The evaluation of impairment following traumatic brain injury must be ongoing, and the clinical picture must be continually updated if treatment is to be focused appropriately. This is particularly true in the early stages of recovery.
- Performance should be observed under multiple conditions.
- A number of skills fall apart under time constraints. This must be considered, before conclusive statements are offered regarding ability.
- Fatigue should always be considered as a contributing factor to poor performance.
- The manner of test response is as important as the test answers. Both should be recorded. Particular attention should be paid to the patient's recognition and self-correction of errors, the effectiveness of cues and the ability to use feedback, and the use of self-employed strategies to improve performance.
- The patient's level of arousal, verbalized anxiety and complaints, and acknowledged areas of strength and weakness should all be noted.
- Family members and friends should be interviewed specifically in regard to the patient's communication style, sociableness, and language interests (for example, reading, writing, debate, public speaking).
- Conversational skills cannot be assessed accurately in a clinician-patient dialogue. They must be assessed with partners other than a clinician and in variety of contexts.

SUMMARY AND COMMENT

The nature of impairment following traumatic brain injury is complex and, in many ways, unlike other conditions with which rehabilitation clinicians are confronted. A working knowledge of cognitive processes is essential to the delineation of impairment, to effective treatment planning, and to interdisciplinary team communication. Although numerous theoretical models have been proposed to explain various aspects of cognition, it is not essential that the clinician promote a particular model, but rather that the cognitive processes be understood. This chapter reviewed a number of models of cognitive processes, and then delineated how these may be affected following traumatic brain injury based on a review of the literature. Attention, memory, problem solving and reasoning, and executive functions are all important aspects of cognition that must be considered. These cannot be viewed as unitary constructs, as each cognitive area is composed of many aspects. It is important to understand these aspects largely as skills, for it is at the skill level that we most often intervene. Functions of the frontal lobes have been discussed for their important role in the overall regulation of cognitive functions and behavior. Additionally, they are particularly susceptible to damage in traumatic brain injury.

The confusion regarding the terminology in the field and the relevance of the aphasia literature also were discussed. Information was presented in a manner that should help clinicians new to the field understand some of the controversy regarding terminology in relation to the brief history of traumatic brain injury rehabilitation.

Finally, given the traditional training of most speech-language pathologists, a note about site of lesions and localization of functions is indicated. The absence of a lesion on a diagnostic imaging study does not rule out the behaviors observed, it only indicates that they may or may not be attributed to a particular region of the brain. It must be emphasized that although neuroimaging techniques and electrophysiology have advanced considerably, they must still be seen as relatively gross measurements in relation to the complex brain functions. The effects of cortical, subcortical, and brain stem disruption following severe traumatic brain injury are vast and complex. An array of impairment should be expected, with some shared commonalities among patients, and some general expectations in relation to the severity of the injury. Hagen[18] has stated aptly that the "variability is their commonality."

REFERENCES

1. Teasdale G, Jennett B. Assessment of coma: a practical scale. *Lancet.* 1974; 2:81–84.
2. Jennett B. Assessment of the severity of head injury. *Journal of Neurology, Neurosurgery, and Psychiatry.* 1976;39:647–655.
3. Jennett B, Teasdale G. Aspects of coma after severe head injury. *Lancet.* 1977; 2:878–881.
4. Yen JK et al. Numerical grading of clinical neurological status after serious head injury. *Journal of Neurology, Neurosurgery, and Psychiatry.* 1978;42:1125–1130.
5. Levin HS, Benton AL, Grossman RG. *Neurobehavioral Consequences of Closed Head Injury.* New York, NY: Oxford University Press; 1982.

6. Newcombe F. The psychological consequences of closed head injury: assessment and rehabilitation. *Injury.* 1982;14:111–136.
7. Brooks, DN. *Closed Head Injury: Psychological, Social, and Family Consequences.* Oxford, England: Oxford University Press; 1984.
8. Levin HS. Part II: neurobehavioral recovery. In Becker D, Povlischock JT (eds). *Central Nervous System Trauma Status Report.* Bethesda, MD: National Institute of Neurological and Communicative Disorders and Stroke; 1985:281–299.
9. Fisher JM. Cognitive and behavioral consequences of closed head injury. *Seminars in Neurology.* 1985;5:197–204.
10. Prigatano G et al. *Neuropsychological Rehabilitation after Brain Injury.* Baltimore, MD: Johns Hopkins University Press; 1986:2–17.
11. Levin HS. Neurobehavioral sequelae of head injury. In Cooper PR (ed). *Head Injury, 2nd ed.* Baltimore, MD: Williams and Wilkins; 1987:442–463.
12. Prigatano, G. Neuropsychological deficits, personality variables, and outcome. In Ylvisaker M, Gobble EM (eds). *Community Re-entry for Head Injured Adults.* Boston, MA: College-Hill Press; 1987:1–23.
13. Rosenthal M, Bond MR. Behavioral and psychiatric sequelae. In Rosenthal M, Griffith ER, Bond MR, Miller JD (eds). *Rehabilitation of the Adult and Child with Traumatic Brain Injury, 2nd ed.* Philadelphia, PA: FA Davis; 1990:179–192.
14. Brooks DN. Cognitive deficits. In Rosenthal M, Griffith ER, Bond MR, Miller JD (eds). *Rehabilitation of the Adult and Child with Traumatic Brain Injury, 2nd ed.* Philadelphia, PA: FA Davis; 1990:163–178.
15. Gualtieri CT. *Neuropsychiatry and Behavioral Pharmacology.* New York, NY: Springer-Verlag; 1991:1–25.
16. Hagen C. Language disorders secondary to closed head injury: diagnosis and treatment. *Topics in Language Disorders.* 1981;1:73–87.
17. Holland AL. When is aphasia aphasia? The problem of closed head injury. In Brookshire RH (ed). *Clinical Aphasiology Conference Proceedings.* Minneapolis, MN: BRK Publishers; 1982:3345–349.
18. Hagen C. Language disorders in head trauma. In Holland AL (ed). *Language Disorders in Adults: Recent Advances.* San Diego, CA: College-Hill Press; 1984:245–281.
19. Wiig EH, Alexander EW, Secord W. Linguistic competence and level of cognitive functioning in adults with traumatic closed head injury. In Whitaker HA (ed). *Neuropsychological Studies of Nonfocal Brain Damage: Dementia and Trauma.* London, England: Springer-Verlag; 1988:186–210.
20. Kennedy MR, DeRuyter F. Cognitive and language bases for communication disorders. In Beukelman DR, Yorkston KM (eds). *Communicative Disorders Following Traumatic Brain Injury: Management of Cognitive, Language and Motor Impairments.* Austin, TX: Pro-Ed; 1991:123–190.
21. Ylvisaker M, Urbanczyk B. Assessment and treatment of speech, swallowing, and communication disorders following traumatic brain injury. In Finlayson MAJ, Garner SH (eds). *Brain Injury Rehabilitation: Clinical Considerations.* Baltimore, MD: Williams and Wilkins; 1994:157–186.
22. Wepman JM. Aphasia: language without thought or thought without language? *ASHA.* March 1976;131–136.
23. Rosenbek JC. When is aphasia aphasia? In Brookshire RH (ed). *Clinical Aphasiology Conference Proceedings.* Minneapolis, MN: BRK Publishers; 1982:360–366.

24. Hartley LL. *Cognitive-Communicative Abilities Following Brain Injury: A Functional Approach.* San Diego, CA: Singular Publishing; 1995.
25. Ben-Yishay Y. *Working Approaches to Remediation of Cognitive Deficits in Brain Damaged Persons.* New York, NY: New York University Medical Center; 1980:1–2.
26. Knight RT. Evoked potential studies of attention capacity in human frontal lobe lesions. In Levin HS, Eisenberg HM, Benton AL (eds). *Frontal Lobe Function and Dysfunction.* New York, NY: Oxford University Press; 1991:138–153.
27. Whyte J, Rosenthal M. Rehabilitation of the patient with head injury. In DeLisa J (ed). *Rehabilitation Medicine: Principles and Practices.* Philadelphia, PA: JB Lippincott; 1988:585–611.
28. Whyte J. Attention and arousal: basic science aspects. *Archives of Physical Medicine and Rehabilitation.* 1992;73:940–949.
29. Adamovich BB, Henderson JA, Auerbach S. *Cognitive Rehabilitation of Closed Head Injured Patients: A Dynamic Approach.* San Diego, CA: College-Hill Press; 1985.
30. van Zomeren AH, Brouwer WH, Deelman BG. Attentional deficits: the riddles of selectivity, speed, and alertness. In Brooks, DN (ed). *Closed Head Injury: Psychological, Social, and Family Consequences.* Oxford, England: Oxford University Press; 1984:74–107.
31. Nissen MJ. Neuropsychology of attention and memory. *Journal of Head Trauma Rehabilitation.* 1986;1:13–21.
32. Mesulam MM. Attention, confusional states, and neglect. In Mesulam MM (ed). *Principles of Behavioral Neurology.* Philadelphia, PA: FA Davis; 1985:125–168.
33. Reed SK. *Cognition: Theory and Applications.* Monterey, CA: Brooks/Cole Publishing; 1982.
34. Sohlberg MM, Mateer CA. *Introduction to Cognitive Rehabilitation: Theory and Practice.* New York, NY: Guilford Press; 1989:111–135.
35. Sohlberg MM, Mateer CA. Effectiveness of an attention-training program. *Journal of Clinical and Experimental Neuropsychology.* 1987;9:117–130.
36. Ponsford J, Kinsella G. Evaluation of a remedial programme for attentional deficits following closed-head injury. *Journal of Clinical and Experimental Neuropsychology.* 1988;10:693–708.
37. Treisman AM. Strategies and models of selective attention. *Psychological Review.* 1969;76:282–299.
38. Weber AM. A practical clinical approach to understanding and treating attentional problems. *Journal of Head Trauma Rehabilitation.* 1990;5:73–85.
39. Lezak MD. *Neuropsychological Assessment, 2nd ed.* New York; NY: Oxford University Press; 1983:7–40.
40. Gronwall DMA. Paced auditory serial-addition task: a measure of recovery from concussion. *Perceptual and Motor Skills.* 1977;43:67–373.
41. Broadbent DE. A mechanical model for human attention and immediate memory. *Psychological Review.* 1957;64:205–215.
42. Deutsch JA, Deutsch D. Attention: some theoretical considerations. *Psychological Review.* 1963;70:80–90.
43. Shiffrin RM, Schneider W. Controlled automatic human information processing: II. Perceptual learning, automatic attending, and a general theory. *Psychological Review.* 1977;84:127–190.

44. Stroop JR. Studies of interference in serial verbal reactions. *Journal of Experimental Psychology.* 1935;18:643–662.

45. Whyte J. Neurologic disorders of attention and arousal: assessment and treatment. *Archives of Physical Medicine and Rehabilitation.* 1992;73:1094–1103.

46. Shallice T, Burgess P. Higher-order cognitive impairments and frontal lobe lesions in man. In Levin HS, Eisenberg HM, Benton AL (eds). *Frontal Lobe Function and Dysfunction.* New York, NY: Oxford University Press; 1991:126–138.

47. Mack JL. Clinical assessment of disorders of attention and memory. *Journal of Head Trauma Rehabilitation.* 1986;1:22–33.

48. Goldman R, Fristoe M, Woodcock R. *Goldman-Fristoe-Woodcock Auditory Skills Battery.* Minnesota, MN: American Guidance Service; 1974.

49. Hasher L, Zacks RT. Automatic and effortful processes in memory. *Journal of Experimental Psychology: General.* 1979;108:356–388.

50. Craik FIM, Lockhart RS. Levels of processing: a framework for memory research. *Journal of Verbal Learning and Verbal Behavior.* 1972;11:671–684.

51. Zechmeister EG, Nyberg SE. *Human Memory: An Introduction to Research and Theory.* Monterey, CA; Brooks/Cole Publishing Company; 1982.

52. Squire LR. *Memory and Brain.* New York, NY: Oxford University Press; 1987.

53. Warrington EK. Neurological disorders of memory. *British Medical Bulletin.* 1971;27:243–247.

54. Baddeley AD, Hitch GJ. Working memory. In Bower GA (ed). *The Psychology of Learning and Motivation, vol 8.* New York, NY: Academic Press; 1974:47–85.

55. Parenté R, Anderson-Parente JK. Retraining memory: theory and application. *Journal of Head Trauma Rehabilitation.* 1989;4:55–63.

56. Parenté R, DiCesare A. Retraining memory: theory, evaluation, and applications. In Kreutzer J, Wehman P (eds). *Cognitive Rehabilitation for Persons with Traumatic Brain Injury.* Baltimore, MD: Paul H Brookes; 1991:147–162.

57. Harris JE. External memory aids. In Neisser U (ed). *Memory Observed: Remembering in Natural Contexts.* San Francisco, CA: WH Freeman; 1982:337–342.

58. Wickelgren W. Chunking and consolidation: a theoretical synthesis of semantic networks, configuring in conditioning, S-R versus cognitive learning, normal forgetting, the amnesic syndrome and the hippocampal arousal system. *Psychology Review.* 1979;86:44–60.

59. Squire LR. Mechanisms of memory. *Science.* 1986; 232:1612–1619.

60. Tromp E, Mulder T. Slowness of information processing after traumatic head injury. *Journal of Clinical and Experimental Neuropsychology.* 1991;13:821–830.

61. Winograd T. Frame representations and the declarative-procedural controversy. In Bobrow D, Collins A (eds). *Representation and Understanding: Studies in Cognitive Science.* New York, NY: Academic Press; 1975:185–210.

62. Linton M. Transformations of memory in everyday life. In Neisser U (ed). *Memory Observed: Remembering in Natural Contexts.* San Francisco, CA: WH Freeman; 1982:77–91.

63. Sperling G. The information available in brief visual presentations. *Psychological Monographs.* 1960;74:(11)498.

64. Posner MI et al. Retention of visual and name codes of single letters. *Journal of Experimental Psychology Monograph.* 1969;7:91–13.

65. Paivio A, Begg I. Pictures and words in visual search. *Memory and Cognition.* 1974;2:515–521.

66. Neisser U, Becklen R. Selective looking: attending to visually specified events. *Cognitive Psychology.* 1975;7:480–494.
67. Standing L, Conezio J, Haber RN. Perception and memory for pictures: single-trial learning of 2500 visual stimuli. *Psychonomic Science.* 1970;19:73–74.
68. Shepard RN. Recognition memory for words, sentences, and pictures, *Journal of Verbal Learning and Verbal Behavior.* 1967;6:156–163.
69. Strauss E, Butler R. The effect of varying types of interference on haptic memory in the Korsakoff patient. *Neuropsychologia.* 1978;16:81–90.
70. Butters N et al. Material-specific memory deficits in alcoholic Korsakoff patients. *Neuropsychologia.* 1973;11:291–299.
71. Oscar-Berman M, Goodglass H, Cherlow D. Perceptual laterality and iconic recognition of visual materials by Korsakoff patients and normal adults. *Journal of Comparative and Physiological Psychology.* 1973;82:316–321.
72. Cermak LS, Real L, DeLuca D. Korsakoff patients' nonverbal versus verbal memory: effects of interference and mediation on rates of association. *Neuropsychologia.* 1977;15:303–310.
73. Reige W. Inconsistant nonverbal recognition memory in Korsakoff patients and controls. *Neuropsychologia* 1977;15:269–276.
74. Cermak L, Tarlow S. Aphasic and amnesic patients' verbal vs. nonverbal retentive abilities. *Cortex.* 1978;14:32–40.
75. Samuels I et al. A comparison of subcortical and cortical damage on short-term visual and auditory memory. *Neuropsychologia.* 1971;9:293–306.
76. Milner B. Visual recognition and recall after right temporal-lobe excision in man. *Neuropsychologia.* 1968;6:191–209.
77. Milner B. Memory and the medial temporal regions of the brain. In Pribram KH, Broadbent DE (eds). *Biological Bases of Memory.* New York, NY: Academic Press; 1970:29–50.
78. Patten BM. Modality specific memory disorders in man. *Acta Neurology Scandinavia.* 1972;48:69–86.
79. Flavell JH, Wellman HM. Metamemory. In Kail RV, Hagen JW (eds). *Perspectives on the Development of Memory and Cognition.* Hillsdale, NJ: Lawrence Erlbaum Publishers; 1977:3–33.
80. Hart JT. Memory and the feeling-of-knowing experience. *Journal of Educational Psychology.* 1965;56:208–216.
81. Hart JT. Memory and the memory-monitoring process. *Journal of Verbal Learning and Verbal Behavior.* 1967;6:685–691.
82. Hart JT. Second-try recall, recognition, and the memory-monitoring process. *Journal of Educational Psychology,* 1967;58:193–197.
83. Shimamura AP, Janowsky JS, Squire LR. What is the role of frontal lobe damage in memory disorders? In Levin HS, Eisenberg HM, Benton AL (eds). *Frontal Lobe Function and Dysfunction.* New York, NY: Oxford University Press; 1991:173–195.
84. Meacham JA, Leiman B. Remembering to perform future actions. In Neisser U (ed). *Memory Observed: Remembering in Natural Contexts.* San Francisco, CA: WH Freeman; 1982:327–336.
85. Brown R, Kulik J. Flashbulb memories. In Neisser U (ed). *Memory Observed: Remembering in Natural Contexts.* San Francisco, CA: WH Freeman; 1982:23–40.
86. Neisser U. Snapshots of benchmarks? In Neisser U (ed). *Memory Observed: Remembering in Natural Contexts.* San Francisco, CA: WH Freeman; 1982:43–48.

87. Bransford JD, Stein BS. *The Ideal Problem Solver: A Guide for Improving Thinking, Learning, and Creativity.* New York, NY: WH Freeman; 1984.

88. Szekers SF, Ylvisaker M, Cohen SB. A framework for cognitive rehabilitation therapy. In Ylvisaker M, Gobble EM (eds). *Community Re-entry for Head Injured Adults.* Boston, MA: College-Hill Press; 1987:87–136.

89. Sternberg RJ, Gastel J. If dancers ate their shoes: inductive reasoning with factual and counterfactual premises. *Memory and Cognition.* 1989;17:1–10.

90. *Webster's New World Dictionary of the American Language, 2nd college ed.* New York, NY: World Publishing; 1972.

91. Ylvisaker M, Szekers SF. Metacognitive and executive impairments in head-injured children and adults. *Topics in Language Disorders.* 1989;9:34–49.

92. Vogenthaler DR. An overview of head injury: its consequences and rehabilitation. *Brain Injury.* 1987;1:113–127.

93. Stuss DT, Benson DF. *The Frontal Lobes.* New York, NY: Raven Press; 1986.

94. Sohlberg MM, Mateer CA, Stuss DT. Contemporary approaches to the management of executive control dysfunction. *Journal of Head Trauma Rehabilitation.* 1993;8:45–58.

95. Duke LW et al. Cognitive rehabilitation after head trauma. In Long CJ, Ross LK (eds). *Handbook of Head Trauma: Acute Care to Recovery.* New York: Plenum Press; 1992:165–190.

96. Prigatano GP. The relationship of frontal lobe damage to diminished awareness: studies in rehabilitation. In Levin HS, Eisenberg HM, Benton AL (eds). *Frontal Lobe Function and Dysfunction.* New York,NY: Oxford University Press; 1991:381–397.

97. Mesulam MM. Patterns in behavioral neuroanatomy: association areas, the limbic system, and hemispheric specialization. In Mesulam MM (ed). *Principles of Behavioral Neurology.* Philadelphia, PA: FA Davis; 1985:1–70.

98. Stuss DT, Mateer CA, Sohlberg MM. Innovative approaches to frontal lobe deficits. In Finlayson MAJ, Garner SH (eds). *Brain Injury Rehabilitation: Clinical Considerations.* Baltimore, MD: Williams and Wilkins; 1994:212–237.

99. Newcombe F. Frontal lobe disorders. In Greenwood R, Barnes MP, McMillan TM (eds). *Neurological Rehabilitation.* Edinburgh, Scotland: Churchill-Livingstone; 1994:377–386.

100. Chapman SB, Levin HS, Culhane KA. Language impairment in closed head injury. In Kirshner H (ed). *Handbook of Neurologic Speech and Language Disorders.* New York, NY: Marcel Dekker; 1995:387–414.

101. Ritchie WR. The traumatic amnesias. *International Journal of Neurology.* 1968;7:55–59.

102. Schacter DL, Crovitz HF. Memory function after closed head injury: a review of the quantitative research. *Cortex.* 1977;13:150–176.

103. Auerbach SH. Neuroanatomical correlates of attention and memory disorders in traumatic brain injury: an application of neurobehavioral subtypes. *Journal of Head Trauma Rehabilitation.* 1986;1:1–12.

104. Ward C. Learning and skill acquisition. In Greenwood R, Barnes MP, McMillan TM (eds). *Neurological Rehabilitation.* Edinburgh, Scotland: Churchill-Livingstone; 1994:111–123.

105. Ben-Yishay Y, Diller L. Cognitive deficits. In Rosenthal M, Griffith ER, Bond MR, Miller JD (eds). *Rehabilitation of the Adult and Child with Traumatic Brain Injury.* Philadelphia, PA: FA Davis, 1982:167–183.

106. Sbordone RJ. A conceptual model of neuropsychologically-based cognitive rehabilitation. In Williams JM, Long CJ (eds). *The Rehabilitation of Cognitive Disabilities*. New York, NY: Plenum Press; 1987:3–25.

107. Lezak MD. Newer contributions to the neuropsychological assessment of executive functions. *Journal of Head Trauma Rehabilitation*. 1993;8:24–31.

108. Schwartz MF et al. Cognitive theory and the study of everyday action disorders after brain damage. *Journal of Head Trauma Rehabilitation*. 1993;8:59–72.

109. Levin HS et al. The contribution of frontal lobe lesions to the neurobehavioral outcome of closed head injury. In Levin HS, Eisenberg HM, Benton AL (eds). *Frontal Lobe Function and Dysfunction*. New York, NY: Oxford University Press; 1991:318–338.

110. Ylvisaker MS, Holland AL. Coaching, self-coaching, and rehabilitation of head injury. In Johns DF (ed). *Clinical Management of Neurogenic Communicative Disorders, 2nd ed.* Boston, MA: Little Brown and Company; 1985:243–257.

111. Baxter R, Cohen S, Ylvisaker M. Comprehensive cognitive assessment. In Ylvisaker M (ed). *Head Injury Rehabilitation: Children and Adolescents*. San Diego, CA: College-Hill Press; 1985:247–274.

112. Halper AS, Cherney LR, Miller TK. *Clinical Management of Communication Problems in Adults with Traumatic Brain Injury*. Gaithersburg, MD: Aspen Publications; 1991:27–54.

113. Hartley LL, Levin HS. Linguistic deficits after closed head injury: a current appraisal. *Aphasiology*. 1990;4:353–370.

114. Thompsen IV. Evaluation and outcome of aphasia in patients with severe closed head trauma. *Journal of Neurology, Neurosurgery, and Psychiatry*. 1975;38: 713–718.

115. Sarno, MT. The nature of verbal impairment after closed head injury. *Journal of Nervous and Mental Disease*. 1980;168:685–692.

116. Sarno MT, Buonaguar A, Levita E. Characteristics of verbal impairment in closed head injured patients. *Archives of Physical Medicine and Rehabilitation*. 1986;67:400–405.

117. Hart T, Hayden ME. The ecological validity of neuropsychological assessment and remediation. In Uzzell B, Gross Y (eds). *Clinical Neuropsychology of Intervention*. Boston, MA: Martinus Nijhoff Publishing; 1986:21–50.

118. Nelson NW, Schwentor BA. Reading and writing disorders. In Beukelman DR, Yorkston KM (eds). *Communication Disorders Following Traumatic Brain Injury: Management of Cognitive, Language, and Motor Impairments*. Austin, TX: Pro-Ed; 1991:191–249.

119. LaPointe LL, Horner J. *Reading Comprehension Battery for Aphasia*. Tigard, OR: CC Publications; 1979.

120. Goodglass H, Kaplan E. *Boston Diagnostic Aphasia Examination*. Malvern, PA: Lea and Febiger, 1983.

121. Milton SB, Prutting CA, Binder GM. Appraisal of communicative competence in head injured adults. In Brookshire RH (ed). *Clinical Aphasiology Conference Proceedings*. Minneapolis, MN: BRK Publishers; 1984:114–123.

122. Hartley LL. Assessment of functional communication. In Tupper DE, Cicerone K (eds). *The Neuropsychology of Everyday Life: Assessment and Basic Competencies*. Boston, MA: Kluwer Academic Publishers; 1990:125–168.

123. Mentis M, Prutting C. Cohesion in the discourse of normal and head-injured adults. *Journal of Speech and Hearing Research*. 1987;30:88–98.

124. Hartley LL, Jensen PJ. Narrative and procedural discourse—after closed head injury. *Brain Injury.* 1991;5:267–285.

125. Ehrlich JS. Selective characteristics of narrative discourse in head-injured and normal adults. *Journal of Communication Disorders.* 1988;21:1–9.

126. Coelho CA, Liles BZ, Duffy RJ. Discourse analyses with closed head injured adults: evidence for differing patterns of deficits. *Archives of Physical Medicine and Rehabilitation.* 1991;72:465–468.

127. Hartley LL, Jensen PJ. Three discourse profiles of closed-head-injury speakers: theoretical and clinical implications. *Brain Injury.* 1992;6:271–282.

6

Cognitive-Communicative Rehabilitation: Theoretical and Clinical Considerations

Numerous approaches to the remediation, or rehabilitation, of cognitive impairments have been suggested. Some provide an operational framework for the delivery of all cognitive remediation, and others offer specific strategies or treatment activities tailored to a particular problem, for example, visual-spatial neglect. Although models of rehabilitation and health care delivery have been discussed, the reader will find that approaches to cognitive rehabilitation are interrelated, if not mutually deterministic. How one chooses to approach the issue of disability (that is, from a biologic versus sociologic, or impairment versus handicap level) will influence one's approach to cognitive rehabilitation, to some extent. This may be conceptualized as a macroview of rehabilitation. Similarly, if one has an established paradigm for the delivery of cognitive remediation services, it may influence one's view of disability and rehabilitation, sometimes without being recognized as an influence. This, in turn, may be thought of as a microview of rehabilitation. As an example, a deficit-oriented approach that seeks to break down cognitive processes to the lowest level is consistent with a biomedical model of rehabilitation and impairment level of disability. Other connections between approaches to rehabilitation and models of rehabilitation will become apparent. In the author's opinion, much of what has been presented in the literature regarding the rehabilitation of cognitive-communicative impairment following traumatic brain injury represents a microview of and biologic approach to traumatic brain injury rehabilitation.

Terminology in rehabilitation also reflects one's view of the aim or purpose of treatment. *Cognitive rehabilitation (CR)*, *cognitive remediation (CR)*, *cognitive retraining (CR)*, and *cognitive rehabilitation therapy (CRT)* appear to be used interchangeably in the literature. A limited review[1,2,3,4,5,6,7,8,9,10,11,12,13,14,15] of fifteen articles, chapters, and texts, each with one of the preceding terms in the title, indicated that there is an implied, shared understanding of terminology; only five of the authors[2,6,7,8,13] provided a definition or frame of reference for the chosen term. To demonstrate the scope encompassed by the terminology, several of the definitions are presented. Beginning with the greatest degree of specificity, "cognitive rehabilitation . . . refers to the thera-peutic process of increasing or improving an individual's capacity to process and use incoming information so as to allow increased functioning in every-day life. This includes both methods to restore cognitive function and compensatory techniques."[8] Another, less specific, definition offers the ex-planation that "cognitive retraining can be defined as those activities that improve a brain-injured patient's higher cerebral functioning or help the patient to better understand the nature of those difficulties while teaching him or her methods of compensation."[9] Difficulties are not specified, but the implied referent is impairment of higher cognitive functioning, typically thought of as problem solving, reasoning, and executive functions.

Gordan[13,16] and Wilson[7] each use the term *intervention* to define re-mediation and rehabilitation (respectively), without defining intervention. Consequently, their characterizations are lacking in specificity as well:

> Cognitive remediation is a form of intervention in which a constellation of procedures are applied by a trained practitioner (usually a neuropsychologist, speech-language pathologist, or occupational therapist) to provide brain-injured individuals with the skills and strategies needed to perform tasks that are difficult or impossible for them due to the presence of underlying cognitive deficits.[13,16]
>
> Cognitive rehabilitation attempts to remediate, ameliorate or alleviate cognitive deficits that have resulted from brain injury. The term "cognitive rehabilitation" can apply to any intervention strategy or technique which intends to enable clients or patients and their families to live with, manage, bypass, reduce, or come to terms with cognitive deficits precipitated by injury to the brain.[7]

Although it is not essential that terms be defined in every article address-ing cognitive rehabilitation, it is important that the reader know if the author intends a broad (restoration, alleviation, and compensation) or nar-row (remediation of specific processes) focus. Because this text is meant to increase general awareness about the field, as well as be instructive, both broad and narrow approaches are reviewed. Wilson's definition introduces some additional terms that warrant discussion.

In the medical literature, *rehabilitation* refers to the restoration of func-tion, the reduction or minimization of impairment, the prevention of further deterioration, and ultimately the amelioration of disability.[17]

The term *remediate* specifically means to correct, and it therefore seems to carry with it the greatest challenge to clinicians. *Ameliorate* means to make better or more tolerable, to improve. *Alleviate* also tends to imply less change than *remediate*, in that it means to make more bearable, to lessen, or to relieve. *Alleviate* is often used in medicine (for example, alleviate symptoms), but it seems to be used less in clinical rehabilitation. This is perhaps because clinicians think that it implies less than they "should" be doing. Yet, refer-ring back to the goals of rehabilitation, there is no semantic or ethical basis for the idea that alleviation and amelioration are not appropriate goals of rehabilitation. *Accommodate* means to make fit or suitable, and, by so doing, to bring into agreement. One legitimately could ask, "Should agreement occur between an individual and a particular task, the daily living environment, the work place, and/or society?" In rehabilitation, *accommodate* is frequently used in reference to environmental and architectural barriers that must be changed "to accommodate" the individual with a disability. *Compensate* is used routinely in rehabilitation, and as defined by Webster[18] it means "to supply an equivalent; [and] to offset error, defect or undesired effect; [also] to counterbalance." From a clinical perspective, compensation has been defined as "the deliberate application of a procedure that enables a patient to obtain a goal the realization of which would otherwise be prevented by impaired functioning."[19]

Benedict[10] has suggested that cognitive rehabilitation is directed at one of two goals: remediation or compensation. Remedial intervention seeks to restore function according to the concept that neuronal recovery is associated with the "exercise of neuronal circuits."[10] (Recovery is discussed in the next section.) On the other hand, interventions aimed at compensation "concede the unrecoverable loss of function, and assist patients with behavioral strategies that circumvent impaired functions."[10] In this author's opinion, it is erroneous to conceptualize the goals of rehabilitation in terms of this limited dichotomy. First, persons with traumatic brain injury experience numerous areas and degrees of impairment and can have a wide repertoire of residual skills. Treatment must be tailored to address these variations in skills. Second, restoration of function is not always possible, but compensation is not necessarily the logical or most beneficial option. Again, the individual's needs, skills, and support systems are determining factors.

The reader is encouraged to consider these concepts in relationship to the various approaches to cognitive-communicative rehabilitation presented below. For the clinician, it is important to continually review one's own thoughts about the nature and purpose of the interventions provided. For the rehabilitationist, it is important to consider when remediation is the most appropriate goal, when amelioration and alleviation are needed, and when compensation is indicated. These courses of action are not always readily apparent,[20] and in fact require careful analysis and decision making on the part of the clinician and patient.

RECOVERY THEORIES AND REHABILITATION

Theories regarding the recovery of function must be considered when thinking about the neurophysiologic substrates to cognitive rehabilitation, although a review of the literature indicates that no single theory of recovery has figured prominently in any one proposed approach to cognitive rehabilitation. Rather, the lack of sound evidence regarding change in neural structure has been cited as a criticism of cognitive rehabilitation; that is, the lack of evidence that cognitive rehabilitation produces structural change has been offered as proof of its ineffectiveness.[13] However, as Gordon[16] has pointed out, cognitive rehabilitationists have never made claims that changes in neural structures result from cognitive rehabilitation, only that changes in cognitive processes have been demonstrated. Theories of the recovery of function are important to understand, because it is often necessary to account for natural or spontaneous recovery, as opposed to treatment, as potentially the sole contributor to cognitive-communicative improvement. Conceptually, if one thinks that cognitive rehabilitation is a viable method of improvement of function, one must also hold some view regarding the plasticity and adaptability of the central nervous system. Therefore, a brief discussion of the theories of recovery commonly considered in the literature is presented below.

First, it is important to note that theories of recovery describe, or attempt to account for, phenomena related to early neurologic recovery, often referred to as spontaneous or natural recovery. Second, a definition of recovery is warranted. Almi and Finger[21] define *recovery* as "a theoretical construct that implies a complete regaining of identical functions that were lost or impaired after brain damage." Further, an absolute definition is needed to circumvent the problem associated with degrees of recovery, that is, the extent to which the regaining of some function(s) constitutes recovery.

The concept of *plasticity* assumes that the central nervous system has properties that allow for the reorganization of the brain at a neurophysiologic and anatomic level following brain injury, and that this reorganization results in improved function or functional recovery. Not all theories of recovery assume plasticity, per se; some posit instead the transient effects of the injury on neural functioning. In general, these transient effects can be referred to as *neural shock*. Recovery occurs as the shock effects diminish. Specifically, neural shock theories propose that not all neurons are damaged permanently, and that those closest to the site of injury and related through interconnections suffer only temporary impairment. Perhaps the most well known of these theories is von Monakow's *diaschisis*, which is a passive phenomenon (as opposed to the result of edema or some other pathologic symptom) that represents shock along neural connections.[22] Diaschisis is a similar construct to Luria's concept of *inhibition*, which refers to a diffuse suppression of those axons not affected permanently by the injury. Recovery would occur as a result of these axons becoming "deinhibited."[7]

Denervation supersensitivity refers to the possibility that following axonal injury some receptor sites become supersensitive and able to receive weakened input.[21] Recovery is a function of these receptors becoming supersensitive to neurotransmission from partially denervated neural tissue. Supersensitivity phenomena have been observed to occur in the peripheral nervous system.[8]

Axonal regeneration theories suggest that recovery is due to an active process of axonal sprouting that results in the growth of new synapses by healthy axons, also referred to as *collateral sprouting* and *reactive synaptogenesis*.[21] Axonal growth following injury has been observed in animal studies, making this a known, rather than hypothetical, phenomenon.[8]

According to these models of recovery, the basis of rehabilitation is that the recovery process is facilitated by the stimulation of neural activity, which is accomplished by pharmacologic and functional treatment. (*Functional*, in this sense, refers to cognitive, perceptual, communicative, and motor functions). Theories of axonal growth and receptor site sensitivity certainly appear to provide the strongest basis for early neuropharmacologic intervention.

As described by Ben-Yishay and Diller,[3] the recovery theory of *compensation* is based on the principles of central nervous system organization put forth by Hughlings Jackson. According to these authors, Jackson's theory is that the ontogenetically older, lower-level systems of the central nervous system are capable of assuming some functions of higher level systems because they carried out similar functions at an earlier point in development. Under intact nervous system conditions, the lower levels are inhibited by higher cortical levels, but they are "released" in the presence of cortical damage and thus become able to assume some functions normally managed by the damaged regions. This theory assumes hierarchical anatomical organization as well as a hierarchy of functions.[23] Damage to the central nervous system results in a regression (to an earlier developmental level) of skills.[3,23]

The concepts of *redundancy* and *duplication of function* propose that recovery occurs because functions (cognitive, perceptual, motor, et cetera) are represented in more than one area in the brain. Following injury to certain areas of the brain, other areas are available to assume the functions of the damaged regions. Recovery is a result of the undamaged neural structures carrying out functions that they are programmed to mediate. One of the most commonly held views of recovery, and the basis of much of rehabilitation, is that of *reorganization*[7,20] or *substitution*.[3,8,23] The premise behind these theories is that undamaged regions of the brain can assume or take over the functions of the damaged regions, a process that occurs spontaneously (that is, is not dependent on treatment). Rehabilitation that operates on this premise seeks to establish new pathways to perform old functions, as well as to reorganize functions in such a way that they can be carried out by undamaged regions. These theories are based on a strong assumption "that the [central nervous system] CNS in its normal state is underutilized, and that a reserve exists that allows for the substitution . . . [Additionally, there is] certain flexibility across functions within the CNS."[23] Hence, *reduplication* or *redundancy* may be seen either as a requisite to substitution theory,[23] or as a counter theory (explanation) for the recovery process.[8] The difference between substitution and redundancy is that the former requires the establishment of new pathways; in the latter, the pathways are already available and programmed to assume the functions of the damaged regions. The distinction between substitution and reorganization is less clear. Reorganization implies a dynamic process in which both functions and neural structures are altered to optimize neurologic and long-term functional recovery. Although an attempt is made here to present these as separate constructs, the theoretical distinction is impractical because the underlying premise—that undamaged regions of the brain can assume functions once carried out predominantly by the injured areas—is the same for all three theoretical constructs. Consequently, the terms *redundancy, substitution,* and *reorganization* are used imprecisely in the literature.

Melodic Intonation Therapy, a treatment technique well known to speech-language pathologists, is an example of a technique based on the substitution of function concept.[24] This therapy approach operates on the assumption that an intact right hemisphere can facilitate language production. Most treatment programs based on substitution theory are similar to Melodic Intonation Therapy in that an exact substitution of function is not expected (that is, the assumption is not that language functions can be transferred to the right hemisphere in the presence of left hemisphere damage). An example of a treatment technique that substitutes one modality for another is that of letter tracing (tactile) used to improve reading (visual) ability in dyslexia.

The term *substitution* also has been used to refer to the substitution of behavioral strategies that rely less on damaged areas of the brain and more on intact areas.[3] The idea here is not so much that the intact area of brain takes over the same function, as that residual strengths (cognitive, sensory, motoric, et cetera) or intact abilities can be used or substituted for the impaired abilities by requiring different behavioral responses (for example, using an augmentative communication system). This also has been described as compensation.[7] In this sense, substitution is a treatment objective rather than a premise of neurologic recovery per se.

As can be surmised, the differences between the last three proposed recovery mechanisms are somewhat subtle, depending upon interpretation. None has been proven empirically.[23] According to these theories then, the goal of rehabilitation is to facilitate the reorganization of the central nervous system, whether by stimulating the "redevelopment" of higher level control, by activating or tapping unused regions, or by reorganizing functions in such a way as to stimulate undamaged cortical regions. Some[25] have argued that recovery theories in general do not provide an adequate or complete explanation of recovery, because they do not account for individual motivational and psychosocial variables.

Sohlberg and Mateer[8] have suggested that there is a broad division among those who provide cognitive rehabilitation. The basis of this division is the timing of intervention. According to Sohlberg and Mateer, some proponents of cognitive rehabilitation advocate that intervention should begin as early as possible, given that its purpose is to stimulate the neurologic recovery process. Others consider that the efforts and effects of remediation can stand alone and that intervention can therefore be initiated at any time. This would appear to be a largely theoretical division, since a number of clinicians work in rehabilitation settings where patients in both early and late stages of recovery are treated. From a research perspective, however, spontaneous recovery must be accounted for, as discussed earlier.

APPROACHES TO COGNITIVE-COMMUNICATIVE REHABILITATION

Several approaches and variants of approaches to cognitive, communicative, and behavioral rehabilitation have been presented in the literature. Not all of these can be discussed within a single text, and certainly not within a chapter. There are, however, predominant influences that have guided current practice in the field, and are pertinent to practicing clinicians and students. Rehabilitation interventions have been influenced largely by theories of neurologic recovery, theories of cognitive development and processes, and theories of learning and behavior.[3,7,6,8] In practice, most treatment approaches incorporate a combination of influences. This, in part, may be because no single area of influence is considered adequate to guide the development of comprehensive programs. For example, theories of neurologic recovery do not include presumptions about the types of activities most likely to provide neuronal stimulation. Theories of cognitive development do not account for disruption to what were at one time operational adult processes. Behavioral theories do not adequately address impaired cognitive ability. The complexity of the neurobehavioral sequelae to traumatic brain injury requires that clinicians have at their disposal a variety of approaches and an understanding of the theoretical underpinnings of each.

Before we can begin a discussion of approaches, some distinctions between abilities, skills, processes, and functions need to be made. Frequently these terms are used interchangeably in clinical settings, but, in the context of specific approaches, it should not be assumed that they represent the same concept. Additionally, the same term can be used by different authors to refer to different concepts. Often, in the literature, the point of reference must be assumed.

Ability seems to be the most straightforward term, in that it suggests the "state of being able."[18] The term can be used in a variety of contexts and still mean the same thing, because it is the broadest in scope. Ability can range from basic physiologic ability, such as being able to be aroused (arousability), to complex cognitive ability, such as being able to program a computer (computer programming ability). *Skill* specifically refers to a learned activity, but also to the effective use of this learning (knowledge) in performance. Proficiency is implied in skill. The term *process* refers to a "natural phenomenon marked by gradual changes that lead toward a particular result."[18] It also refers to a specific method or set of operations used to do something. For example, *information processing* refers to a development that involves changes (information is changed from discrete physical features into something that can be recognized and then used), and it implies a set of operations (sensory recognition, attention allocation, encoding, and consolidation). In the clinical arena, *process* has also come to mean the components or individual operations thought to constitute a larger cognitive activity. As might be expected, the term is used to refer to both the set of operations and the individual operations or components. The term *component processes*[26] is sometimes used to describe what are thought to be discernible units of cognitive activity (for example, attending, learning, and reasoning).

Function is the broad, general term for the natural, required, or expected activity of a person or thing. It particularly refers to the "action for which a person or thing is specially fitted or used or for which the thing exists."[18] In this sense, it seems that function cannot be ascertained without a referent, and, clinically, that referent must be the patient and the patient's environment. Function cannot be determined solely by the clinician. It is the opinion of this author that one cannot develop a functional approach to treatment until the "required" or "expected" activity of the individual—the special fit—has been determined. In theory, context would appear to be a primary determinant of functional training, but not necessarily of skill or process training.

Skills training and *functional training* are sometimes used to mean the same thing; however, this is not necessarily the case. Reading is a skill, but some would not consider paragraph or text reading to be functional tasks for many patients (for example, an individual who needs to do very little reading in the workplace or does not read when at leisure). In this case, addressing reading as a therapeutic goal would not be considered functional training. The term *functional skills training* is sometimes used to circumvent this confusion. Some authors[13] have made a distinction between skills training and cognitive rehabilitation. This is interpreted to mean a distinction between component process training and direct training of functional skills, but the distinction further illustrates the confusion in terminology.

Developmental and Hierarchical Approaches

The *developmental approach* is based on the theory that the recovery of function after brain injury follows the sequence of original cognitive, communicative, and motor skills development. According to this approach, then, rehabilitation "takes the patient through these steps" of development.[14] Neurodevelopment training (NDT) for those with motor skills impairment is one of the best examples of a developmental approach in rehabilitation. Adamovich et al.[4] have presented a developmental approach to cognitive rehabilitation. Although they do not refer to it as developmental, its theoretical underpinnings, as described in their text, come from developmental cognitive psychology. Under their paradigm, assessment and treatment proceed in the following sequence: arousal and alerting, perception and attending, discrimination, orientation, organization (categorization and sequencing), retrieval, and high level thought processes (convergent and divergent thinking, deductive and inductive reasoning, and multiprocess reasoning). In their text, these authors have provided examples of activities designed to tap each of these areas based on a hierarchy of recovery. Adamovich and Henderson[27] also have published a test designed to follow this recovery sequence.

A *hierarchical approach* usually implies a progression from simple processes and tasks to more complex ones. Hence, for this type of approach, tasks must be designed in a carefully graded manner that reflects an understanding not only of the process to be targeted, but also of the task structure and cognitive demands placed on the individual. Ideally, this variable is considered in all approaches. The developmental and hierarchical approaches are quite similar in their orientation to skill development as a highly sequenced, staging process. A developmental approach is a hierarchical approach, but the reverse is not necessarily true. One can carefully grade treatment to target the simplest to the most complex skills within the repertoire of an individual without necessarily recapitulating developmental stages. In the approach employed by Adamovich and colleagues,[4] treatment activities within each stage are organized from simple (those that make the least demands on the patient's processing ability) to complex. Thus, this approach is also accurately described as a hierarchical approach.

Whyte[28] has proposed a hierarchy of cognitive activity that also serves to clarify some terms. The lowest level of activity in this hierarchy is an *operation* (for example, looking, engaging, and disengaging alertness). A *process* is more complex, and may involve many operations (for example, visual scanning). *Skills* are next in the hierarchy and involve the coordination of different processes. (Examples include reading, driving, arithmetic calculation, writing, and typing.) The term *metaskills* is used to refer to behavior that goes "beyond" one skill and may involve linking skills together, or applying knowledge associated with one skill to other skills (for example, using reading and writing skills to edit a book). The highest level of cognitive activity is a *global function*, which can be assumed to require the integration of all of the preceding activities (work is an obvious example).

Whyte's hierarchy is useful for demonstrating how confusion among terms can cloud the clinical picture. As an example, assume that an interdisciplinary team decides that patient X can best benefit from cognitive rehabilitation that begins at the process level. The speech-language pathologist targets attentional processes at a basic level of focusing and selection, but the occupational therapist uses skills, processes, and operations interchangeably

and therefore focuses treatment on paragraph reading. The result is a dispar-
ity in treatment that is intended to reduce confusion and cognitive overload,
but that may in fact worsen it.

Process Specific Approach

The *process specific approach* to cognitive rehabilitation is based on Kaplan's
approach to neuropsychologic assessment, which seeks to analyze separate
aspects of cognitive functioning that may be affected differentially by brain
injury.[8] Complex cognitive functions, such as attention, are considered to be
composed of smaller units or processes that can be systematically evaluated
and treated if impaired. Key to this approach is the systematic and comprehensive assessment of cognitive functions in such a way that impairment in
component processes is identified.

Bracy[29] has presented a list of twenty-four basic processes or abilities
needed to learn and generalize complex behaviors that range from the
ability to accurately sense (receive) environmental stimuli to the ability to
profit from feedback. He employs a hierarchical approach to the rehabilitation of these processes (for example, basic sensory awareness, focused attention to sensory input, sustained attention for extended periods). Bracy[30] has
also developed a number of software programs that he employs in his
process training.

Sohlberg and Mateer[8] have offered a comprehensive review of a process
specific approach to cognitive rehabilitation. They review six principles of
rehabilitation that constitute the process-specific approach they use.

(1) A *theoretically motivated* model defines each cognitive process area.
(2) Therapy tasks are administered *repetitively*.
(3) Goals and objectives are *hierarchically* organized.
(4) Remediation involves *data-based* and directed treatment.
(5) The use of *generalization probes* provides measurements of treatment
     success.
(6) Ultimate measures of success must be *improvements in level of
     vocational ability and independent living*.

As noted by Sohlberg and Mateer, these principles are principles of
rehabilitation that should be followed regardless of the specific approach one
takes. Regarding different processes, they have outlined treatment procedures that can be used to address the following areas: attention, memory,
visual processing, executive functions, and problem solving. They have
described in detail a number of techniques they employ, particularly for
attention training. (Refer to Chapter Five for their breakdown of the five
components of attention.)

The appropriateness of these techniques must be determined by the
clinician's knowledge of the patient, the nature of the clinical setting, the
discharge goals and environment, financial resources and motivation, and

emotional variables. The methods presented by Sohlberg and Mateer are systematic, particularly the attention training, but they require the clinician to provide a dedicated amount of treatment time and a strong commitment to measurement. The authors have also provided the attention training module in a packaged therapy kit, which can be purchased.[31] However, as with all packaged treatment materials, these are only as effective as the knowledge base of the clinician. The author knows of no workbook, software program, or training kit that is appropriate for all individuals with traumatic brain injury. Moreover, although it is widely agreed that attentional problems are a predictable accompaniment to traumatic brain injury, attentional training should in no way be assumed to be requisite treatment for all patients. Careful evaluation is indicated to delineate the type and extent of cognitive-communicative impairment in relation to other behaviors (for example, the psychological/emotional domain).

The idea that cognitive functions can be divided into subfunctions, subskills, component processes, or operations is the basis of much of cognitive rehabilitation and is not new with the work of Sohlberg and Mateer—although their work represents one of the more systematic approaches presented in the literature. The attentional training and problem-solving models employed by Ben Yishay and colleagues[3,32] at the New York University Medical Center approach each of these complex functions by addressing different components or stages. For example, the problem-solving model they employ (based on Luria's model)[3] is composed of eight stages: formulate problem, analyze conditions, formulate plan, choose tactics, execute plan and monitor, compare solution to problem, and integrate into personal knowledge base. Theoretically, individuals could have difficulties at different stages, and each stage could be addressed independently. In general, hierarchical approaches are also based on the assumption that complex cognitive functions are supported by certain basic cognitive abilities that must be addressed first in the treatment sequence.

Several variations of cognitive information processing, or the process approach, have been presented in the literature. Duke et al.[14] have described a cognitive behavioral approach that focuses on the distinction between automatic and controlled processing. They argue that learning is accomplished through controlled processing, and that the ability to adapt and generalize to new situations is a function of controlled processing. The executive system directs the controlled aspects of attention allocation and memory selection. The units of memory that are automatically stored and retrieved are schemata. These can be influenced, however, by encoding, which can be manipulated as a controlled process (for example, rehearsal, elaboration, imagery). Retrieval also can be a controlled process when an active search of memory is conducted. Although the structure of memory cannot be altered by intervention, the way information is stored and retrieved can be.

Following brain injury, both automatic and controlled processes can be deficient. During the active period of neurologic recovery, the recovery of automatic processes correlates with the extent of neurologic recovery. Duke et al.[14] suggest that intervention that stimulates, but makes low demands on attention and executive control, is indicated to facilitate recovery. Automatic processes may not recover fully, and following the acute stage of neurologic recovery, intervention in the form of stimulation is of limited benefit.

Theoretically, controlled processes will recover in a hierarchical manner beginning with sensory awareness, followed by the control of attention allocation, then the ability to manipulate information in short-term or working memory (that is, associating current perceptual information with prior knowledge). The last functions of controlled processing to recover are the planning and execution of complex thoughts and behaviors. Executive control is presumed to develop or recover over an extended period of time, and the restoration of executive control should be the focus of intervention. Lower skills are necessary for information processing and can be expected to improve as executive control improves. Depending upon the stage of recovery, executive control training might focus on the control of attentional processes, memory, or problem solving and reasoning.

Those who support the use of a process or component approach to the remediation of cognitive-communicative impairment hold the premise that skills acquired in cognitive process training can be generalized to a variety of activities and settings, because the skills transcend any one task or group of tasks. In other words, cognitive processes are considered to be the foundation to purposeful behavior, not isolated skills. Although many programs have documented success in the rehabilitation of some cognitive processes,[5,8,32,33] the concept that specific cognitive functions can be rehabilitated is not without criticism. Specifically, the rehabilitation of memory through drill and practice type activities has come under considerable scrutiny for its lack of effectiveness and carryover to daily functioning.[7,8,33,34,35,36] Ruff et al.[37] reviewed the literature that has addressed attention retraining and memory retraining interventions. Although they found that the data from several studies were not convincing, they concluded that a modular approach to attention training warranted continued use and evaluation. Their recommendations for memory retraining were that clinicians need to look to newer theoretical models of memory (such as the division into procedural and declarative systems) and avoid the tendency to base training on older models that have led to the overuse of strategies such as visual imagery, rehearsal, and elaboration—none of which has proven to be particularly effective.

Cost effectiveness and efficiency are sometimes cited as reasons that the remediation of specific cognitive processes should be abandoned in favor of skill development. The lack of ecological validity and the failure to demonstrate that improvement in a single cognitive process can translate into functional gains have also been offered as criticisms of the cognitive process approach.[13,38] "The disadvantage of attempting to remediate basic cognitive functioning is that this type of intervention is of unproven efficacy, so that a good deal of the patient's time and effort may be devoted to a pointless task and result in no actual functional improvement."[39] Many of these criticisms are offered on behalf of the functional approach to rehabilitation, which is discussed next.

Functional Approaches

Perhaps one of the most popular approaches to rehabilitation is the *functional approach* or the functional skills approach. A proponent of functional intervention, Giles,[34] has stated that "the focus of rehabilitationists should not be on recovery in and for itself, but on the improvement of real world functional performance." Terms such as "real world," "daily living," "real life," and "natural environment" are used in conjunction with "functional" to shift focus away from the clinical setting.

Use of the functional approach, or at least of its terminology, has no doubt been encouraged by the proliferation of functional assessment scales (discussed in the preceding chapter) and, in particular, outcome studies using the *Functional Independence Measure (FIM)*. The Functional Independence Measure is thought to include a list of "activities generally considered to be essential for survival"[40] in normal daily performance. It is heavily weighted toward motoric activities (for example, eating, grooming, bathing, dressing), although cognitive-communicative variables are included. The widespread use of the Functional Independence Measure might be seen to reflect current thinking about functional activities and rehabilitation. Many of the activities measured are the same ones targeted in functional skills training. Activities of daily living and functional skills often are used synonymously and are not necessarily limited to self-care skills, but can include activities and skills such as driving, money management, reading, writing, cooking, washing, and so on.

From a functional perspective, the goal of rehabilitation may be to improve the performance of personally relevant and needed skills. Generally, functional rehabilitation is seen as an end-stage approach, in that the skill (final output) that is needed is taught directly. However, this is true only if one considers functional rehabilitation and functional skills training to be the same. Returning to our definition of function, the term *skills* is not included. In the author's opinion a functional approach to rehabilitation is different from functional skills training, or training in the activities of daily living. Skill training is limited to the single skill that is taught. Although there may be generalization of knowledge from a trained skill to similar skills, a primary criticism of skill training is lack of generalization.[23] On the other hand, a functional approach to rehabilitation is not limited to skills training in and of itself. Cognitive processes may be addressed at a component level, but the context in which they are addressed must take into account the eventual *expected activities* of the individual. Rehabilitation, whether of skills or cognitive processes, cannot occur in a clinical vacuum; it must be designed to bridge, even to lessen, the distance between the treatment environment and the natural environment. From this perspective, attention process training as a primary therapeutic intervention may or may not be functional, depending upon the most pressing needs of the individual. Similarly, skill training alone may be insufficient. For example, a student struggling to return to school needs to be trained in attention and learning skills. To neglect these in favor of teaching daily activities should, from a *functional perspective*, be considered negligent. The expected activity of a student primarily is to learn. If the student needs to use public transportation, bus riding skills also might be appropriate to teach.

Some have taken issue with the idea of functional activities training being viewed as cognitive rehabilitation. Fryer and Fralish[15] have suggested that training in functional activities can be considered cognitive rehabilitation when:

(1)   the skill to be focused upon is identified for and used by the person undergoing rehabilitation;
(2)   instrumental skills and the developed activities are clearly specified and explained;
(3)   the hierarchical mastery of skills is charted by the individual; and,
(4)   feedback is provided and the individual is able to reflect upon the task completed.

A review of the literature will reveal that there is an apparent division within the field of traumatic brain injury rehabilitation, concerning the most effective approach to rehabilitation. Should clinicians address basic cognitive processes that are thought to underlie a variety of skills, or should they teach individuals as many activity skills as possible? According to Wood,[41] the dichotomy among rehabilitation practitioners is between those who promote procedural learning in training and those who use a declarative model of learning. Because "procedural learning assimilates information in a form closely related to the way it is intended to be used," there is a greater likelihood that the skills (knowledge) will be used. On the other hand, declarative learning relies on the ability to understand relationships between events within an individual's own world, which may be impossible for someone with a severe brain injury.

As suggested by Fryer and Fralish,[15] and implied by others, there is an apparent concern that activity performance and skill training are often considered to be the same in rehabilitation settings. This author is in agreement that the mere performance of activities, under the guise of skill training, is unacceptable. Functional activities conducted in this manner deserve no less criticism than do repetitive cognitive exercises using computer programs. Any type of activity used in treatment must be chosen because it provides support to the overall, conceptually, and theoretically well-founded approach to rehabilitation.

Approaches Based On Learning and Behavior Theory

Learning can be conceived of as "a relatively permanent change in behavior resulting from practice or experience."[42] Consequently, behavioral change is dependent upon learning ability. Traditionally, learning theories have sought to explain the way individuals learn in response to environmental cues and motivators. Behavioral analysis specifically seeks to define the conditions under which designated (targeted) behaviors occur and are learned. When relationships between environmental events and behavior (response or set of responses) are formed or understood, the process is referred to as *associative learning*. Associations or relationships can be formed between two events, or components, of the learning situation: either between the stimulus that signals a need for a response (the antecedent) and the behavior itself (response), or between the behavior and the consequences produced by or resulting from the behavioral response (the consequence).

Conditioning refers to an applied behavioral construct that operates on the premise that associative learning can be manipulated by making changes in the conditions. *Stimulus control* is a type of conditioning designed to alter behavior through the manipulation of antecedent events. Antecedent events occur within the environment and cue or "prompt" us to respond in a certain manner. Our response is based on learned associations. For example, when one member of a family begins to set the table for a meal, other members are "cued" to respond in a certain manner. Depending upon the behavioral responses learned in association with this cue, one might offer to assist the cook, begin to solicit beverage requests from others, or have a seat at the table and wait for the meal to be served. Being prepared to respond to this situation requires the ability to discriminate the relevant cues signaling that a meal is about to be served. "Stimulus-control techniques rely upon people being able to discriminate those aspects of the environment which act as cues for behavior."[43] Following brain injury, the ability to detect environmental signals or cues for behavioral responses can be diminished; therefore, it may be necessary to teach individuals to detect and then respond to these signaling events. This is referred to as *discrimination training*. Its goal is to increase the likelihood that a desired response will be elicited by a particular stimulus, and to decrease the likelihood that the same response will be elicited by another, irrelevant stimulus. Stimulus control has been achieved when a particular stimulus consistently elicits a desired, predictable response. Several techniques have been described that can be used to improve stimulus control.[43,44,45]

Conditioning techniques that focus on the manipulation of consequences in the *antecedent-behavior-consequence (A-B-C)* paradigm are referred to as *response-consequence* learning methods. These methods operate on the premise that the frequency of a response to specified events can be increased by consequences that are experienced as rewarding. The reverse premise also holds true: responses that do not lead to rewarding consequences, or do lead to punitive consequences, will be diminished. Unfortunately, in the rehabilitation setting, conditioning based on the latter idea (withholding rewards or providing negative consequences) appears to be applied most often[41] (for example, withholding "smoke breaks" from the individual who is repeatedly late to therapy sessions, instead of rewarding promptness).

Reinforcement is a procedure that is employed to modify the relationship between an event and its consequences. Reinforcers, or reinforcing events, are those that increase the likelihood that a behavior will be repeated.[38] Similarly, events that are not reinforcing (for example, unpleasant situations, pain, punishment) tend to decrease the likelihood that a behavior will be repeated. Reinforcers may be internal and inherent in a response itself, or external to the response. Wood[41] has pointed out that reinforcement offers a powerful tool for behavioral change when understood and used effectively. It is important in behavior modification and rehabilitation because it is thought to aid learning.[42]

Reinforcers are important not only because they provide gratification, but because they serve as feedback regarding the success or lack of success associated with a particular response.[41] To be effective, reinforcers must be of value to the patient, not to the clinician or the rehabilitation team. They must be carefully selected with an understanding of the patient's motivation and ability to distinguish between pleasant and unpleasant consequences, both of which may be impaired following brain injury.[41] Wood and Burgess[46] also note that, following a brain injury, an individual's ability to understand social praise may be diminished, and that reinforcers, accompanied by social praise, can serve a dual purpose: to reward a desired behavior, and to reestablish the value of social praise in and of itself. They suggest that tangible reinforcers always be paired with social praise.

Differential reinforcement is a technique that can be employed to diminish undesirable behaviors by increasing the frequency of occurrence of other behaviors through reinforcement (*differential reinforcement of other behaviors* or *DRO*). Differential reinforcement operates on the premise that the undesirable behavior will be extinguished because it is elicited less frequently (than the newly rewarded behavior) and not reinforced. Behaviors chosen for reinforcement should be incompatible (interfering) with the production of the undesirable or target behavior, in order to optimize the success of differential reinforcement.[41] It is not always possible to choose a highly desirable alternate behavior for reinforcement, but it is important to choose one that is innocuous and does not further impede daily functioning.

Psychodynamic and Neuropsychological Approaches

The *psychodynamic approach* has perhaps been employed the longest in traumatic brain injury rehabilitation, but to a limited degree.[14] This approach emphasizes the important role of psychosocial and emotional variables in recovery and outcome. From this perspective, the individual must be viewed as more than a collection of cognitive and physical limitations, distinct from the previous person and the new postinjury person. Interpersonal relationships and intrapersonal characteristics become core features for treatment, instead of secondary aspects that merely "get in the way" of successful rehabilitation. This approach is conceptually the same as the holistic approach advocated by Ben-Yishay,[47] which has been in operation since 1975; the milieu-oriented neuropsychological approach promoted by Prigatano;[5] and the health promotion neuropsychological paradigm described by Stanczak.[48]

Following the psychodynamic or neuropsychologic approach, specific areas of cognitive impairment are addressed, typically as component processes, but not to the exclusion of issues of self-awareness, motivation, and the ability to interrelate with others. The psychosocial variables, not the overt cognitive and physical impairments, are viewed as the hallmarks of the condition. Problems in motivation and self-awareness are considered to be directly related to the brain injury. Whether viewed as a direct consequence of brain injury or as problems exacerbated by the injury, they are not overlooked as pre-existing behaviors that hold little promise for improvement through rehabilitation. Improving self-awareness and self-regulation, through feedback and through alternative "sets" or perspectives from which to view actions and behavior, is paramount, and ideally it is incorporated into all treatment sessions. Additionally, interdisciplinary programs should provide group treatment sessions where specific behaviors are addressed by team members and the individuals with traumatic brain injury. Many[5,32,47] assert that mixed groups with clinicians and patients provide essential opportunities for individuals with brain injury to develop and practice the behaviors necessary for successful interrelating and the establishment of relationships.

Prigatano[5] has presented four major goals of neuropsychological rehabilitation:

> First, the brain-injured patient may be more confused in his or her thinking than is obvious by direct examination . . . Consequently, the first major goal of cognitive rehabilitation is to reduce the overall or generalized cognitive confusion . . . Next, cognitive retraining should enhance the patient's awareness of his or her residual strengths as well as deficits . . . Third, the patient must be helped to recognize the need for compensatory

behaviors . . . The fourth step is to help the patients deal with their cognitive deficits not only in the presence of a given therapist but also as the deficits emerge in interpersonal behavior.

As can be seen, a primary goal in this type of approach to rehabilitation is the development of self-awareness. Other types of intervention, such as behavior modification or cognitive component training and skill training, may be employed, but none of them represents the underlying premise of the psychodynamic approach: fundamental changes in self-concept occur as a result of brain injury, and these changes must be addressed foremost, if rehabilitation is to succeed.

Which Approach?

In the literature, many authors claim that their particular approach is soundly grounded in theory from the cognitive sciences,[8,34] but the intent of these assertions must be questioned, given the shortage of universally agreed upon theories of human information processing, cognitive development, and neurologic recovery. This caution does not mean that theoretical guidance is not critically important; it is only intended to point out that there are more theories than approaches, and many can offer guidance. For example, some behavioral theorists have come to recognize the importance of cognitive processes in learning and behavioral change.[41] Although at one level this makes behavioral theory more appealing, at least to the practicing clinician, at another level a pure interpretation of behavior as the product of conditioning becomes clouded by the poorly understood cognitive variables that mediate behavior. Similarly, rehabilitation approaches that only consider cognitive processes, in isolation from behavioral variables, are incomplete, although perhaps "purer" and more scientific. The fact that many programs are based on information from both the cognitive and behavioral sciences cannot be disputed, and certainly a program or treatment approach that has a theoretical basis is preferable to one that does not. In the typical rehabilitation setting, however, the needs of the individual—learning style and potential, post-treatment environment, support networks, and available resources—must be considered in the approach(es) employed. Some individuals will progress best using a procedural learning approach. Others may benefit most from the direct intervention of cognitive processes. Regardless of the theoretical approach, the systematic application of rehabilitation procedures must always be chosen over random selection from a potpourri. Clinicians must not only be extremely knowledgeable about the basis of different approaches, but must also be flexible enough to vary approaches from one group to another, according to the patients' characteristics and needs. Careful evaluation and monitoring of treatment performance *and* daily functioning are essential to demonstrating the effectiveness of any approach.

SPECIFIC INTERVENTION STRATEGIES AND MODELS

Behavioral Strategies

Numerous strategies from behavioral and learning theory can be implemented in rehabilitation regardless of the specific approach; that is, rehabilitation in general may be conceptualized as behavior modification. Rehabilitation clinicians typically are not trained in specific behavior modification techniques, yet many of the following techniques are employed routinely in rehabilitation settings. *Cues* or *prompts* are events that occur in the environment naturally, or may be generated artificially, in order to increase the production of a behavior. Prompts and cues are antecedent events, and although in the clinical setting they are generally thought of as controlled events administered by the clinician, the majority of cues or prompts are naturally-occurring environmental events that elicit behavioral responses. Removal of certain antecedent events that "cue" an individual to respond can serve the reverse function of diminishing behaviors.

Clinicians who work with behavioral analysts, but themselves are not trained formally in behavioral analysis, often become frustrated when asked to identify antecedent conditions that lead to (provoke) undesirable behaviors (for example, an outbreak of profanity). Indeed, in rehabilitation settings, where multiple stimuli bombard patients with diminished tolerance, antecedent conditions are often difficult to identify. Sometimes they are personally embarrassing to clinicians, who may learn that a behavior within their own repertoire serves as the antecedent to the patient's undesirable behavioral response. It is important that the clinician be able to depersonalize the negative behaviors of the patient, in order to maintain a therapeutic relationship. If this is not possible, the clinician should withdraw from the patient's rehabilitation program. Seldom is it beneficial for the patient or the clinician to "wait it out" and hope that the situation will improve in time; valuable time will be wasted.

Shaping of responses or behaviors refers to the gradual development of a desired behavior(s) through systematic reinforcement of close approximations of the behavior.[42,43] Shaping is an appropriate technique to employ when a behavioral response is nonexistent, or occurs with very low frequency, and therefore has little opportunity to be reinforced. The desired response can be "shaped" by reinforcing responses that closely resemble, or are components of, the desired behavior. For example, a speech-language pathologist wants a patient by the name of John to join a communication group that is addressing turn taking, but John is unable to remain seated in a room for more than five minutes without walking around and interjecting comments. In this scenario, the clinician might first address the behavior of sitting in a chair for six minutes, instead of attempting to reduce the frequent interruptions John makes. Often in rehabilitation, clinicians attempt to modify the final desired behavior (in this case following turn-taking cues), when in fact the behavior is not present, and therefore cannot be differentially reinforced.

The importance of task analysis cannot be overemphasized in the application of learning procedures. *Task analysis* refers to the process of breaking down tasks into components, which can be viewed as distinct units for learning purposes. Tasks and activities have stimulus and response characteristics. The task of feeding oneself requires the recognition of food and the use of fingers and/or utensils to put the food in the mouth. Although stimulus properties should be considered carefully, a task analysis typically involves dividing the response characteristics into steps or units. In task performance, however, the completion of one step often signals or triggers the initiation of the next step, so that the steps become linked together, like a chain. *Chaining* refers to the process of linking the units together to complete a task, such as dressing. Chaining can be employed as a learning technique to teach the component parts of a task that is too complex to be learned as a whole. *Forward chaining* refers to this strategy when it is used to teach a skill beginning with the first step and proceeding to the last step; each step follows the mastery of the preceding step. *Backward chaining* is used when the sequence is reversed and training begins with the last step and proceeds to the initial step. The choice of which type of chaining to employ in teaching complex tasks should be based, in part, on the difficulty an individual has in understanding the sequence of steps, since backward chaining is more difficult to conceptualize.[43]

When cues or prompts are gradually decreased in frequency of use, in order to encourage a particular response, the technique is called *fading*. In the beginning phase of training, the desired behavior is reinforced until the individual has learned to respond consistently in the presence of the cues. Once the desired or near desired level of performance has been achieved, the cues are provided with a decrease in frequency (at either a predetermined or random rate). Fading can also be accomplished by lengthening the interval between the stimulus presentation and the cue or prompt.[39]

Sometimes responses can be increased by using the *encore procedure*, or in speech-language pathology terms, the "say it again" technique. This technique is applied when an infrequently demonstrated behavior or skill is elicited without prompting; the behavior is first rewarded, and then the individual is requested to repeat the response, which then is reinforced again.

Overlearning simply means to teach a skill or task beyond the point of initial acquisition to the point that it is nearly automatic, or overlearned. Overlearning increases the likelihood that a skill can be used under a variety of circumstances (but only if the circumstances present low decision-making demands). Overlearning might be the best technique to apply when safety behaviors are required and the skill will be used under similar conditions repeatedly. For example, the ability to dial a family member's phone number might be an appropriate "skill" to teach to a near automatic level.

"Most behaviors that we rely on for independence are carried out more or less automatically as habit patterns" or overlearned skills.[41] Habits make low demands on the cognitive system because of the automaticity with which they can be carried out. Decision making and the need to evaluate alternative strategies for task performance and problem solving are reduced by having an available repertoire of habits from which to draw. This is important to consider for individuals who have reduced decision-making capacity, judgment, and self-monitoring. Wood[41] argues that "These factors make it imperative that social and functional skills acquired in rehabilitation are consolidated as habit behaviors."

Highlighting is a strategy for increasing the ability to discriminate among the different properties of stimuli by exaggerating or enhancing the features of crucial elements. Pointing out environmental cues such as signs, buildings, or landscaping to improve spatial orientation is a type of highlighting. Highlighting strategies can range from simple alteration of stimulus materials, such as using colors or bold type to improve visual recognition, to more complex strategies that can be employed by patients themselves, such as underlining key phrases in written text.

Giles and Clarke-Wilson[42] have presented two other types of learning strategies that can be employed in traumatic brain injury rehabilitation to improve performance: the incorporation of goal statements as a part of treatment and the use of regular debriefing. *Goal statements* serve to orient individuals to the "to be learned" aspects of the treatment activity, and so may assist them in focusing attention on relevant stimuli. Additionally, goal statements serve as cues to desired behavioral responses. They should be incorporated into the beginning of each treatment session and interspersed throughout as needed. *Debriefing* is the act of informing individuals about their performance. Specific feedback should be given at the end of each task and at the end of each treatment session, so that individuals know the results of their efforts.

Transfer and Learning Paradigms

Parenté and colleagues[49,50] have reviewed transfer of learning paradigms in relationship to memory retraining. Transfer models have predictive value for the transfer of skills from one situation to another based on the nature of treatment or stimulus parameters (tasks) and the response or performance parameters. Cognitive response sets are the way individuals "are taught to mentally organize or encode task elements;"[50] thus, responses imply more than the motoric output of performance. Knowledge of learning paradigms can have great bearing on the appropriateness of treatment in relationship to "real life" skills needed for daily living, academics, or work.

Six learning paradigms have been discerned, and these are presented in Table 6.1. Letters of the alphabet represent the task and response elements in the models.

The greatest amount of transfer can be expected when treatment tasks and responses are identical to the tasks and responses required to function (perform) in the daily environment (for example, home or work). This model is indicated by the AB:AB relationship, where the first A represents the treatment task, the first B represents the response to that task, and the second set of letters represents the task (A) and response (B) required in the environment. The letters are the same as to indicate that the environmental situation is identical to the training situation, something that is rarely achieved in the rehabilitation setting.

When training is completed in the environment in which a skill is required and used, transfer of learning is not an issue. (This is not to say that learning is not an issue.) On-the-job training, training in the home, and community setting in which the individual lines, and training in the academic setting using required educational materials represent instances of a true AB:AB paradigm. Although learning in the environment in which a skill is to be used is ideal in order to limit problems associated with the transfer of learning, it is not always feasible or advantageous. For many individuals with traumatic brain injury, learning is inhibited by over-stimulation and inconsistency. When environments are highly distractible with little order, and clinicians have limited ability to control the amount and degree of stimulation, learning is not facilitated. If the environment

Table 6.1
Transfer of Learning Paradigms.

Treatment		Environment			
Task	Response	Task	Response	Relationship	Degree of Transfer
A	B	A	B	identical	most
A	B	A'	B'	similar	++
A	B	C	B	different task	+
A	B	C	D	different task and response	least
A	B	A	D	different response	none
A	B	A	Br	reorganized response	none

Adapted from Parenté R, DiCesare A. Retraining memory: theory and applications. In Kreutzer J, Wehman P (eds). *Cognitive Rehabilitation for Persons with Traumatic Brain Injury*. Baltimore, MD: Paul H, Brookes; 1991: 147–161.

cannot be modified to increase order and reduce distractions and over-stimulation, alternative environments should be used for training until skills have at least partially been acquired.

Treatment approaches that use simulated work activities or academic exercises approach the AB:AB model, but unless the performance or learning environment is truly controlled and identical to the real or transfer environment, the model is not AB:AB. Simulated activities are better represented by the AB:A'B' relationship, where the treatment variables are similar to the environmental variables, both in terms of the tasks presented and of the response required. An example of this would be teaching an individual to use a word processing program, in an office environment that is within the rehabilitation setting but closely approximates the actual work environment. The computer hardware and word processing program would need to be the same in both settings, and the types of word processing "assignments" performed in rehabilitation would have to match the tasks the individual would be expected to perform in the post-treatment work environment. The individual's general approach to the word processing tasks at work would be identical to that taught in the treatment setting. Because of the limited resources of rehabilitation settings, most cannot reproduce multiple home, school, or work settings; thus, this model, also, is difficult to employ with all individuals.

In the AB:CB model, treatment tasks are different from the tasks occurring in the daily environment, but both sets of tasks require the same responses. In the above word processing example, the computer hardware might be different, but the word processing package and the types of assignments would remain the same from the treatment to the work setting. Another example of this model uses different types of reading material, but the approach to the material (for example, highlighting, identification of main ideas, note taking) remains the same. When the task elements remain the same, but the response requirements differ, the model is AB:AC, which has a low expectancy for skill transfer. This model is followed too frequently in rehabilitation, particularly with the use of computer programs or paper and pencil tasks that have little to no relevance to the daily environment (for example, rotating visual images on the screen, listing items in a category, matching colored cubes).

Two additional models offer a negative (as opposed to low) prediction of transfer. The AB:AD model indicates that a different response set is required in the daily environment from the one reinforced in the treatment setting, even though the task is the same. This model also appears to be followed too frequently in the rehabilitation setting, particularly when clinicians fail to learn about the post-treatment environment, or to educate families adequately about the training strategies used and the expected responses. For example, an individual with dysphagia who has been taught to compensate by using a spoon and drinking with a straw, may be expected, in the home, to eat with a fork and drink from a large glass.

The last model is the AB : AB^r, which, like the preceding model, predicts no transfer of skills, and potentially creates great confusion for the patient. The author has found that it is particularly important to avoid this type of learning condition for students who hope to return to an academic setting following or during treatment. The small "r" indicates that a reorganization of the mental response set is required by the same task. For example, a speech-language pathologist may teach a student to read one paragraph, write down the main idea, and then proceed to the next paragraph in the same manner. If the student then returns to school and is told by the teacher to read an entire chapter, and then reread for main ideas, the student will become confused and may not be able to apply either technique effectively.

As can be seen from the above examples, some form of transfer paradigm is always followed, regardless of the nature of the task. Knowledge of these paradigms places the choice of learning contingencies in the hands of the clinician and patient, instead of leaving it open to random selection. It is easy to assume that functional skills training always employs an AB : A′B′ paradigm, yet the skills taught in the clinical setting do not always match those needed in an individual's home/work/school environment. Consequently, the "cognitive distance" for transfer may be greater than that implied by the AB : A′B′ paradigm. What is functional for the individual must always be established, and it must be defined by the post-treatment environment rather than by the clinician's perspective. Individuals can be taught a variety of activities or skills that transfer from one setting to another, but if these skills do not maximally increase functioning they remain of little use, and a great deal of energy may be expended needlessly. For example, the types of activities performed in sheltered workshops (such as, sorting and packaging) are easier to teach than the more complex problem-solving skills, but if an individual refuses to work in that environment, treatment time has been wasted—regardless of whether or not the therapy team finds it to be a best-fit scenario. As important as the discharge environment is to successful learning, in reality, it is not always known in advance.

Intervention Using a Multimodel Approach

Gross and Schutz[51] have discussed five models that can be applied in neuropsychological intervention, depending on the patient's learning ability and residual skills. Their work indicates that the order of learning demands and ability is hierarchical.[7] The lowest level model is the *environmental control model,* which assumes that "one method of increasing (behavioral) adjustment is to modify the person's physical and social environment."[51] This model would be the most appropriate for patients with the lowest level of learning ability. The next level is the *S-R (stimulus-response) conditioning model,* which is most effective with individuals who have learning potential but cannot generalize. It is consistent with other models of associative learning and behavior modification. The third model focuses on *training skills and abilities*. This model assumes that one can learn to modify behaviors through instruction and skill practice. Skills must be broken down into processes for training. Thus, this model is consistent with the process approach. It should be used with individuals who are able to learn and generalize, but have difficulty self-monitoring.

The *strategy substitution model* "assumes a failure may be viewed specifically in the context of a particular way a task is attempted and thus may not reflect the client's ability to perform the task."[51] The process of choosing alternative strategies for improved task performance is the focus of training. The "choosing" belongs to the patient; therefore, the ability to self-monitor is required.

The last model proposed is the *cognitive cycle model*. It attempts to establish new cognitive processing abilities analogous to the executive system, and it therefore requires the greatest number of intact abilities. The cognitive cycle model basically follows a model of normal problem solving and includes five stages: self-identification of goals, production of conditional predictions, plan for action, initiation of the activity, and analysis of feedback.

Gross and Schutz seem to support the view offered by Prigatano[5] and others[47,48] that an individual must develop an understanding of a new self-concept in order to gain full awareness of an impairment. Admittedly, this requires a "substantial set of cognitive skills" that may not be available.[51] The appeal of these models is that the authors have attempted to account for individual differences following brain injury and to recognize that these must be addressed in distinct, if not unique, ways. Seldom is this obvious need addressed in the cognitive rehabilitation literature.

Compensation Training

Compensatory training, as a form of intervention, is certainly not something new, or something that has come about with traumatic brain injury rehabilitation. Assistive devices, defined as any invention specifically designed to help accomplish a task, have long been employed by occupational and physical therapists to help individuals perform daily activities. Augmentative communication systems, designed to assist individuals with various communication impairments, have also been employed for decades. There are numerous industries that exist for the purpose of marketing and manufacturing "assistive devices" for the populace at large. Several of these are listed in Table 6.2; some of them we use regularly in rehabilitation.

The need to develop cognitive compensatory aids for many patients with traumatic brain injury is perhaps what has brought compensatory training into the common vocabulary of virtually all rehabilitation disciplines. Many of the considerations that must be reviewed regarding restorative training must also be considered in compensatory training.

Table 6.2
Common Assistive Devices Used by the Public.

Alarm clocks	Large button telephones
Beepers/pagers	Shoulder phone rests
Watches	Magnifying glasses
Calendars/schedules	Eye glasses
Shopping lists	Hearing aids
Post-its	Needle threaders
Labels	Rubber jar grips
Tape recorders	Velcro-closure shoes
Calculators	No-spill coffee mugs

Compensation training can be divided into two broad categories: training in the use of devices (external aids) and training in the use of internal strategic plans for circumventing problems. External aids include those that simplify tasks, those that replace functional requirements, and those that are actual prostheses. Although external aids would appear to be the easiest to employ, their use often requires self-initiation, and hence recognition of the need to use an aid. Both of these considerations are important matters in compensation training.

Barco et al.[52] have identified four types of compensation based on the level of awareness needed by the patient, in order for the strategy to be successful. The first type is referred to as *external compensation*, meaning that it is outside of the patient's initiation. External compensation techniques include cuing from someone other than the patient, and modification of the environment. This author has used the term *accommodation* to refer to environmental modifications that are done to optimize an individual's functioning in the home, work, academic, and community settings. Preferential seating is an example of a type of classroom accommodation that is provided for individuals with hearing impairments or other disabilities. In order for clinicians to make appropriate environmental accommodations, of course, they must have access to the settings in which individuals are expected to function. Frequently, several home visits, work visits, or school visits are indicated for individuals who require this level of restructuring. The use of cuing techniques from others requires willingness both on the part of the "cuer" and on the part of the patient "being cued;" otherwise, confrontational situations arise frequently. External compensation is indicated for individuals who have marginal awareness of their difficulties or of the need to circumvent problems.

Situational compensation can be employed with individuals who have awareness of their difficulties but do not recognize problem situations as they arise or while they are happening. Compensation strategies that can be habitualized and triggered by a situation should be chosen for use. The individual should be taught to apply the strategy habitually to a certain set of situations, thus eliminating the need to search for alternate solutions or recognize different problems. An example would be teaching an individual to always check the refrigerator door for messages upon entering the house.

Recognition compensation is best used with individuals who can recognize problems as they occur, but who cannot anticipate problem situations. Specific strategies should be taught for managing different situations, but several different strategies should not be chosen for the same problem, or the chance of confusion will increase.

The last type of compensation discussed by these authors is *anticipatory compensation*. As its name implies, this type requires that an individual have awareness of difficulties, and an ability to identify potential problem situations. The need to employ a compensation strategy is triggered by the awareness that a problem is about to occur. This is preferable for the obvious reason that problems may be avoided or minimized. Individuals who demonstrate this level of awareness are apt to be able to learn a number of strategies, and thus will have greater flexibility.

A number of issues become important when considering the type of strategy or external aid to use in compensation training. Several authors have cautioned that compensation training can be poorly conceived and overdone.[20,39] "Unfortunately, patients are often taught techniques without adequate consideration being given to whether the likely improvement in the patient's quality of life warrants the effort required for them to learn the compensatory technique."[39] Given the cognitive limitations of many individuals for whom greater independence is desired, compensation often seems a logical choice; however, "adding compensatory procedures to the ordinary demands on these (cognitive) resources can have the effect of making a marginally functional person less functional."[20]

Neither determining the most suitable candidates for compensation training nor selecting the best strategy to use is an easy choice. In addition to understanding the degree and nature of an individual's cognitive-communicative disability, clinicians should ask the following questions before initiating training. Although the questions refer to strategies, they are pertinent to external aids as well.

What is the individual's attentional capacity?
What is the individual's ability to learn?
What is the individual's level of motivation?
How realistic is the individual's personal appraisal of limitations?
How aware is the individual of others in the environment?
What are the individual's goals, and how realistic are they?
Does the individual use self-generated strategies?
   If so, are these effective?
   If not, can they be modified to be made effective?
What specific need(s) will the strategy meet?

How much effort is needed to use the strategy?

How much effort is needed to learn the strategy?

How will use of the strategy be reinforced?

Where can the strategy be applied?

Will the strategy generalize to novel situations?

Will the strategy capitalize upon strengths?

Is the team (clinicians, patient, and family) in agreement?

Will the strategy be accepted and reinforced by others in the post-treatment environment?

If these questions are answered thoughtfully, the difficulty in choosing a strategy can be diminished. Clinicians often think that because we are the "professionals" we are the best suited to design compensatory aids for someone else's use. A personal example is offered to illustrate how erroneous this line of thinking can be. Over a period of several months, this author observed that a member of her family had accumulated a drawer filled with note cards about different things to do or remember at work. Many of the cards appeared to contain the same information, in such a way that they could be categorized. To be of assistance, the author purchased an organizer, labeled different sections according to the card categories, and copied what seemed to be frequently needed "facts" into one of the sections. Unbeknownst to the author, however, the cards served many purposes: one was that they could be quickly removed, once the information was no longer needed; another was that they fit easily into a shirt pocket. The ill-fated organizer, on the other hand, did not fit into a shirt pocket and required too much "searching" to find the necessary facts—two good reasons for its limited use and tragic destiny in the trash.

Often, individuals who need some type of compensation or assistance employ aids or implement strategies on their own. It is better to examine these self-generated strategies and then reinforce their use, or modify them if necessary, than to "begin from scratch." These strategies often have the greatest likelihood of generalizing from situation to situation and of being used consistently. The use of different strategies for specific problems is discussed in greater detail in the next two chapters.

The Use of Computers in Rehabilitation

Many have used the term *cognitive retraining* to refer to the use of computer programs, sometimes to the extent that cognitive retraining has been called computer retraining. The increasingly popularity of personal computers, at the time when clinicians were searching for innovative ways to treat the cognitive deficits following traumatic brain injury, may account for this interchange of terms. Current terminology seeks to clarify this confusion, and the term *computer-assisted cognitive rehabilitation (CACR)*[20,53] is typically used for this purpose. Although it seems somewhat of a leap in logic, the popular analogy between brains and computers may have added to the lay person's perception of the usefulness of computers in the rehabilitation of "thinking abilities." It is not such a stretch, however, to recognize the extent to which computer models of information processing, from the cognitive sciences (artificial intelligence), have influenced intervention.[53] Even so, it seems illogical to think that computer programs are suitable to use in the remediation of all cognitive impairment, when "cognition," by its very nature, is dynamic and interactive. Nonetheless, personal experience with numerous rehabilitation facilities has left no doubt in this author's mind that clinicians have used computers in unethical ways. These include using computers to: replace therapy sessions missed or canceled by clinicians, increase the utilization of aides or nonprofessionals who typically are less expensive than licensed clinicians, spread a clinician among several patients working in a "computer lab," provide patients with "busy work" under the guise of additional practice, or mislead consumers who may have little knowledge of computers or cognitive processes.

The fervor for computer-assisted cognitive rehabilitation witnessed in the early to mid-eighties appears to have diminished somewhat. In part, this may be due to an increase in consumers' recognition of potential abuses, but it is also related to the lack of hard proof that benefits result from cognitive rehabilitation in general, or from computer-assisted cognitive rehabilitation in particular.[53] Nonetheless, computer-assisted therapy, whether for physical rehabilitation or for cognitive-communicative rehabilitation, is not without its benefits when used knowledgeably and judiciously.

First, it is important to consider the computer program itself. Many clinicians order software with little idea about the contents and structure of the program and then "try it out" with a patient. This type of trial and error, in and of itself, is not necessarily without some therapeutic benefit, depending upon the goals, skill level, and awareness of the patient. As a general rule, however, valuable therapy time can be wasted in this way. Most publishers of therapeutic software provide for a 30-day review period. Clinicians should take advantage of this and "test" numerous software programs, then select for purchase only those that truly meet the needs of the patient population being treated. Ylvisaker and colleagues[20] have suggested that there are five categories of programs based on the components addressed: basic-level cognitive components (for example, reaction time), visual-perceptual components (for example, scanning), cognitive-language organizing processes (for example, categorization), higher-level cognitive language components (for example, reasoning), and academic/integrative tasks (for example, mathematics).

Second, it is important to determine which patients will benefit from computer use. Although computers can be motivating for some, they are not motivating for all. Consideration also should be given to the amount of time that may have to be devoted to helping someone become comfortable with a computer. Most importantly, the cognitive-communicative needs of individuals are variable. Not all patients can benefit from computer-assisted rehabilitation. A computer program will do little for the individual whose greatest need is to be able to follow conversation in a group setting.

In addition to providing a source of motivation for some individuals, computers have provided benefits for clinicians as well. Computers have proven to be very useful in helping clinicians track performance data. Many programs also are useful for the ability to present precisely controlled stimuli, particularly if the rate of presentation needs to be controlled. Feedback from computers is immediate and impartial, which can sometimes work to the clinician's benefit in therapeutic relationships where rapport is not well established. Additional benefits are that computers can provide practice opportunities that might otherwise be avoided, and can provide structured activities for the patient to complete as home assignments with little monitoring from others.

Variables that Affect Treatment Performance and Daily Functioning

In many ways, the highly structured clinical setting is ideal for persons who have sustained a brain injury: distractions can be removed, rest breaks can be granted, structure is imposed. Because of the highly structured environment in which clinicians work, it is easy for them to assume that treatment materials are somehow automatically modified to best meet the individual's needs (for example, workbooks, computer programs, textbooks). The so-called cookbook approach follows this assumption. There is also a tendency to assume that somehow individuals will leave the treatment setting and automatically adjust to a less structured, often chaotic environment. Both of these tendencies should be resisted.

Table 6.2 provides an overview of some of the treatment and performance variables that can be modified or manipulated to improve performance, or at least be recognized as variables contributing to performance. Although these are easiest to control in the clinical setting, consideration of performance variables should in no way be limited to the clinical setting. In the "real world," extremes of stimulus input, distraction, and the effects of internal variables are most likely to occur, at least part of the time. Trying to find a restaurant on a city street in New York with five hungry children is an example of such an extreme. Although clinicians may be sensitive to the effects of many of these variables, we do not always share this knowledge with our patients to help them become self-regulating or modifying.

Clinicians can serve patients better by helping them identify the variables that most affect performance, and by teaching them ways to manipulate the environment for maximum performance. This is a form of awareness training that can begin at the earliest stages by simply trying to help patients

Table 6.3
Variables to Consider in Modifying Treatment.

STIMULUS/PERFORMANCE (TASK) VARIABLES
speed or rate of presentation
order of presentation
length of information in each stimulus item
complexity of information: simple to abstract
single or multiple choice responses
clinician personality/attitude

INTERNAL VARIABLES
sleep/restfulness
anxiety/worry
stimulants (e.g., caffeine)
depressants
physical discomfort/pain

EXTERNAL VARIABLES

Grades of Distraction:
low-low (one to one/quiet setting)
low-high (one to one/competition with environmental stimuli)
high-low (competition with others/quiet setting)
high-high (competition with others/competition with environmental stimuli)

Types of Distraction (pleasant or unpleasant):
Visual   Gustatory
Auditory   Tactile
Olfactory

---

identify internal variables that potentially affect performance (for example, "My leg hurts, and I'm thinking about that instead of this task."). Providing feedback, and at the same time seeking information from the patient about performance, can help improve self-awareness (for example, "That seemed really hard for you. What do you think might have changed so that this task was more difficult than the previous one?"). Not only can the careful gradation of stimulus variables assist clinicians in recognizing the limits of information processing, but it can also help patients identify them as well. When too many variables are altered simultaneously, as is often the case in "packaged" materials, it becomes difficult to determine the exact nature of performance breakdowns that might be attributable to stimulus variables or to response requirements.

Frequently, in communication therapy, we train our patients to ask for repetition or rephrasing in order to improve comprehension, for example, "Can you repeat that, one sentence at a time, or slow down?" (rate), or, "Can you rephrase that?" (length or complexity reduction), or "Let's go into

this office to talk. I'm having difficulty understanding you in the hall."
(distraction elimination). Awareness training involves recognition that a
breakdown has occurred, identification of those variables that might have
caused the breakdown, and then a reduction in those variables. Patients can
learn to recognize some of these variables.

Clinicians are aware of their own internal states, and often make assumptions or ask questions about the internal states of their patients, but they
may fall short in helping patients to recognize internal variables with the
intent of making modifications. Granted, in the real world, we often have to
work through, or in spite of, uncontrolled performance variables. With an
intact nervous system, this can be accomplished without undue difficulty.
Following brain injury, however, a cognitive system may be compromised
to such an extent that it cannot be expected to "override" stimulus-
performance variables. This additional demand may push the system to the
level of dysfunction that results in safety risks, poor academic performance,
or poor performance on the job. In the author's opinion, it is better to
identify and try to eliminate as many detrimental variables as possible,
to promote maximum achievement. Accordingly, accommodation is an
important rehabilitation concept.

GENERAL PRINCIPLES TO CONSIDER IN DELIVERING TREATMENT

Regardless of the primary approach taken by the clinician, a number of
principles apply to all conditions. Some of the more important ones to
consider are presented below.

- The choice of treatment tasks must not be random, but based on
  comprehensive evaluation (observation, formal testing procedures,
  interview, subjective complaints, family reports, et cetera).
- It is essential to perform task analyses prior to the initiation of
  treatment.
- Treatment always can be modified across at least two dimensions:
  stimulus demands and performance demands.
- Reinforcement is beneficial to the extent that it is immediate, that it
  is clearly associated with a particular behavior, and that it provides
  the learner with *specific* information about the accuracy of a response.
- Reinforcement should be considered for its potential value in
  motivating individuals and helping them to maintain a positive
  attitude.
- The use of reinforcement schedules can serve to unify staff toward
  common treatment goals and improve consistency in the use of
  feedback from multiple disciplines.
- The effects of treatment must be monitored formally (evaluated) on
  a regular basis.

- Treatment that proves to be ineffective should be discontinued.
- Rehabilitation is functional only if the post-treatment demands of the individual are known and used to guide treatment.
- The patient must be a partner in treatment with the clinician.

SUMMARY

This chapter has provided a discussion of most of the approaches, and the underlying theoretical assumptions, used in cognitive-communicative rehabilitation. These have included recovery theories, developmental and hierarchical approaches, cognitive processes and process-specific approaches, functional and skills training approaches, learning and behavioral approaches, and the holistic or psychodynamic approach. It was pointed out that functional rehabilitation frequently is considered to be the same as skills training, although this author prefers a broader view, incorporating the idea that the "expected" activity of individuals in their post-treatment environment should define what is functional and determine the focus of rehabilitation.

A number of behavioral techniques were discussed, because these are not usually included in the training programs of rehabilitation clinicians, except perhaps psychologists. Specific strategies that can be used to improve behavioral responses and learning were presented (for example, prompting, fading, highlighting). Six paradigms illustrating the conditions under which the transfer of learning is (or is not) optimized were discussed, because of their importance in helping clinicians choose the most optimal conditions for learning.

In conclusion, for rehabilitation to be functional, it must be based on the knowledge of recovery, cognitive processes, learning theory, and behavior modification. In the broadest sense, rehabilitation can be thought of as nothing less than the application of specific techniques to promote behavioral change. Learning is essential for changing behavior in all conditions. When learning is impaired, as it most often is following traumatic brain injury, the clinician must have knowledge of the processes that support learning, in order to affect any change. Accordingly, the rehabilitation of cognitive-communicative impairment cannot be accomplished using a single approach. Clinicians must arm themselves with all available resources, but these should be applied with discrimination, in a systematic manner, and in accordance with a well-founded rationale.

REFERENCES

1. Diller L. A model for cognitive retraining in rehabilitation. *Clinical Psychologist.* 1976;29:13–15.
2. Gianutsos R. What is cognitive rehabilitation? *Journal of Rehabilitation.* 1980;July:36–40.

3. Ben-Yishay Y, Diller L. Cognitive remediation. In Rosenthal M, Griffith ER, Bond MR, Miller JD (eds). *Rehabilitation of the Head Injured Adult*. Philadelphia, PA: FA Davis; 1983:367–380.

4. Adamovich BB, Henderson JA, Auerbach S. *Cognitive Rehabilitation of Closed Head Injured Patients: A Dynamic Approach*. San Diego, CA: College-Hill Press; 1985.

5. Prigatano GP et al. *Neuropsychological Rehabilitation after Brain Injury*. Baltimore, MD: Johns Hopkins University Press; 1986:51–66.

6. Moehle KA, Rasmussen JL, Fitzhugh-Bell KB. Neuropsychological theories and cognitive rehabilitation. In Williams JM, Long CJ (eds). *The Rehabilitation of Cognitive Disabilities*. New York, NY: Plenum Press; 1987:57–76.

7. Wilson B. Models of cognitive rehabilitation. In Wood RL, Eames P (eds). *Models of Brain Injury Rehabilitation*. Baltimore, MD: Johns Hopkins University Press; 1989:115–141.

8. Sohlberg MM, Mateer CA. *Introduction to Cognitive Rehabilitation: Theory and Practice*. New York, NY: Guilford Press; 1989:111–135.

9. Klonoff PS et al. Cognitive retraining after traumatic brain injury and its role in facilitating awareness. *Journal of Head Trauma Rehabilitation*. 1989;4:37–45.

10. Benedict RH. The effectiveness of cognitive remediation strategies for victims of traumatic head-injury: a review of the literature. *Clinical Psychology Review*. 1989;9:650–626.

11. Boake C. A history of cognitive rehabilitation of head-injured patients, 1915 to 1980. *Journal of Head Trauma Rehabilitation*. 1989;4:1–8.

12. Gianutsos R. Cognitive rehabilitation: a neuropsychological specialty comes of age. *Brain Injury*. 1991;5:353–368.

13. Gordon WA, Hibbard MR. The theory and practice of cognitive remediation. In Kreutzer JS, Wehman PH (eds). *Cognitive Rehabilitation for Persons with Traumatic Brain Injury: A Functional Approach*. Baltimore, MD: Paul H Brookes; 1991:13–22.

14. Duke LW et al. Cognitive rehabilitation after head trauma. In Long CJ, Ross LK (eds). *Handbook of Head Trauma: Acute Care to Recovery*. New York, NY: Plenum Press; 1992:165–190.

15. Fryer J, Fralish K. Cognitive rehabilitation. In Deutsch PM, Fralish KB (eds). *Innovations in Head Injury Rehabilitation*. New York, NY: Matthews Bender; 1994:7.1–7.35.

16. Gordan WA. Cognitive remediation: an approach to the amelioration of behavioral disorders. In Wood RL (ed). *The Neurobehavioral Sequelae of Traumatic Brain Injury*. New York, NY: Taylor and Francis; 1990:175–193.

17. Haas J. Ethical considerations of goal setting for patient care in rehabilitation medicine. *American Journal of Physical Medicine and Rehabilitation*. 1993;72:228–232.

18. *Webster's Ninth New Collegiate Dictionary*. Springfield, MA: Merriam-Webster; 1985.

19. Crosson B et al. Awareness and compensation in postacute head injury rehabilitation. *Journal of Head Trauma Rehabilitation*. 1989;4:46–54.

20. Ylvisaker M et al. Topics in cognitive rehabilitation therapy. In Ylvisaker M, Gobble EM (eds). *Community Re-entry for Head Injured Adults*. Boston, MA: College-Hill; 1987:137–220.

21. Almi CR, Finger S. Toward a definition of recovery of function. In Finger S,

LeVere TE, Almli CR, Stein DG (eds). *Brain Injury and Recovery: Theoretical and Controversial Issues.* New York, NY: Plenum Press; 1988:1–14.

22. Glassman RB, Smith A. Neural capacity and the concept of diaschisis: functional and evolutionary models. In Finger S, LeVere TE, Almli CR, Stein DG (eds). *Brain Injury and Recovery: Theoretical and Controversial Issues.* New York, NY: Plenum Press; 1988:45–69.

23. Ruff RM, Baser CA. An experimental comparison of neuropsychological rehabilitation. In Kreutzer JS, Wehman P (eds). *Community Integration Following Traumatic Brain Injury.* Baltimore, MD: Paul H Brookes; 1990:85–102.

24. Albert M, Sparks R, Helm N. Melodic intonation therapy for aphasia. *Archives of Neurology.* 1973;29:130–131.

25. Goldstein G, Ruthven L. *Rehabilitation of the Brain-Damaged Adult.* New York, NY: Plenum Press; 1983.

26. Szekers SF, Ylvisaker M, Cohen SB. A framework for cognitive rehabilitation therapy. In Ylvisaker M, Gobble EM (eds). *Community Re-entry for Head Injured Adults.* Boston, MA: College-Hill Press; 1987:87–136.

27. Adamovich BB, Henderson J. *Scales of Cognitive Ability for Traumatic Brain Injury.* Austin, TX: Pro-Ed; 1992.

28. Whyte J. Outcome evaluation in the remediation of attention and memory deficits. *Journal of Head Trauma Rehabilitation.* 1986;1:64–71.

29. Bracy OL. Cognitive rehabilitation: a process approach. *Cognitive Rehabilitation.* 1986;4:10–17.

30. Bracy OL. *Psychological Software Services.* Indianapolis, IN: Neuroscience Publishers.

31. Sohlberg MM, Mateer CA. *Attention Process Training (APT).* Puyallup, WA: Association for Neuropsychological Research and Development; 1986.

32. Ben-Yishay Y. *Working Approaches to Remediation of Cognitive Deficits in Brain Damaged Persons.* New York, NY: New York University Medical Center; 1980: Monograph 61.

33. Wilson BA. *Rehabilitation of Memory.* New York, NY: Guilford Press; 1987.

34. Giles GM, Clark-Wilson J. Functional skills training in severe brain injury. In Fussey I, Giles GM (eds). *Rehabilitation of the Severely Brain Injured Adult: A Practical Approach.* London, England: Croom Helm; 1988:69–101.

35. Glisky EL, Schacter DA. Remediation of organic memory disorder: current status and future prospects. *Journal of Head Trauma Rehabilitation.* 1986;3:54–63.

36. Schacter DL, Glisky EL. Memory remediation: restoration, alleviation and the acquistition of domain-specific knowledge. In Uzzell BP, Gross Y (eds). *Clinical Neuropsychology of Intervention.* Boston, MA: Martinus Nijhoff; 1986:257–282.

37. Ruff RM et al. Effectiveness of behavioral management in rehabilitation: cognitive procedures. In Wood RL (ed). *The Neurobehavioral Sequelae of Traumatic Brain Injury.* New York, NY: Taylor and Francis; 1990:305–334.

38. Hart T, Hayden ME. The ecological validity of neuropsychological assessment and remediation. In Uzzell BP, Gross Y (eds). *Clinical Neuropsychology of Intervention.* Boston, MA: Martinus Nijhoff; 1986:21–50.

39. Giles GM. Functional assessment and intervention. In Finlayson MAJ, Garner SH (eds). *Brain Injury Rehabilitation: Clinical Considerations.* Baltimore, MD: Williams and Wilkins; 1994:124–156.

40. Cook L, Smith DS, Truman G. Using Functional Independence Measure profiles as an index of outcome in the rehabilitation of brain-injured patients. *Archives of Physical Medicine and Rehabilitation.* 1994;75:390–393.

41. Wood RL. Neurobehavioral paradigm for brain injury rehabilitation. In Wood RL (ed). *The Neurobehavioral Sequelae of Traumatic Brain Injury.* New York, NY: Taylor and Francis; 1990:3–17.

42. Giles GM, Clark-Wilson J. *Brain Injury Rehabilitation: A Neurofunctional Approach.* London, England: Chapman and Hall; 1993.

43. Wood RL. Conditioning procedures in brain injury rehabilitation. In Wood RL (ed). *The Neurobehavioral Sequelae of Traumatic Brain Injury.* New York, NY: Taylor and Francis; 1990:153–174.

44. Malec J. Training the brain-injured client in behavioral self-management skills. In Edelstein BA, Couture ET (eds). *Behavioral Assessment and Rehabilitation of the Traumatically Brain-Damaged.* New York, NY: Plenum Press; 1984:121–150.

45. Jacobs HE. Yes, behaviour analysis can help, but do you know how to harness it? *Brain Injury.* 1988;2:339–346.

46. Wood RL, Burgess PW. The psychological management of behaviour disorders following brain injury. In Fussey I, Giles GM (eds). *Rehabilitation of the Severely Brain-Injured Adult: A Practical Approach.* London, England: Croom Helm; 1988:43–68.

47. Ben-Yishay Y et al. Neuropsychologic rehabilitation: quest for a holistic approach. *Seminars in Neurology.* 1985;5:252–259.

48. Stanczak DE, Hutcherson WL. Acute rehabilitation of the head-injured individual: toward a neuropsychological paradigm of treatment. In Long CJ, Ross LK (eds). *Handbook of Head Trauma: Acute Care to Recovery.* New York, NY: Plenum Press; 1992:125–136.

49. Parenté R, Anderson-Parenté JK. Retraining memory: theory and application. *Journal of Head Trauma Rehabilitation.* 1989;4:55–65.

50. Parenté R, DiCesare A. Retraining memory: theory, evolution, and applications. In Kreutzer J, Wehman P (eds). *Cognitive Rehabilitation for Persons with Traumatic Brain Injury.* Baltimore, MD: Paul H Brookes; 1991:147–161.

51. Gross Y, Schutz LE. Intervention models in neuropsychology. In Uzzell BP, Gross Y (eds). *Clinical Neuropsychology of Intervention.* Boston, MA: Martinus Nijhoff; 1986:179–204.

52. Barco PP et al. Training awareness and compensation in postacute head injury rehabilitation. In Kreutzer J, Wehman P (eds). *Cognitive Rehabilitation for Persons with Traumatic Brain Injury.* Baltimore, MD: Paul H Brookes; 1991:129–146.

53. Levin, W. Computer applications in cognitive rehabilitation. In Kreutzer J, Wehman P (eds). *Cognitive Rehabilitation for Persons with Traumatic Brain Injury.* Baltimore, MD: Paul H Brookes; 1991:163–178.

7

Acute Rehabilitation

The stages of rehabilitation have been defined in terms of neurologic recovery and time postinjury, behavioral recovery, and practice setting (for example, hospital, rehabilitation unit, community re-entry, et cetera). From the standpoint of intervention, the term *early recovery* usually refers to the period beginning with the loss of consciousness and ending at the point when the patient first demonstrates alertness and purposeful responsiveness. The length of this recovery period is highly variable from individual to individual, and is dependent upon numerous factors, including the severity of the brain injury, complicating medical conditions, the influence of drugs and alcohol at the time of injury, and individual personality features. The presence of coma is not in and of itself an indicator that the patient is in the early neurologic recovery phase, given that severely injured individuals may remain in coma for months to years (that is, beyond the period of spontaneous recovery). The behavioral characteristics (that is, the extent of purposeful responses) may go unchanged during this period of months or years. Therefore, intervention based solely on behavioral observation, without consideration of length of time postinjury and overall neurologic status, may not be indicated. In other words, the provision of an aggressive coma stimulation program (discussed in the next section) based solely on the observation of nonpurposeful responding behavior would be questionable, clinically and ethically. Additionally, the assumption that an early intervention program is associated only with hospital settings is inaccurate. The management of coma (acute, prolonged, and persistent vegetative) may take place in an intensive care unit, a hospital ward, a nursing home, or even in the individual's home. All of these variables must be considered in determining the type and intensity of treatment.

In the past, much emphasis has been placed on the importance of early, aggressive treatment,[1,2,3,4] although the research in this area is limited. However, the long-term needs of individuals with traumatic brain injury are immense. It is not known, at this time, whether intensive treatment (usually six to seven hours of therapy daily) up front has a greater impact on long-term (five or more years) progress and outcome than does extended rehabilitation of less intensity, or intermittent periods of rehabilitation for years. Data of this nature are just beginning to appear in the literature.[5] These points are made because the financial resources of individuals also must be considered in treatment decisions. The author knows personally of cases where individuals were maintained in coma stimulation programs for months, exhausting all funding sources for rehabilitation services, at which point they emerged from coma and needed rehabilitation. Financial considerations dominate the health care arena and, unless one has the luxury of working in a fully funded research facility, they significantly impact treatment decisions at all stages.

EARLY STAGES OF RECOVERY

Early intervention by rehabilitation clinicians has a threefold purpose: prevention of postinjury complications, such as contractures, skin breakdown and aspiration pneumonia; stimulation to increase neuronal activity; and maximizing the patient's comfort. All of these have the goal of preventing deterioration and promoting recovery.

Some[6,7] have indicated that the earliest point for rehabilitation to begin is when the patient is in the intensive care unit. The type of intervention that can and should be provided in the intensive care unit will depend on the individual setting. Many intensive care units are ill prepared to have numerous clinicians and family members at the patient's bedside, in addition to the staff required for the numerous medical services typically being provided. Most would agree that sensory stimulation of any type should be conducted only with *medically stable* individuals. Patients are usually in the intensive care unit because their condition has not stabilized. Therefore, caution must be the guide used when providing sensory stimulation to acutely injured persons, who have limited energy reserves that are needed for life preservation. It is not unusual, however, for patients to begin to display increased arousal in the intensive care unit. In Chapter Four, Pierce discussed in detail the neurologic signs to observe during this period.

Providing treatment in the intensive care unit is not for the timid. For the new clinician, it can be an intimidating place, given the rapid pace at which decisions sometimes must be made and the presence of numerous technological instruments (for example, ventilator, intracranial pressure monitor, intravenous drip, electrocardiac monitor, oxygen supply, suctioning pump). Clinicians working in this setting must become technologically competent to monitor the equipment during any activity. Additionally, clinicians will ideally be working with the patients' families in any stimulation program and most likely will establish therapeutic relationships with key family members. Families may have ongoing questions about the purpose of different mechanical devices and how they may or may not be affecting the patient's progress. Clinicians should be prepared to answer their questions in lay terms. This requires a certain degree of familiarity with the intensive care unit, which the clinician can only truly gain from direct experience.

Although the organization of intensive care units varies from facility to facility, their purpose and nature typically do not. The intensive care unit offers an expensive type of health care. In the author's experience, patients are transferred out of intensive care units as early as possible, usually once medical stability has been maintained for a certain period of time (determined by the attending physician), and hourly monitoring is no longer indicated. A stay in the intensive care unit is followed by transfer to what is sometimes referred to as a "step-down unit," indicating a lower level of medical supervision than intensive care, but a higher level than on an acute hospital floor. If this level of care is not indicated, or the hospital does not offer this "transition level," then transfer is directly to an acute hospital floor that may be primarily neurosurgical, neurological, medical, or orthopedic, depending upon the most pressing needs of the patient or according to the primary physician's specialty. Occasionally, patients are maintained in intensive care until judged stable and then are transferred directly to a rehabilitation unit, if it offers good medical support. Additionally, some rehabilitation units or facilities with good medical support admit patients who have not regained consciousness fully but are otherwise medically stable.

This discussion should lead the reader to the understanding that the setting in which early intervention takes place is variable. As stated in Chapter Two, some facilities have an acute care team that is responsible for providing services in the "acute" setting, which includes intensive care. Other facilities establish a traumatic brain injury team that works with this diagnostic group exclusively throughout the stay in the facility, regardless of the point in recovery. Because of the complexity of the population, however, it is recommended that a core team of professionals be established to provide care at even the earliest stages. A stream of unfamiliar clinicians will do little to provide the consistency needed by the patient, family, and other medical staff. Because the medical status of a patient can change rapidly in the acute stages, it is imperative that the clinician obtain up-to-date information prior to the initiation of any intervention. This requires the ability to read the medical chart for pertinent information (for example, changes in neurologic signs, documentation of seizures, changes in medication, changes in vital signs, changes in alertness), a skill that is acquired with practice. The detailed description of neurological signs and evaluation provided in Chapter Four is intended to assist the clinician in this area. More importantly, however, the initiation of intervention in the acute stages of recovery requires good communication with the nursing staff, who have primary responsibility for the patient's general care, and who will have the most current information.

The rationale behind preventive measures and comfort measures is apparent. Speech-language pathologists are not involved in a large number of preventive measures, although in some settings they may provide suctioning, particularly in conjunction with swallowing therapy (discussed later). This is a technical procedure for which one should obtain direct training from nursing, respiratory therapy staff, or through formal education, as discussed by Pierce in Chapter Four. All clinicians, however, should be able to recognize the potential need for suctioning in order to inform nursing or respiratory therapy.

Stimulation Therapy

The primary focus of cognitive-communicative intervention by speech-language pathologists in the acute stages of care is the provision of sensory stimulation, referred to as *coma stimulation therapy* or *coma arousal therapy*. This is a highly controversial service and, like other forms of cognitive intervention, it is not the exclusive domain of speech-language pathologists. The purpose of sensory stimulation at a physiologic level is to increase neuronal activity and improve arousal. At a behavioral level, the purpose is to improve the recognition of environmental events and shape adaptive responses.[8] There are several rationales that can be offered for the provision of sensory stimulation. The most sound, however, are based on data obtained from animal studies. First, several researchers[9,10,11] have demonstrated the beneficial effects of early sensory stimulation and motor training on the recovery of animals following experimental lesions. Second, a number of sensory deprivation studies[12,13,14,15] have demonstrated cortical changes (for example, increases in the size of dentritic spines, changes in the number of synapses and synaptic vesicles, et cetera) in animals exposed to a sensory rich environment, in comparison to animals deprived of environmental enrichment. Moore[16] has indicated that sensory deprivation, such as occurs when an individual is placed in the relatively isolated intensive care unit, has deleterious effects on the already compromised central nervous system. Therefore, stimulation is needed to counter these effects.

The reader is again reminded that multiple connections exist between the *reticular activating system (RAS)* and the *cortex*, and that the reticular activating system relays information to the cortical regions. The exact nature of this information is unknown; it may be alerting signals or information about the intensity or amount of stimuli. Because of its wide distribution, the reticular activating system may be particularly vulnerable to the effects of medications, abnormal sleep patterns, and sensory deprivation.[16] Farber[17] has postulated that the reticular activating system is affected by sensory deprivation in a way that raises the activation threshold of the reticular neurons, thereby reducing the amount of information flow to the cortex. Sensory stimulation may serve to lower this activation threshold, and hence increase cortical activation.

The preceding rationales form the theoretical basis for sensory stimulation. There is an emerging literature from clinical research on the therapeutic benefit of sensory stimulation. It is difficult to consider these studies collectively because of differences in the programs, measures of responsiveness, measures of outcome, populations studied, and so on. Perhaps one of the earliest studies to report the effects of sensory stimulation on arousal and outcome was conducted by the pioneer advocates of stimulation therapy, LeWinn and Dimancescu.[18] These authors used an intense (six hours per day), multisensory stimulation approach with 16 individuals with severe brain injuries and compared them to a matched group of individuals who did not receive stimulation therapy. Their claims of a reduction not only in morbidity but also in mortality, as a result of the stimulation program, may have set the course of stimulation therapy off to a dubious start. To this author's knowledge, no studies since have made similar claims, nor have these authors replicated their original findings.

Several studies[19,20] have examined the effect of sensory stimulation on physiologic functions such as heart rate, respiratory rate, and intracranial pressure, and have found that auditory stimulation tends to elicit changes in these functions. Intracranial pressure changes have been documented during conversation stimulation, with a decrease in pressure when conversation had a neutral content. For patients with Glasgow Coma Scale scores above seven, an increase in pressure was observed during emotionally-charged conversation. These studies provide minimal support for the long-term therapeutic benefit of sensory stimulation, but do suggest that loud or exciting auditory input should be avoided with critically ill persons in whom an increase in any of these functions may be undesirable. Several authors[21,22] have found that positioning of patients facilitates responsiveness and that physical stimulation that elicits motor responses is more effective than passive techniques.[23] In addition to pulse rate, respiration, blood pressure, and intracranial pressure, electroencephalographic recordings have been used to monitor responsiveness to stimulation in the comatose patient,[23,24] but these have been found to be less reliable in indicating arousal than behavioral responses.[24]

One of the most carefully designed studies available for review, by Jones and colleagues,[25] found, in a single case study, an increase in arousal with auditory stimulation that was provided by a tape of familiar voices, in comparison to two tapes of music and nature sounds. These authors used objective procedures in both the presentation of stimulation and the assessment of arousal and responses. Prerecorded audio tapes, that could be controlled without adding extraneous auditory stimulation, were used to present the four types of auditory stimuli. Physiologic measures (with instrumentation) were taken, and behavioral responses were video recorded for independent ratings by unbiased clinicians. In addition to the finding that familiar voices caused an increase in pulse rate, respiratory rate, and behavioral responses, the authors also found variations in the reliability of measures of physiologic changes. (Pulse rate appeared to be the most reliable measure in all conditions, while respiratory rate monitoring was influenced by extraneous body movements, and measures of galvanic skin responses lacked the sensitivity to detect subtle changes; thus, the latter could not be used.) The authors concluded with interpretative caution that human speech, in and of itself, may increase arousal since the variable of unfamiliar voices was not included in their study. However, several other authors[3,8,26] have recommended the incorporation of familiar voices and people into the clinical management of individuals in coma.

One of the findings of Kater[2] was a better outcome for patients who have an initial Glasgow Coma Scale score above seven at the initiation of treatment with stimulation therapy, than for those individuals with a lower score. This is not a surprising finding if the Glasgow Coma Scale score is taken as an indication of initial severity of the injury, in which case it would be difficult to attribute the improved outcome to sensory stimulation therapy alone, if at all. However, additional studies[27,28] have indicated that, even after several months of coma, patients who score higher on some type of assessment scale (for example, Glasgow Coma Scale, Rancho Scale) tend to have better long-term outcomes (that is, do not remain in a true, unresponsive, vegetative state), even though classified as "vegetative." These findings tend to support the work of Bricolo and colleagues[29] and Rappaport et al.[30] that suggests there are subgroups within the "slow-to-recover" or persistent vegetative population, some of whom gain the ability to execute commands and communicate.[29]

In studies by Radar, Alston, and Ellis[31] and Pierce and colleagues,[32] coma stimulation procedures were not found to have a significant effect on overall responsiveness, or on disability outcome. As is the case with many studies, the results of these studies cannot be compared because of differences in programs and measures used to assess changes. Ellis and Radar[33] have noted that a major problem for the research in this area is the lack of standardized procedures for assessing changes in behavioral responses over time, particularly when these changes may be subtle.

To circumvent this problem, Ansell and Keenan[27] developed the *Western Neuro Sensory Stimulation Profile (WNSSP)* as a "formal objective measure of cognitive function in severely impaired head-injured adults ... [and] to monitor behavioral changes in patients who remain at Rancho levels II and III for extended periods of time." Their measure consists of 32 items divided across six subscales: Arousal/Attention, Auditory Comprehension, Visual Comprehension, Visual Tracking, Object Manipulation, and Tactile/Olfactory Response. Following a validation and reliability study with 50 patients, the authors concluded that this tool is useful for demonstrating small behavioral changes, and that it may therefore serve to distinguish "those patients with the potential to improve from those who will probably remain in a vegetative state." They also found it to be useful not only in demonstrating change but in identifying patterns of performance (for example, strong and weak modalities) that could be used to guide treatment planning.

In a similar manner, Radar and Ellis[28] have developed the *Sensory Stimulation Assessment Measure (SSAM)* to use in the early assessment of patients with severe brain injuries who do not communicate or follow commands consistently. Their measure is an extension of the Glasgow Coma Scale categories and includes a greater number of response measures within each of the three categories of eye opening, motor, and vocalization/verbalization responses. A protocol of stimulation techniques for the five senses is followed, and responses are scored using the extended assessment scale. These authors conducted a validity and reliability study with 20 patients who had resumed the sleep-wake cycle but did not follow commands consistently or communicate. Their conclusions were similar to those of Ansell and Keenan above in that they found the assessment tool to be useful in documenting behavioral changes (both in quantity and quality), planning and monitoring treatment, and providing indications of later impairment.

It should be noted that a number of these studies have been conducted on the slow-to-recover group of individuals who have sustained traumatic brain injury. This is also the group of patients for whom Smith and Ylvisaker[8] have cautioned that stimulation therapy may not be appropriate. The stimulation programs discussed in the next section are intended to be applied in the early stages of neurologic recovery, although there is no recommended cut-off point at which this type of therapy should be discontinued in patients who demonstrate poor responsiveness. As with all interventions, however, either treatment parameters are changed or treatment is discontinued when measurable progress is no longer demonstrated. Although all patients display ups, downs, and periods of plateau, the goal of "improved responsiveness" must be refined and continually upgraded if progress is being demonstrated (that is, increases in the frequency of responses and improvement in the quality of responses should be measured). The previously discussed assessment instruments are useful for this purpose.

A few studies have examined the effects of early (initiated within a few days postinjury), formalized sensory stimulation programs on reducing coma length and the length of stay in hospitals or rehabilitation centers. In general, findings indicated a reduction in the length of coma[3,34] and in the length of hospitalization[34] for patients who received this type of intervention compared to those who did not. Further, Mackay and colleagues[34] found that patients who participated in an acutely administered stimulation program (within a few days of admission), when compared to a group who did not, achieved better placement outcomes (that is, were able to return home instead of needing continued supportive nursing care).

Other rationales for the initiation of sensory stimulation are that it provides a means for formal observation of behavioral changes over time, so progress is monitored, and that "it provides a structured system of intervention that the family can use without reverting to more primitive attempts at intervention."[33] The importance of family involvement in purposeful activities is stressed in Chapter Eleven of this text. The decision to involve families in sensory stimulation may be best made on an individual basis. However, due to costs, this author strongly recommends the use of family members and nursing support personnel in the provision of sensory stimulation over long recovery periods, if stimulation is in fact indicated.

The claims that sensory arousal therapy promotes recovery from coma and affects long-term outcome are not well substantiated. Nonetheless, clinical reports have indicated a reduction in length of hospitalization and length of coma. There is no doubt that studies have shown that sensory stimulation can improve responsiveness in patients who have remained in coma for over a year; however, the long-term benefits have not been demonstrated. There are few data to indicate that individuals in the slow-to-recover group who receive stimulation therapy progress to the point of being able to participate in a traditional rehabilitation program, experience a reduction in the level of care, or return home. As with all types of rehabilitation intervention, these data are needed if treatment effectiveness is to be demonstrated.

Types of Sensory Stimulation Programs

Few articles have described in detail the treatment and measurement parameters used in their programs. Several types of sensory stimulation programs have been mentioned, however, and these are reviewed.

One of the most frequently used approaches, as presented in the literature, appears to be the *multisensory approach*. The stimulation modalities used most often are visual, auditory, gustatory, olfactory, tactile, and kinesthetic. Approaches of this nature may or may not base the stimulation on a hierarchy, and may or may not alternate sessions (for example, auditory in the morning, visual in the afternoon). The term, however, implies that all sensory modalities are stimulated during each session, with numerous sessions per day. A variety of stimulation techniques would be used in this approach, such as placing different smells under the nose, placing different tastes on the tongue and lips, applying different temperatures and textures to the skin, applying massage, performing range of motion exercises, tracking a light or finger, presenting speech and nonverbal sounds to alternate ears, and so on. A criticism of this approach is that it provides a bombardment of stimuli to the patient, who begins with limited information processing capacity and is then overloaded.[35]

Wood[35,36] has recommended that, instead of coma arousal, *sensory regulation* should be the goal of the rehabilitation team. He is critical of the commonly held notion that patients are understimulated in the acute care setting (sensory deprived) where all care procedures must be considered as sources of sensory stimulation (for example, range of motion, skin care, grooming), in addition to the continuous background noise of television, radio, and staff chatter to which patients are exposed. "To suggest that periods of sensory stimulation added to this continuous stimulation under the guise of 'therapy' will significantly alter the information processing capabilities of a vegetative patient is so absurd that it borders on clinical naivety."[35] Wood does not discourage the use of stimulation procedures, per se, but rather stresses the importance of reducing the amount of stimulus bombardment that naturally exists in the acute care and rehabilitation settings by structuring the environment, providing rest periods in which sleep can occur (30 to 45 minutes), regulating the nature of communication with the patient, and establishing optimal conditions when presenting sensory information to improve responses.

Another approach to sensory stimulation is what this author will call the *familiar routines approach*. This approach seeks to take the patient through familiar sensory and motor experiences in the same sequence that they may have been experienced in a routine 24-hour day prior to the injury. The rationale is that simulating familiar experiences capitalizes upon habitual, overlearned behaviors that are more permanently stored in memory and more readily accessible, than are new, unfamiliar behaviors. This approach also has a developmental aspect to it, in that the individual is being "taken back" through earlier stages of experience. For example, if an individual had a morning routine that started with washing the face, then drinking coffee and reading the paper, followed by brushing the teeth and getting dressed, this routine would be simulated in the hospital, approximating the times of day when these activities were performed prior to the injury. In this scenario, the coffee and toothpaste would presumably stimulate olfaction and gustatory sensation and response, reading the paper to the patient would provide auditory stimulation and perhaps visual, and physically assisting the patient through these activities would provide kinesthetic and tactile stimulation. Kater[2] advocates the use of familiar overlearned behaviors to stimulate arousal in a coma stimulation program, on the basis of ease of memory access as presented above.

A third approach is the *structured stimulation approach* which has been described by Smith and Ylvisaker[8] and thus will be highlighted only. Their approach is based on and organized according to several underlying principles. First, following the writings of Moore,[16] they conceptualize that the phylogenetically older systems of the nervous system (limbic system, midbrain, brain stem) may remain more intact following injury than do the more recently developed cortical regions. Therefore, stimulation therapy begins with the more "primitive" senses mediated by these lower levels: movement, smell, and touch. Second, according to the early writings of Hebb,[37] each individual has a range of tolerance for stimulation. Treatment aims to fall within that range, that is, to stimulate cortical activity but not cause habituation to the stimulation, which occurs with continuous and repetitive stimulation. Relying on information from animal studies,[38] they suggest that treatment should progress gradually and systematically from unisensory to multisensory. Additionally, the authors note that stimulation may have either inhibitory effects or excitatory effects, and that these may be patient specific. Stimulation that tends to inhibit responsiveness should be avoided with patients who exhibit low arousal, lethargy, and hypotonicity. Similarly, patients in an excited state should not be excited further by stimulation. Finally, Smith and Ylvisaker support the idea that a familiar environment is more beneficial to the patient, and particularly, that meaningful stimulation may contribute to cortical activity.

Drawing upon the previously-cited research, and adhering to the principles outlined above, the following conclusions regarding sensory stimulation programs are presented:

- All individuals should be approached as if they understand everything. Clinicians should introduce themselves and explain all procedures. Conversations with other staff or family should be kept to a minimum in the presence of the patient.
- Stimulation sessions should be brief and offered in as distraction-free an environment as possible.
- The continuous playing of televisions and radios has the effect of habituation instead of stimulation and should be limited. Continuous talking has the same effect. Speech should be delivered at a slow, deliberate rate and controlled for length and complexity.
- Initially one sensory modality should be used, first stimulating those senses mediated by subcortical regions.
- The patient's emotional and physiologic status (blood pressure, pulse, respiration, and intracranial pressure) should be monitored carefully, especially to avoid excitation.
- Items familiar to the patient should be used in treatment sessions.
- Family members should be trained to carry out sensory stimulation, particularly during routine activities such as bathing and grooming.
- Treatment should progress to the point of assisting patients in active participation in activities that involve sensory-motor integration, not merely passive stimulation.
- Clinicians should be responsive to (that is, reinforce) the patient's natural attempts at communication and other behaviors that indicate intent and should seek to shape these behaviors in a purposeful direction, not to establish new, unfamiliar responses.
- Clinicians, speech-language pathologists in particular, should serve as role models for peers and family by demonstrating therapeutic communication with the patient.

Clinicians are cautioned to be careful in their terminology and explanation of the benefit of coma stimulation therapy so as not to mislead family members or create false hope. Families are often desperate for hope and may grasp at any technique that sounds like an active process designed to speed recovery. At this point, explanations that state the purpose of coma stimulation is to arouse the individual from coma or to speed the coma recovery process are unfounded and can be misleading.

Augmentative Communication and Hearing

As patients begin to emerge from coma and show signs of increased responsiveness, it may be necessary to establish a nonverbal means for communication for them. At this stage, no attempts should be made to establish an elaborate communication system, because the individual's long-term needs cannot yet be predicted, nor can an accurate assessment of cognitive-communicative ability be made. DeRuyter and Kennedy[39] have recommended that the most natural response systems be attempted first, as these will have the greatest amount of success. For yes/no responses these include head nods and gestures, but not necessarily the commonly prescribed "thumbs up" or "thumbs down" gestures. Patients should be observed carefully to determine which body movements they can make or may already be using when attempting to respond. In terms of a hierarchy for yes/no responding, if head nods and gestures do not work, then color cards for pointing or eye-gaze can be attempted, followed by eye blinks, and then some type of buzzer response.[39] Chapter Nine addresses the assessment and treatment of motor speech disorders at great length.

By virtue of damage to the head, otological and audiological problems should be suspected following a traumatic injury. (Refer to Chapter Four for the incidence of hearing impairment.) Sakai and Mateer[40] have reviewed the causes and types of hearing impairment that often follow closed head injury. In brief, these include conductive loss associated with ossicular chain injury, blood in the middle ear or canal, perforation or laceration of the tympanic membrane, inflammation, and infection. Sensorineural hearing loss may occur as the result of disruption and loss of hair cells, disruption of the membranous labyrinth, or damage to the eighth cranial nerve. Central nervous system impairment involving the temporal lobes can, of course, also be a cause for audiological impairment. Given the susceptibility of the hearing system, evaluation should be considered as soon as possible. Cowley et al.[6] have recommended that assessment begin in the intensive care unit with portable audiometric equipment. *Auditory brain stem evoked responses (ABR)* can be used to determine the integrity of the brain stem auditory pathways, but these provide little information to aid in the management of peripheral hearing impairment. In some settings, speech-language pathologists may be responsible for arranging audiological services and hence should be aware of the potential needs.

Swallowing and Feeding

The incidence of swallowing disorders following traumatic brain injury is unknown[41] but has been estimated to be as high as 78 percent in acute hospital settings,[42] although lower estimates of 27 percent[43] and 26 percent[44] have been reported in acute rehabilitation facilities. The importance of maintaining adequate nutrition in patients who have suffered a traumatic brain injury, and in many cases multiple trauma, was discussed in Chapter Four. As should be evident, the early evaluation and management of potential swallowing disorders is an important aspect of the speech-language pathologist's role in the early stages of recovery. With some exceptions, the management of dysphagia following traumatic brain injury is not unlike that of other conditions. It would do an injustice to the complexity of swallowing and its evaluation to delineate evaluation and treatment procedures in a cursory fashion, when several texts have been devoted to the subject. (These are included in Appendix B along with other selected readings.) Therefore, only a few key issues will be discussed.

In addition to neurologic impairment, swallowing may be affected in other ways following a traumatic brain injury in combination with direct injury to the face and neck resulting in fractures or even puncture wounds.[41] Logemann and colleagues[41] have noted that problems in laryngeal elevation and cricopharyngeal functions generally are the result of physical damage rather than of neurological impairment. The most common swallowing motility problems noted by Lazarus and Logemann,[45] who evaluated patterns of swallowing impairment in 53 patients with traumatic brain injury, were problems of a delayed or absent swallowing reflex problems (delayed for absent) (81 percent), followed by reduced lingual control (53 percent), and then reduced peristalsis (32 percent).

As with other conditions, swallowing assessment should not be performed until patients are awake, alert, and able to follow commands. Logemann[46] has suggested that, following a thorough review of the patient's medical history, the following observations should be made upon entering the patient's room to perform a bedside assessment:

> (1) status of lip closure, (2) oral v nasal breathing, (3) level of secretions, (4) patient awareness of secretions, (5) patient management of secretions (ie, swallowing, coughing, wiping the mouth), (6) patient awareness of the clinician's approach, and (7) the nature and content of initial verbalization by the patient.

As stated previously, treatment for dysphagia following traumatic brain injury does not differ significantly from that offered to other populations, and consists of either teaching compensatory strategies (for example, altering food consistencies, temperatures, volume, and speed of intake; positioning; and adaptive postures) or implementating techniques to change the physiology of the swallowing process at either the oral or pharyngeal stages (for example, stimulation, exercises, and swallowing maneuvers). There are, however, unique challenges presented by this population. In the early stages, arousal and attention problems typically prohibit the initiation of any type of oral feeding. Following a study of 39 patients with severe brain injuries, Mackay and Morgan[47] indicated that oral intake could not be initiated successfully until Rancho Level IV, and that oral feeding was not achieved successfully until Rancho Level VI, regardless of the presence of a swallowing problem.

The cognitive impairments that accompany traumatic brain injury may prohibit the use of multistep sequence procedures, particularly if there are insufficient staff or family members to assist at all meals. Additionally, severe motor impairments, such as spasticity, may make it difficult, if not impossible, for some individuals to use techniques such as taking small sips or "small spoonfuls," independently. Therefore, a close working relationship among team members becomes imperative to the careful exploration of all avenues (assistive devices, alternate positioning) for oral intake.

An important consideration in the early stages of recovery is the family's need to nurture and be of assistance. It is not unusual for family members to initiate feeding (unbeknownst to staff) when patients begin to show purposeful responses. This possibility should not be overlooked, and counseling regarding the need to wait for diagnostic evaluation, to establish safety, should be provided.

Perhaps some of the more difficult decisions regarding nutritional management and oral intake must be made with those individuals who, for whatever reasons, are admitted to acute or even postacute rehabilitation facilities eating regular diets, despite an obvious swallowing problem and suspected aspiration. Once the nature of the swallowing problem has been documented and alterations in oral intake are indicated, it is often quite difficult to obtain compliance with modified diets and/or the use of compensatory techniques because of the patient's cognitive and behavioral limitations, and the fact that he or she prefers eating a regular diet. In these cases, it is essential to obtain the full cooperation and support for the therapeutic program from the team, and in particular from family members. Regardless of when a swallowing problem is detected, family members should always be considered vital to the effective implementation of any treatment program.[48]

MIDDLE STAGES OF RECOVERY

In the middle stages of recovery, individuals have emerged from coma and characteristically emerge into a "new world" with confusion, disorientation, and sometimes agitation. From a behavioral perspective, the middle stages generally are classified as Rancho Levels IV, V, and VI,[49] although it is well accepted that not all patients traverse through all eight Rancho levels. Still, the scale provides a characterization of behaviors that is understood by multiple disciplines and provides a common vocabulary for discussing patients in a hospital setting. Regarding stage of neurologic recovery, the time frame is variable, but generally the middle stages can be expected to occur within the first six months. The setting where one finds individuals in the middle stages of recovery is also quite variable, and can range from an acute rehabilitation facility to an outpatient setting or home. In the past several years, acute rehabilitation hospitals have experienced a noticeable decline in admissions, and patients are discharged to their homes earlier than was the case in the 1980s.[50] The home health care field has been reported to be one of the fastest growing rehabilitation industries because of the cost reductions associated.[51] Therefore, therapists may find themselves working independently in an individual's home, and the coordination of multiple services may be lacking. All of the issues discussed below are pertinent to the home setting and to other types of rehabilitation settings.

Monitoring Post-Traumatic Amnesia

The duration of *post-traumatic amnesia* is an important variable to monitor as soon as patients begin showing signs of responsiveness. Initially, post-traumatic amnesia was assessed by testing memory retrospectively; however, the unreliability of patients' recall of the last event prior to the injury, as well as the difficulty in reporting when continuous memory is restored make this a highly subjective method. Several prospective measures have been described, but perhaps the most widely used is the *Galveston Orientation and Amnesia Test (GOAT)*, developed by Levin and colleagues.[52] It is a ten-item questionnaire that asks questions regarding basic biographical information (name, address, place of birth), to determine temporal orientation (time, day, date, month, year), current location, date of admission, how admitted, and last preinjury memory and first postinjury memory. The Galveston test has been criticized for its heavy reliance on temporal orientation, given that a number of hospitalized individuals without brain injuries lose track of time and dates.[53] It has also been criticized for the tendency to underestimate the length of post-traumatic amnesia[54] and for the fact that patients can fail the two memory items yet achieve scores that indicate the resolution of post-traumatic amnesia.[53]

Forrester et al.[53] have proposed an alternative test called the *Julia Farr Centre Post Traumatic Amnesia Scale* which they claim separates memory from orientation questions so that each can be scored separately. Their rationale is that orientation frequently returns before memory and, therefore, it is unnecessary to test memory function in patients who are disoriented. "[G]iven that patients in post-traumatic amnesia have short attention spans and difficulty maintaining concentration, the use of redundant questions should be avoided." The Julia Farr Centre Post Traumatic Amnesia Scale has six orientation questions that concern autobiographical information (name, marital status, children, and occupation), and orientation to place and to the "general passage of time." Once orientation has been determined, the ability to "lay down" new memories can be assessed using a five-item memory scale (memory for a name, gesture, and three pictured objects).

Orientation is a frequent component of treatment at this level and should be facilitated in all activities. Corrigan and associates[55] advocate the use of an orientation group, both to improve orientation and to monitor post-traumatic amnesia. To test for the latter, they use the *Orientation Group Monitoring System (OGMS)*, which has been correlated with the Galveston Orientation and Amnesia Test and tends to yield a longer period of post-traumatic amnesia.[54] The reasons for this variance have to do with the criteria used to determine the resolution of the amnesia. The Galveston test relies on a single score compared to a normative range. The Orientation Group Monitoring System scores seven dimensions of behavior using a one to three rating of correctness. Then subscores are computed for each of these dimensions and are averaged into a weekly aggregate score used to determine clearing of post-traumatic amnesia. The seven cognitive dimensions rated are: orientation to time and place, identification of staff and group peers, associative learning, attention to the activities, episodic recall for events of the preceding day, and the use of environmental cues to facilitate orientation. The advantages of the Orientation Group Monitoring System method would seem to be that it provides a higher degree of certainty that post-traumatic amnesia has ended, because responses are assessed over a longer period, and it is economical in that it can be incorporated into treatment.

The importance of assessing the duration of post-traumatic amnesia is not only that it has been shown to be a good prognostic indicator[52] and a sign of progress when amnesia ended, but also that termination is an indication that new learning can occur, and the focus of intervention can change to incorporate more active learning. An additional reason to take frequent measures of cognitive functions during the acute stage of post-traumatic amnesia is to detect and document cognitive deterioration that may be due to medical complications or medications. The Orientation Group Monitoring System has been found to be a sensitive index to subtle cognitive deterioration associated with medical factors.[56]

During post-traumatic amnesia, it is important that tasks that fall outside of the scope of the individual's attention and memory abilities not be made a routine part of therapy. It serves no purpose to push patients to recall daily events or facts (that is, frequent quizzing) when they are still in post-traumatic amnesia, and it may add to their confusion and lower self-esteem. Clinicians and family members should view themselves more as information providers than information seekers during the acute recovery period.

Agitation

As stated in the opening paragraph, confusion is a hallmark of the middle stages of recovery. Confusion reflects an impairment in attention, which is indeed extremely limited following the emergence from coma and, in many cases, for some time thereafter. Agitation is not a predictable accompaniment to traumatic brain injury. Research in this area indicates a somewhat broad range of incidence. Levin and Grossman[57] studied admissions to a neurosurgical service and found that approximately one third of the patients admitted went through a period of agitation. Other studies[56,58,59] have indicated higher rates of up to 55 percent when the incidence of restlessness and agitation are combined. Corrigan and Mysiw,[56] who reported the highest percentage of agitated patients, concluded, however, that agitation cannot be considered a discrete stage of recovery that all individuals with traumatic brain injury experience. They also noted that agitation was much less likely after post-traumatic amnesia had ended, and was clearly associated with levels of cognitive functioning.

Many agitated patients can participate in structured tasks for brief periods (minutes). Typically, simple activities that require a motor response and have low cognitive demands are best for engaging the patient (for example, matching activities). A few trials may be all the patient can manage before needing to change the task. It may be necessary to follow brief periods of cognitive activity by a ten minute period of "walking the halls" or some other type of physical activity.

When patients are sitting and visibly restless, they should not be forced to remain seated for a "few more minutes," but rather, should be encouraged to stand and walk, if necessary. Individuals with brain injury who are restless are similar to the rest of us who experience restlessness; the need to move is a strong urge. They differ, however, in their ability to inhibit this urge. At this level, it is difficult for restless or agitated individuals to maintain composure, and this should not be an expectation. When restlessness or agitation is obvious, clinicians should be extremely sensitive to the fact that patients' behaviors may be highly unpredictable, and testing the limits of attention should be avoided. When treating individuals who are confused and restless in small treatment settings, the door should remain open. Patients who are restless often can sit for a few minutes at a time but then may suddenly stand and wish to move about. If doors are closed and space is limited when individuals experience the need to move about, restlessness can escalate into agitation or even aggression. Clinicians should be prepared for this possibility in order to act calmly.

Corrigan and Mysiw[56] noted that as patients' confusion level improved, agitation dissipated. Corrigan[60] has developed the *Agitated Behavior Scale* which can be used to evaluate the presence and extent of agitation in patients. This tool is useful in treatment planning because it provides objective data from systematic monitoring of the patient instead of relying on subjective impressions that often vary among staff members. As patients demonstrate a decrease in confusion and restlessness, treatment can take a more structured format.

In the most extreme cases, patients are highly confused, have no memory, and are severely agitated. Although most would argue that pharmacologic interventions that negatively affect cognitive processing and recovery should be avoided, pharmacologic management is not always contraindicated.[59] Agitation can be very disturbing to family members and taxing on staff. Further, extremely agitated individuals are at increased safety risk. As discussed in Chapter Four, medications vary greatly in their sedating effects. Additional research needs to be conducted in this area to determine the beneficial and negative effects of various medications.

Staff play a vital role in helping family members understand and manage agitated states. As role models and comforters, staff can follow and share with families the following "tips" for working with highly confused patients:

- Maintain consistent structure across all disciplines and in the environment.
- Avoid unnecessary change.
- Accompany patients at all times.
- Safeguard against patients' wandering out of the building.
- Alternate periods of activity with periods of rest.
- Be prepared to alternate between cognitive activities and physical activities.
- Do not be confrontational.
- Use unambiguous language.
- Limit choices to two alternatives to promote a sense of control and independence but do not force decisions.
- Do not take verbal or physical aggression personally, if patients display these.

The Treatment Agenda

Structure and Routines

Armed with this information, the clinician can now understand the importance of structure and routine during the middle stage of recovery. One of the most important goals of rehabilitation in the acute stages of recovery is to provide the structure that individuals are unable to self-impose. This implies not merely restructuring patients' rooms, but also restructuring communication, staff and family interactions, task demands, the treatment environment, and so on. The importance of routine also cannot be overemphasized, for two reasons. First, patients need consistency in order to place fewer demands on their cognitive system, and to optimize learning through repetition. Second, staff generally function as a prosthetic memory for patients during this stage. If schedules are unpredictable and staff members change, patients will be presented with confusing information that will serve only to further increase their internal state of confusion. One need only observe a busy physical therapy gym to realize that in a typical day staff often rely on their patients to know where and when their next appointment is. "Uhm. Let's see, Jim, where do you go now? I don't seem to have your schedule." When working with confused individuals, staff must be vigilant about knowing, having, and "sticking to" patients' schedules.

The introduction of external orientation aids to the patient's environment is an important aspect of treatment. The initial goal is not to generate spontaneous use of such aids, but rather to provide individuals with the information necessary to be oriented. Watches/clocks, calendars, schedules, pictures, name tags, and labels should be used routinely with patients in the middle stages of recovery. It is important, however, that patients' rooms not be so cluttered with pictures, calendars, or schedules that salient cues cannot be discerned. Clear, printed labels can be used to identify the location of items, but that should not be overdone.

Patients should be given a logbook (also called a memory notebook, journal, or diary) in which activities and events of the day can be recorded. Initially, recordings are entered by staff and family, but this responsibility should gradually be turned over to the patient, as indicated by clinical improvement. For consistency, team members should decide the nature of the information (for example, highlights or details) to be entered into the logbook and the frequency with which it will be entered (for example, hourly, at mealtime).[61] The logbook should accompany the patient at all times and can include a schedule and pertinent identifying information (for example, name, family members, birth date). In some cases, it may be preferable to provide the patient with a more conspicuous schedule. For individuals in wheelchairs, schedules are often attached to the arm of the chair or to a lap board, but for ambulatory individuals the location of schedules can present a problem. For some individuals a schedule card can be placed in the shirt pocket, but this method requires that all of the person's day clothing have a shirt pocket, and it still requires a search for the card. As a solution to the "search" problem, this author, working with an occupational therapist, devised an arm band with Velcro fasteners and an open pocket which could hold a three by five index card. The patient's schedule was printed on the card, and stickers were used to update the day and date so that it was not necessary to reproduce the card every day. For severely disoriented individuals, aids such as this can prove useful because they are conspicuous and serve to "remind" staff and families as well as the patient.

As has been stated, in the middle stages of recovery, orientation of the patient becomes a primary focus for all therapists. Structured treatment may be carried out in group and individual sessions. Orientation sessions should not be limited to a period of question asking, but rather should provide patients with the level of cuing needed to begin to orient themselves. These treatment sessions should not take place in sterile rooms where cues are unavailable. Throughout the course of the day, most individuals rely on clocks, watches, beepers, calendars, and memo books to "be oriented," and glance out the window to monitor the passage of time. Part, if not all, of orientation treatment should be geared toward helping individuals identify and use these external aids on a routine basis.

During the middle stage of recovery the control and modification of treatment parameters, as discussed in Chapter Six (see Table 6.3) are extremely important. All aspects of treatment should occur along a continuum and include the adjusting of activities from multiple choice to open ended; from simple to complex; from unisensory to multisensory; from one-to-one to small group; from no time requirement to gradually imposed time limits; from familiar, repetitive stimuli to novel stimuli; from no demands on short-term memory and retrieval to independent recall; from no demands on initiation to independent initiation; and so on.[61] Levels of assistance and cuing (for example, maximum verbal assistance with visual cues to maximum verbal assistance without visual cues) can be used to document progress and upgrade goals.

As confusion begins to clear and patients are able to tolerate up to 20 to 30 minutes of activity, attention training using a program such as that of Sohlberg and Mateer may be initiated. The advantage of their program is that the stimuli have been carefully graded, an important variable for treatment at this stage in particular. However, all aspects of the program may not be appropriate, and stimulus items should be carefully evaluated. Training can and should be discontinued if it becomes too taxing for any individual. Certain computer programs that target simple visual reaction time or selective attention may also be used, especially those that have carefully graded stimuli. Visual cancellation tasks are commonly used to address attention at this stage. The use of words, as opposed to letters or symbols, has the advantage of addressing reading at a very basic level and, unless the individual will need to scan letters or symbols for employment, words may be considered more "functional."

Ylvisaker and Urbanzyck[62] stress the importance of activities that "promote reorganization of the semantic knowledge base." The *semantic feature analysis task* developed by Ylvisaker and colleagues[63] is an example of an activity designed to reinforce and tap the organizational aspects of semantic memory. Using a feature analysis guide, individuals (in group or individual sessions) systematically search through memory for various features of a word (concept), such as its physical properties, use, action, and associations. Activities that employ word associations and organizational categories are appropriate to use at this level because the stimuli can be carefully manipulated to meet the needs and level of functioning of the individual. Gillis and Dixon[64] found that, in a population of patients with closed head injury, oppositional associations were easier than either semantic or rhyming associations. It should be noted that activities of this nature may be best represented visually, in order to lower the cognitive demands of the task (that is, items do not have to be retained in short-term memory while making decisions). Clinicians are cautioned, however, that frank reading problems and visual perceptual problems must be ruled out as contributors to poor performance when using printed materials to address word associations, categorization, sequencing, and so forth. Matching activities can assist in ruling out these problems and they make low demands on the patient's attention during the early stages of recovery.

Other types of activities that can be utilized with patients at the acute stage include discrimination of like features among objects (pictured or real) or words, sequencing of common activities or procedures, following simple written directions, reading simple paragraphs to detect key points, and brief note taking. At this stage of recovery, it is imperative that clinicians assume responsibility for the cognitive complexity of stimulus items and treatment activities. This author has found that it is often necessary to modify commercially-available treatment materials (software and workbooks) or to develop appropriate materials from scratch. Frequently, packaged activities target a range of complexity within a single task. Hence, performance cannot be associated with a specific level of stimulus complexity.

Discourse analysis, for the purpose of intervention, may be appropriate for individuals on the high end of progress (that is, no longer in post-traumatic amnesia, purposeful with little confusion and no agitation). During this period, however, the constellation of symptoms will most likely not be stable. Linguistic recovery, on the other hand, can be monitored successfully by means of discourse analysis (refer to Chapter Five). At this stage, treatment of communication in the realm of conversational discourse and pragmatics should be deferred, and the primary focus should be treatment designed to improve attention, orientation, and organization.

Compensatory Strategies

In the early stages of rehabilitation, the use of compensatory strategies (as opposed to aids) is not warranted in most cases, for several reasons. All of the guidelines for compensation training discussed in Chapter Six apply. Frequently, at this stage, individuals do not possess sufficient learning ability to acquire a new strategy, and the extent of cognitive-communicative disability still may be largely unknown as recovery continues. Individuals do not possess the executive skills needed to implement effective strategy usage and may not have the necessary skills to think critically about the type of strategy they would be willing to use, or to forecast its potential use. At this stage, compensation is external and includes environmental modification, modification of communication, and the use of aids.

SUMMARY

The acute rehabilitation period begins with interventions aimed at the prevention of postinjury complications, stimulation of cognitive and cortical activity, and maintenance of the patient's comfort. Rehabilitation may begin as early as the intensive care unit stay, but care must be taken that the patients' medical condition is not disturbed or complicated by movement or excitation. Clinicians working in the intensive care unit must be knowledgeable about the technological supports and monitoring equipment frequently present, and close communication with the medical staff and family members is important.

Sensory stimulation, known as coma stimulation or coma arousal therapy, is controversial. The theoretical and clinical rationales for therapy of this nature were reviewed in this chapter. This included a review of the relevant research from animal studies, theories of the role of the reticular activating system in arousal, and a discussion of the clinical research conducted in this area. Four types of coma intervention were considered: multisensory stimulation, sensory regulation, familiar routines, and structured sensory stimulation.

Confusion is the hallmark of recovery immediately postcoma. Agitation is a frequent, related behavioral symptom, but occurs in less than 50 percent of the population. Thus, it is not necessarily a discrete stage in the recovery from traumatic brain injury. It is a disturbing characteristic, nonetheless, and some guidelines for managing the confused and agitated patient were presented. The importance of structure and routine were emphasized repeatedly, since these are central components of intervention during the early and middle stages of recovery. The treatment of orientation, attention, and organization was discussed as the primary focus of formal therapy during the acute stage of rehabilitation.

REFERENCES

1. Cope DN, Hall K. Head injury rehabilitation: benefit of early intervention. *Archives of Physical Medicine and Rehabilitation.* 1982;63:433–437.
2. Kater KM. Response of head-injured patients to sensory stimulation. *Western Journal of Nursing Research.* 1989;11:20–33.
3. Mitchell S et al. Coma arousal procedure: a therapeutic intervention in the treatment of head injury. *Brain Injury.* 1990;4:273–279.
4. Spettell CM et al. Time of rehabilitation admission and severity of trauma: effect on brain injury outcome. *Archives of Physical Medicine and Rehabilitation.* 1991;72:320–325.
5. Spivak G et al. Effects of intensity of treatment and length of stay on rehabilitation outcomes. *Brain Injury.* 1992;6:419–434.
6. Cowley RS et al. The role of rehabilitation in the intensive care unit. *Journal of Head Trauma Rehabilitation.* 1994;9:32–42.
7. Mackay-Fahan L et al. From shock trauma to community living: acute rehabilitation intervention at Saint Francis Hospital and Medical Center. *Cognitive Rehabilitation.* 1987;6:6–11.
8. Smith GJ, Ylvisaker M. Cognitive rehabilitation therapy: early stages of recovery. In Ylvisaker M (ed). *Head Injury Rehabilitation: Children and Adolescents.* San Diego, CA: College-Hill Press; 1985:275–286.

9. Rosenzweig MR, Bennett EL, Diamond MC. Cerebral changes in rats exposed individually to an enriched environment. *Journal of Comparative and Physiological Psychology.* 1972;80:304–313.

10. Will BE et al. Relatively brief environmental enrichment aids recovery after post weaning brain lesions in rats. *Journal of Comparative and Physiological Psychology.* 1977;91:33–50.

11. Finger S, Stein DG. *Brain Damage and Recovery: Research and Clinical Perspectives.* New York, NY: Academic Press; 1982.

12. Walsh RN et al. Environmentally induced changes in the dimensions of the rat cerebrum. *Developmental Psychobiology.* 1971;4:115–122.

13. Globus D et al. Effects of differential experience on dendritic spine counts in rat cerebral cortex. *Journal of Comparative and Physiological Psychology.* 1973;82:1756–181.

14. Cragg BG. Plasticity of synapses. *British Medical Bulletin.* 1974;30:141–145.

15. Ferchmin PA, Bennett EL, Rosenzweig MR. Direct contact with enriched environment is required to alter cerebral weights in rats. *Journal of Comparative and Physiological Psychology.* 1975;88:360–367.

16. Moore JC. Neuroanatomical considerations relating to recovery of function following brain lesions. In Bach-y-Rita P (ed). *Recovery of Function: Theoretical Considerations for Brain Injury Rehabilitation.* Baltimore, MD: University Park Press; 1980:9–90.

17. Farber SD. *Neurorehabilitation: A Multisensory Approach.* Philadelphia, PA: WB Saunders; 1982.

18. LeWinn EB, Dimancescu MD. Environmental deprivation and enrichment in coma. *Lancet.* 1978;2:156–157.

19. Johnson SM, Omery A, Nikas D. Neurologic aspects of critical care: effects of conversation on intracranial pressure in comatose patients. *Heart and Lung.* 1989;18:56–63.

20. LaPuma J et al. Talking to comatose patients. *Archives of Neurology.* 1988;45:20–22.

21. Radar MA, Alston JB, Ellis DW. Sensory stimulation of severely brain-injured patients. *Brain Injury.* 1989;3:141–147.

22. Turner J, Hinkle J. Motor response study. *Journal of Neuroscience and Nursing.* 1987;19:336–340.

23. Weber PL. Sensorimotor therapy: its effect on electroencephalograms of acute comatose patients. *Archives of Physical Medicine and Rehabilitation.* 1984;65:457–462.

24. Sisson R. Effects of auditory stimulation on comatose patients with head injury. *Heart and Lung.* 1990;19:373–378.

25. Jones R et al. Auditory stimulation effect on a comatose survivor of traumatic brain injury. *Archives of Physical Medicine and Rehabilitation.* 1994;75:164–171.

26. Quine S, Pierce JP, Lyle DM. Relatives as lay-therapists for the severely head-injured. *Brain Injury.* 1988;2:139–149.

27. Ansell BJ, Keenan JE. The Western Neuro Sensory Stimulation Profile: a tool for assessing slow to recover head injured patients. *Archives of Physical Medicine and Rehabilitation.* 1989:70:104–108.

28. Radar MA, Ellis DW. The Sensory Stimulation Assessment Measure (SSAM): a tool for early evaluation of severely brain-injured patients. *Brain Injury.* 1994;8:309–321.

29. Bricolo A, Turazzi S, Giannantonio F. Prolonged posttraumatic unconsciousness: therapeutic assets and liabilities. *Journal of Neurosurgery.* 1980;52:625–634.

30. Rappaport M, Dougherty LM, Kelting DL. Evaluation of coma and vegetative states. *Archives of Physical Medicine and Rehabilitation.* 1992;73:628–634.

31. Radar MA, Alston JB, Ellis DW. Sensory stimulation of severely brain-injured patients. *Brain Injury.* 1989;3:141–147.

32. Pierce JP et al. The effectiveness of coma arousal intervention. *Brain Injury.* 1990;4:191–197.

33. Ellis DW, Rader MA. Structured sensory stimulation. In *Physical Medicine and Rehabilitation: State of the Art Reviews, Vol. 4.* Philadelphia, PA: Hanley and Belfus; 1990:465–477.

34. Mackay LE et al. Early intervention in severe head injury: long-term benefits of a formalized program. *Archives of Physical Medicine and Rehabilitation.* 1992;73:635–641.

35. Wood RL. Critical analysis of the concept of sensory stimulation for patients in vegetative states. *Brain Injury.* 1991;5:401–409.

36. Wood RL et al. Evaluating sensory regulation as a method to improve awareness in patients with altered states of consciousness: a pilot study. *Brain Injury.* 1992;6:411–418.

37. Hebb DO. Drives and the conceptual nervous system. *Psychological Review.* 1955;62:243–254.

38. Gotsick JE, Marshall RC. Time course of the septal rage syndrome. *Physiological Behavior.* 1972;9:685–687.

39. DeRuyter F, Kennedy MR. Augmentative communication following traumatic brain injury. In Beukelman DR, Yorkston KM (eds). *Communication Disorders Following Traumatic Brain Injury: Management of Cognitive, Language and Motor Impairments.* Austin, TX: Pro-Ed; 1991:317–365.

40. Sakai CS, Mateer CA. Otological and audiological sequelae of closed head trauma. *Seminars in Hearing.* 1984;5:157–173.

41. Logemann JA, Pepe J, Mackay LE. Disorders of nutrition and swallowing: intervention strategies in the trauma center. *Journal of Head Trauma Rehabilitation.* 1994;9:43–56.

42. Yorkston KM et al. The relationship between speech and swallowing disorders. *Journal of Head Trauma Rehabilitation.* 1989;4:1–16.

43. Weinstein CJ. Neurogenic dysphagia: frequency, progression and outcome in adults following head injury. *Physical Therapy.* 1983;12:1992–1997.

44. Cherney LR, Halper AS. Recovery of oral nutrition after head injury in adults. *Journal of Head Trauma Rehabilitation.* 1989;4:42–50.

45. Lazarus C, Logemann J. Swallowing disorders in closed head trauma patients. *Archives of Physical Medicine and Rehabilitation.* 1987;68:79–84.

46. Logemann JA. Evaluation and treatment planning for the head-injured patient with oral intake disorders. *Journal of Head Trauma Rehabilitation.* 1989;4:24–33.

47. Mackay LE, Morgan AS. Early swallowing disorders with severe head injuries: relationships between RLA and the progression of oral intake. *Dysphagia.* Abstract. 1993;8:161.

48. Hutchins BF. Establishing a dysphagia family intervention program for head-injured patients. *Journal of Head Trauma Rehabilitation.* 1989;4:64–72.

49. Kennedy MR, DeRuyter F. Cognitive and language bases for communication disorders. In Beukelman DR, Yorkston KM (eds). *Communication Disorders*

TRAUMATIC BRAIN INJURY REHABILITATION

Following Traumatic Brain Injury: Management of Cognitive, Language and Motor Impairments. Austin, TX: Pro-Ed; 1991:123–190.

50. Personal Communication. Staff of The Institute of Rehabilitation and Research and Memorial Health Care System. Houston, TX; January 1994.

51. Personal Communication. Marketing Staff of Orthopaedic and Neurological Rehabilitation, Inc. Los Gatos, CA; October 1994.

52. Levin HS, O'Donnell VM, Grossman RG. The Galveston Orientation and Amnesia Test: a practical scale to assess cognition after head injury. *Journal of Nervous and Mental Disease.* 1979;167:675–684.

53. Forrester G, Encel J, Geffen G. Measuring post-traumatic amnesia (PTA): an historical review. *Brain Injury.* 1994;8:175–184.

54. Mysiw WJ et al. Prospective assessment of posttraumatic amnesia: A comparison of the GOAT and the OGMS. *Journal of Head Trauma Rehabilitation.* 1990;5:65–71.

55. Corrigan JD et al. Reality orientation for brain injured patients: group treatment and monitoring of recovery. *Archives of Physical Medicine and Rehabilitation.* 1985;66:626–630.

56. Corrigan JD, Mysiw WJ. Agitation following traumatic head injury: equivocal evidence for a discrete stage of cognitive recovery. *Archives of Physical Medicine and Rehabilitation.* 1988;87–492.

57. Levin HS, Grossman RG. Behavioral sequelae of closed head injury: quantitative study. *Archives of Neurology.* 1978;35:720–727.

58. Reyes RL, Bhattacharyya AK, Heler D. Traumatic head injury: restlessness and agitation as prognosticators of physical and psychologic improvement in patients. *Archives of Physical Medicine and Rehabilitation.* 1981;62:20–23.

59. Brooke MM et al. Agitation and restlessness after closed head injury: a prospective study of 100 consecutive admissions. *Archives of Physical Medicine and Rehabilitation.* 1992;73:320–330.

60. Corrigan, JD. Development of a scale for assessment of agitation following traumatic brain injury. *Journal of Clinical and Experimental Neuropsychology.* 1989;11:261–277.

61. Haarbauer-Krupa J et al. Cognitive rehabilitation therapy: middle stages of recovery. In Ylvisaker M (ed). *Head Injury Rehabilitation: Children and Adolescents.* San Diego, CA: College-Hill Press; 1985:287–310.

62. Ylvisaker M, Urbanzyck B. Assessment and treatment of speech, swallowing, and communication disorders following traumatic brain injury. In Finlayson MAJ, Garner SH (eds). *Brain Injury Rehabilitation: Clinical Considerations.* Baltimore, MD: Williams and Wilkins; 1994:157–186.

63. Ylvisaker M et al. Topics in cognitive rehabilitation therapy. In Ylvisaker M, Gobble EM (eds). *Community Re-entry for Head Injured Adults.* Boston, MA: College Hill Press; 1987:137–215.

64. Gillis RJ, Dixon MM. Linguistic impairment in closed injured patients: the role of the clinical aphasiologist in assessment and treatment. In Brookshire RH (ed). *Clinical Aphasiology Conference Proceedings.* Minneapolis, MN: BRK Publishers; 1982:308–324.

8

Postacute Rehabilitation and Community Integration

As stated in Chapter Two, postacute rehabilitation may transpire in a variety of setting types, including outpatient clinics, community-based facilities, transitional residential facilities, group homes, or the home of the individual injured. Technically, the term *postacute* refers to services offered to individuals who are no longer in need of acute medical management. The point at which these services begin, however, is quite variable. The postacute stage of rehabilitation may begin for some individuals as early as a few weeks postinjury, or as late as several years postinjury for others. Because of this diversity, postacute settings must either have the flexibility and resources to accommodate a variety of needs, or else must establish specific criteria concerning the skills that must be mastered before one is eligible for the program. (For example, Ben-Yishay's program at New York Medical Center has very specific criteria for admission, including at least one year postinjury). All programs should have criteria based on the type of services offered, the ancillary support that is available, the funding base, and the program's mission. Programs that have the staff and equipment to provide a wide range of services, however, may have fairly broad admission criteria. Additionally, many postacute rehabilitation facilities have several programs within the organization (for example, pediatric, vocational, educational, mild brain injury), and can accommodate a wide range of needs. Acute medical management (in hospitals and free standing rehabilitation facilities) is expensive, and one of the motivations for focusing service delivery at the nonresidential, postacute level is cost containment. It is not unusual for postacute rehabilitation programs to admit individuals who are still confused, and those who are "confusable" are common. Therefore, a high degree of structure must still be maintained for many patients at the postacute stage.

Typically, the "pace" of the postacute setting is more relaxed than that of the acute setting, but the intensity may be greater (that is, the amount of treatment, the nature of family concerns, the nature of relationships both with staff and other patients, the lack of support if the patient is at home, and so on). Clinicians working in postacute settings have been known to say, "This is where the real work gets done." Having been a part of several postacute rehabilitation centers, the author can well understand and appreciate that sentiment.

The permanence of the cognitive and psychosocial impairments begins to appear more "in focus" in the postacute setting than in the earlier stages of recovery, when transitions and improvement can be fairly dramatic. The rate of progress slows, and therapeutic gains appear less obvious. Patients are usually in their homes, or at least have been home for periods of time. Family members and friends begin to realize that, unlike coma, the disability that now confronts them is not one from which the individual will recover. This is not to say that progress does not continue, only that the rate is slowed and gaps in skills become more apparent.

An individual's experience in the acute medical setting will often have a significant influence on the individual's, and the family's, view of postacute rehabilitation. If they viewed the experience as one of success, in an environment of caring and competence, they will usually enter the postacute setting with continued motivation, and with optimism for much more improvement. If, on the other hand, their experiences were unpleasant (beyond the trauma itself), and they think that the staff did not do "everything they could" to speed the recovery process and ensure an optimal outcome, they may come to the postacute setting with anger, hostility, and great skepticism toward all health care professionals. Trust may be slow to develop, and disagreements among staff and family members may arise from the beginning.

It is important for clinicians to realize that, at this stage, families are beginning to experience a great sense of loss, often to a greater extent than the individual injured. A commonly shared opinion among rehabilitation clinicians (although perhaps totally unjustified) is that families frequently think of the drive home from the hospital as the road to full recovery. Family members have been known to make comments along the order of "Once he gets home, I know he will be fine." Often, once individuals do go home, the reality of the disability takes hold. Its severity, and the impact it has on the daily functioning of all family members—not just the individual with a brain injury—becomes apparent. It is this "reality" that clinicians must strive to help the individual and the family manage in the least destructive (that is, dysfunctional) manner possible. Chapter Eleven discusses family issues and needs in greater detail.

GENERAL CONSIDERATIONS FOR THE POSTACUTE PHASE

Regardless of the primary setting, at this stage of rehabilitation, programs should design treatment that constantly keeps in view the community in which the injured individual will have to function, including the academic, work, leisure, and home environments. As noted in previous chapters, there is a strong movement in rehabilitation to progress beyond the stimulus-and-performance-bound (some use the word "sterile") clinical environment, to the more natural, personally relevant environment known as community. Community re-entry programs serve a threefold purpose: to specifically address skills needed for functioning as a community member, to help individuals identify and learn to use available resources in the community of residence, and to enhance community acceptance of persons with traumatic brain injury, through education, observation, and first-hand experience. Although a focus on community re-entry by no means can resolve all of the issues faced by individuals with traumatic brain injury—issues such as independent living, employment, and the need for support networks—it does at least take rehabilitation clinicians in the right direction. Many of the problems of transfer and generalization are lessened because the conceptual distance (between training and the environment) is either eliminated or decreased.

It is perhaps unrealistic to expect a community to automatically accept a new member, particularly if that member is perceived to be different. By the same token, it is also unrealistic to expect that individuals with traumatic brain injury, and their personal support networks (which are often limited to family members), can be "rehabilitated" and then dropped into the community to resume or establish a role. Community re-entry programs can help lessen the distance between acceptance and rejection, as well, merely by being *in* and a *part of* the community.

Several authors[1,2,3] have noted that the use of the word "patient" tends to perpetuate the sick role and a role of helplessness that is counterproductive to the goal of independence. Although the term has been used throughout this text for consistency, it is not the preferred term for this stage of rehabilitation, which should be de-emphasizing a medical focus and emphasizing the "person within a community" focus. Alternate terms have been used, such as "client," "trainee," and "student." However, whenever possible (for example, in reports, team conferences, conversations), the individual's name should be used in preference to any label.

At this stage of rehabilitation, many facilities employ a curriculum-based approach. In such an approach, modules or classes are developed to address specific physical, cognitive, communicative, and psychosocial skills. Modules may be divided further into levels or components. General performance criteria are established for each module or level (for example, before exiting the attention-training module, the individual must achieve 100 percent accuracy on all tasks at level two). Typically, the rate of progress can be tailored to meet individual needs, but the content of the module largely remains the same for all individuals. Although there are innumerable time-saving advantages to a curriculum-oriented approach, for the purposes of preparing treatment materials and tailoring goals, it lacks the flexibility (and often staff resources) to truly individualize treatment objectives.

APPROACHES TO MEMORY IMPAIRMENT

As stated in Chapter Six, there is little support for the use of a stimulation approach to improve memory skills (for example, rehearsal and repetition of lists). Some[4,5] have questioned the use of mnemonics as well, although others[6,7] have reported positive treatment effects using encoding strategies or internal memory aids, such as visual imagery. The use of these strategies does not come without a cost, however, and that cost is in the attentional demands needed to employ the strategy, which may be too great for a number of individuals with a traumatic brain injury. Further, much of the research on the use of mnemonics has been conducted with individuals who have normal or near normal intellectual functions, with the exception of memory.[8] This is no small consideration, given the population of concern here.

Before attempting to teach a particular encoding strategy, the clinician must have knowledge of the patient's learning potential and the nature of the memory impairment. Teaching an encoding strategy to an individual whose memory impairment appears to be the result of faulty retrieval will do little to improve the situation. The clinician also should ascertain if the individual has used other learned strategies spontaneously (that is, generalization). Valuable treatment time can be lost, if these variables are not considered carefully (refer to compensation training in Chapter Six).

If it is decided that the enhancement of encoding via internal memory aids is a worthwhile pursuit, the clinician should choose a strategy that is comprehended easily by the individual. If a great deal of time must be spent explaining the strategy to the individual, then the likelihood that it can be employed successfully decreases. The person's ability to comprehend the strategy will certainly influence the ability to learn the strategy. The same applies to the use of retrieval strategies (for example, alphabet search, retracing one's steps, and visualizing the location of items).

Several unique approaches to memory problems, which have been used with small numbers of patients or single subjects, have been described in the literature. Crosson and Buenning[9] developed an individualized memory retraining program, based on his work needs, for an individual with a closed-head injury. Two important points should be made before describing the study. The authors note that their patient's cognitive abilities might be considered "well above those of many head injured victims," and the retraining program was carried out in the patient's home with the assistance of a friend. The memory task itself involved having the friend read paragraphs to the patient, who was then asked to write down what he could recall following each reading. Four conditions were examined, using four paragraphs; three involved the use of strategies to improve storage and recall, and one was used as a control (that is, no strategy was used). The first paragraph was read, and the individual wrote down as much as he could remember without using a strategy. The second paragraph reading involved the use of the strategy to "make a concentrated effort to listen and remember." The third reading condition involved the use of a mnemonic of the patient's choice (visual imagery was suggested). Then, in the fourth condition, the reader was instructed to stop after every fourth line, when the patient was to ask a question that he thought would help him remember the information. After each paragraph reading, the patient wrote down as much as he could remember. This information was taken to the authors' clinic once a week for analysis. When analyzed, the third and fourth conditions resulted in the greatest amount of recall of main ideas. Although the patient's performance on formal memory testing (the Wechsler Memory Scale) improved, the results were not lasting, and the individual did not employ any strategies in his work setting. This study is illustrative of the nature of much of the research on memory remediation, until recently. The results of improved task performance and test performance, without carry over to other settings, are a consistent finding in the literature when transfer and generalization are investigated.[8]

Wilson[10] has used the *preview, question, read, state, and test (PQRST)* model, originally developed as a study model, to improve encoding and recall in a group of eight patients with traumatic brain injury. She found this method to be "significantly superior to rote recall." This author, also, has used the preview, question, read, state, and test method with students who have had traumatic brain injuries, to assist in reading comprehension and recall, and has found it to be helpful, although experimental studies were not performed.

Lawson and Rice[11] employed a method similar to the one above, which they called *executive strategy training*, to improve verbal learning in a student. The first steps of the procedure involve the patient's recognition that there is a memory problem, followed by the recognition that there are strategies that can be used to aid memory. The specific steps of the executive strategy, which can be written on a card to aid recall, are: (W) what are you asked to do?; (S) select a strategy; (T) try out the strategy; and (C) check out how the strategy is working. In Lawson and Rice's study, the student was trained in the use of several mnemonics, prior to the implementation of executive training. He was able to use the mnemonics with improved recall when prompted, but he did not initiate their use; hence, the need for an executive strategy that could facilitate use. The results of the study were that the executive strategy training improved the student's initiative to use some type of mnemonic, and the effects of training were evidenced over a six-month nontreatment interval.

Glisky and Schacter[12] have employed the *method of vanishing cues* to teach a set of vocabulary items associated with computer use (for example, Save: to store items on a disk) to several individuals with varying degrees of amnesia. Initially, letters are provided until the individual is able to guess the response, and then the letters are reduced gradually until no letter cues are needed to remember the computer command. These authors have reported good success with this method, including individuals who were able "to write simple computer programs, edit them, and perform disk storage and retrieval operations." They also report good retention over long intervals (seven to nine months), and the method has been used successfully to teach an individual how to perform her job. These authors clearly note that this type of training is domain-specific learning, and that even small changes between the original training and the test or implementation condition do affect performance negatively. Applying the learning paradigms introduced in Chapter Six, then, the AB:A'B' paradigm will result in the greatest amount of success using this method of memory training.

Sohlberg and Mateer[4,13] have suggested a three-pronged approach to the management of memory disorders. It includes: attention training, for those impairments that result from impaired attentional processes; prospective memory process training, for those individuals who have difficulty with encoding and recall of information; and compensatory training, for those individuals with severe residual memory impairment. (The use of memory notebooks is discussed below.) Their approach to attentional training has been described in Chapter Six, where it was emphasized that attentional problems may underlie memory problems for a number of persons with traumatic brain injury. Their approach to frank memory problems consists of the systematic training of *prospective memory (PROMPT)*. The goal of this approach is "to extend systematically the amount of time an individual is able to remember to carry out specified tasks."[4,13] They begin by giving an individual a simple task (for example, clap your hands) to carry out at a specified time (for example, in five minutes). The time between task assignment and performance is gradually extended in two-minute intervals. They claim some initial success using this approach, evidenced by an increase in the length of time to 15 minutes for three subjects, and improved scores on a standardized memory test.

Memory Notebooks

There are no data to suggest the number of individuals with traumatic brain injury who use memory notebooks (a term used generically here to refer to any type of calendar or scheduling system). Most patients, however, will be given a notebook to use at some point. Although in the acute settings, standard notebooks (for example, three-ring binders) may be used and may be accepted, the sooner an individual can select an organizer of personal choice, the greater the likelihood that it will be accepted for long-term use. In the acute stages of rehabilitation, the memory notebook largely serves as a mechanism to aid orientation, and clinicians assume a great deal of responsibility for helping patients locate information and make entries. As stated in the previous chapter, the spontaneous use of a notebook in the early stages is not expected, because of the patient's general confusion. In the postacute setting, however, the terminal goal is spontaneous use, and the patient's awareness of the need for a memory aid becomes a critical factor in training. "If the client is reluctant to use this type of device, owing to decreased awareness of deficits, decreased motivation or inability to foresee advantages in its use, reality testing of functional memory skills without such a tool is recommended."[14] Reality testing means assisting individuals in the recognition of the impact that a memory disorder has on everyday functioning, by carefully demonstrating instances of failed memory in the context in which they occur. Care must be taken not to embarrass or devalue patients during this process. If an individual recognizes the need for some type of memory "help," then memory notebook training may begin immediately, if deemed appropriate.[14]

The contents of memory notebooks or organizers designed by professionals are generally the same; they include sections such as autobiographical information, calendar, to do list, daily log, assignments, diary or feelings, and names/addresses. Like the physical appearance of the notebook, the interior also should be "personalized" and designed to meet the needs of each individual.[15] Although there is a temptation to include in notebooks everything the individual might want to remember, in many cases this temptation should be resisted. Organizational problems, as well as memory problems, contribute to the ineffective use of notebooks. Notebooks that become too cluttered with information, or have too many sections, may actually result in decreasing the individual's functioning. Before designing a notebook, a priority list of the most important contents should be developed. Too often, the most important question is not asked critically enough: What does the individual need to remember?

Behavioral reinforcement is an important component to memory notebook training. If the individual does not receive reinforcement for its use, more likely than not, it will not be used. Natural success, of course, offers the greatest amount of reinforcement; however, until this is likely, clinicians must take care always to reinforce any spontaneous use of a notebook. Shaping procedures (Chapter Six) may be beneficial in notebook training, in the following manner. An individual first might be reinforced for bringing the aid to each treatment session, then for opening the aid or attempting to locate information, even if the search fails. This should be followed by reinforcement for locating certain types of information (perhaps starting with the date) and then by gradually increasing the amount of information to be located. Several authors[14,15,16] have reported success in memory notebook training.

Sohlberg and Mateer[16] have employed a three-stage approach to memory notebook training that is based on learning theory and relies heavily on procedural learning. The three stages are acquisition, application, and adaptation. The *acquisition* stage involves systematic training in the contents and purpose of the notebook. They use a question/answer format for this stage (for example, What are the five sections in your notebook? What is the "to do" list for? Where do you schedule appointments?). During the *application* stage, role-play situations are used to provide individuals with opportunities to employ the notebook. The final stage, *adaptation*, involves the use of the notebook within the community. The authors established proficiency levels at each stage that had to be reached before an individual could move from one stage to the next. They also developed a four-point scoring system that can be used at the application and adaptation stages. The four scores are: "4, spontaneously and accurately recorded information in appropriate sections; 3, needed cuing for what to write in each section but identified appropriate sections; 2, needed minimal cuing for what sections should be utilized; 1, needed maximum cuing for both what and where to write."

One of the major shortcomings in training individuals to use a memory notebook lies with clinicians, and not with the individuals themselves. Too often, patients are given notebooks with little instruction and then examined for their ability to use them spontaneously. Several authors[4,14,15,16] have stressed the importance of teaching individuals *about* the memory notebook. "Memory book training should include a thorough orientation to the book, development of a system to keep the book close to the individual, learning how to write meaningful information, and development of a system of consistent referral to the book."[14] Because of the slowed rate of learning that is a frequent consequence of traumatic brain injury, numerous sessions may need to be devoted to the orientation of the memory system alone. In a case study presented by Sohlberg and Mateer,[4] one subject required "17 program days" devoted to the acquisition stage of notebook training.

IMPROVING PROBLEM SOLVING AND EXECUTIVE FUNCTIONS

Problem-Solving Models

A number of problem-solving models can be used to teach patients how to approach and solve various problems. The approach does not have to be limited to crisis-type problem situations or to problems in routine daily activities, but can serve as a framework from which to view any number of situations. A model provides a systematic method for analyzing information in a step-by-step fashion, so that it may actually serve to promote understanding at a more global level. Additionally, problem solving occurs throughout the day, so models should not be used only in the "problem solving group" or a specific treatment activity. Rather, the most immediate feedback and sense of success occurs when the model can be applied to situations as they arise.

The model used by Ben-Yishay and his colleagues[17] was presented as an example in Chapter Six. It is a six-stage model that begins with the *formulation of the problem* as it occurs within a context. The second step involves the *analysis of the conditions* of the problem, followed by the *formulation of a strategy or plan* for solving the problem. Step four involves *choosing the tactics to employ* and then *executing the plan* or putting the solution into place. Following the solution, there must be a *comparison of the solution with the problem*—that is, "Did the solution work?"

Ylvisaker and colleagues[18] have proposed a similar model, or step ap-proach, to problem solving, which refines the process a bit by breaking down the cycle further. They incorporate nine steps that begin with *identifying the problem*, then *classifying the problem*, followed by *identifying the goal*. This third step is an important one from the standpoint of motivation. The third step seeks to define what will be gained by solving the problem. It is certainly an acceptable response if the motivation is merely the satisfaction of finding a solution to the problem. However, more often than not, people solve prob-lems because there is a functional gain. For example, referring back to Jane in Chapter Five, if she can determine how to operate the coffee machine, she will be able to have a fresh cup of coffee. Now, for anyone who is a coffee addict, there is the motivation.

Step four requires that the individual *identify information that is relevant* to solving the problem. This is important in helping individuals determine if they in fact have all the necessary information to develop an effective solution. Careful analysis at this stage can obviously save time by preventing the pursuit of "hit and miss" solutions. Steps five and six require *identifying the possible solutions* to the problem and then *evaluating the solutions* in terms of their pros and cons and potential effectiveness. Next is the *determining of the best solution* from the possibilities generated in step five and analyzed in step six. Based on this choice, a *plan is developed to implement the solution*. The final step, nine, is identical to the last step in Ben-Yishay's model, and requires the *evaluation of the results* and the individual's personal satisfaction with the solution applied and its effectiveness.

This author has used a similar model of problem solving, taken from the work of Bransford and Stein[19], and referred to as the IDEAL approach. The use of the acronym has proved helpful in aiding individuals who have difficulty recalling the steps to a model. The first step, common to all models, is *identifying the problem (I)*. The next stage involves *defining the problem (D)*, which is similar to analyzing the conditions or characterizing the problem, in the above models. Bransford and Stein have discussed how differently individuals may conceive a problem. To illustrate this point, they use the example of grease splattering when bacon is fried. Many people can identify this as a problem, but it may be conceptualized, or defined, in different ways: the heat is too high, and therefore the grease splatters; or, hot liquids, such as grease, can burn people. The first definition might lead to the reduction of heat as a solution, and the second to the use of long, heat-resistant gloves to avoid being burned. Sometimes helping individuals conceptualize the nature of problems in a variety of ways (divergent thinking) is a useful step in improving problem-solving abilities.

The next step in the IDEAL model is *exploring alternative approaches (E)*, equivalent to step five in Ylvisaker's model. This stage includes not only the consideration of options, but also an analysis of how the individual is "reacting" to the problem (for example, "let me out of this situation"). The final stages to the model are *acting on the plan (A)* and *looking at the effects (L)*, which are identical to the latter steps in both the other models discussed above.

It is important to understand that problem solving is both a dynamic process and a cycle. All of the steps to problem solving (regardless of the model) may have to be repeated several times before an effective solution is reached, or only one or two steps may have to be repeated. Some individuals may have difficulty at a particular stage of problem solving, in which case breaking that stage down into even smaller steps may be necessary. For example, if someone has difficulty generating multiple solutions for consideration, it may be necessary to help the patient think of similar problems and how they were solved.

In problem solving, or any "high-level" cognitive process, a deficit in other component processes may underlie the difficulty with problem solving or high level ability. Some[4,20] have suggested that remediation should therefore attack the underlying process, which presumably will affect change in the higher level skill. This would be classified as direct training of the underlying process and indirect training of the problem-solving ability.[18] To refer back to the models and approaches to rehabilitation, this is a reductionistic approach. From a functional perspective, one could argue that if training an individual to employ a problem-solving model in fact allows the individual to solve problems with greater ease and proficiency, then treatment is effective. In practice, however, it may be necessary to address several factors that contribute to problem-solving deficiencies simultaneously (for example, attention and the ability to approach problems systematically).

Sohlberg and Mateer[4] have outlined a model for the assessment and treatment of reasoning and problem solving that proceeds from the comprehensive assessment of cognitive process areas (attention, memory, visual processing, language, executive functions, and reasoning/problem solving) to the treatment of the basic or "fundamental" processes (for example, attention, memory, and language), which is followed by comprehensive retesting to determine the effects of treatment. Additional treatment of basic processes is provided, if indicated, before moving to the treatment of problem solving and reasoning, and/or executive functions, again followed by retesting. If performance objectives have been met, treatment progresses to address reasoning, problem solving, and/or executive functions. Treatment is followed by retesting, and can be reinstated at this level, if performance objectives have not been met.

For individuals who progress quickly, this model has a certain degree of appeal; however, for those who do not progress quickly, and who show a splintering among basic skills, the approach becomes less functional. The "recycling" of treatment and assessment until objectives are achieved under each basic process area can be both time consuming and costly. If processes are improved during highly structured tasks, is this improvement transferable to the performance of daily activities? It is this "transferability" that comes into question. These approaches must be carefully evaluated, again with the clinical eye always on the "expected" range of activity of any individual (refer to Chapter Six).

If attentional problems are evident and deemed not to be remediable through direct intervention, part of training in other skill areas will need to incorporate attention compensation training. Individuals do not spontaneously use strategies to remain focused unless there is adequate recognition that attention may be less than optimal for the successful completion of tasks. Much awareness training of attentional processes must be incorporated into treatment, beginning with the ability to identify instances of performance breakdown that may be attributable to fluctuations in attention. Persons may have to be taught "self-talk" compensatory strategies for their attentional problems, in order to stay focused long enough to complete each step in a problem-solving model. (For example, "I need to pay attention. Step one hasn't been completed yet. I'm drifting. Refocus. Step two hasn't been completed yet.") In reality, many of us must use "self-focusing" strategies when we perceive our attention to be drifting.

For many individuals, it is necessary to break problem solving down, as a mental process, into aspects of the process. For example, the ability to consider multiple solutions to a problem involves divergent thinking. Individuals who are in the early stages of postacute rehabilitation may benefit first from treatment using simple divergent thinking activities. A simple divergent thinking task, familiar to all speech-language pathologists, is that of trying to think of as many items in a particular category as possible. Executing a plan to solve a problem often involves several steps. Simple sequencing activities may be employed to assist individuals in this area, if they are not yet ready to learn a multistep problem-solving model.

In reality, the various aspects of cognition cannot be thought of as isolated processes, but various aspects can be approached in a systematic manner. As isolated processes, they are not truly hierarchical in terms of complexity. All aspects of cognition can move quickly to a "higher" level of thinking simply by altering the complexity of the task. For example, a simple divergent thinking task, such as listing items within a category, may be easier than a problem-solving activity that requires a novel solution. Yet, a more difficult divergent task of the same type (for example, listing as many items as you can that are like a cloud), can be more difficult than a simple problem-solving task (for example, Jack had two pennies. Sue gave him another one. How many does he have now?). Again, the clinician is reminded of the importance of understanding the parameters of treatment and knowing how to modify them. There are, however, few norms for tasks such as divergent thinking, verbal analogies, proverb interpretation, and deductive reasoning.

One should never assume that tasks used in therapy can be completely distilled to represent a single process that can be taught. Everything one does relies upon knowledge that results from experience, whether that experience be educational, vocational, or practical. Even if an individual exhibits problems that can be isolated to a particular area, it does not follow that tasks requiring that ability will automatically be suitable for treatment. As an example, consider Mr. Jones, who is a carpenter and demonstrates problems in analogical reasoning, and who has a therapist who decides to address the problems by using verbal analogies as part of treatment. The therapist may begin with simple analogies, such as "up is to down as high is to ???" (low), or "tall is to short as giant is to ???" (dwarf or midget). Perhaps Mr. Jones is able to solve the first analogy and not the second, but with enough practice reaches 80 or 90 percent accuracy at this level. So, the clinician upgrades the difficulty level, and Mr. Jones is able to solve some of the harder analogies, such as "low is to high as basement is to ???" (roof), but is unable to solve others, such as "door is to house as ??? (valve) is to heart." One might assume that if Mr. Jones has learned the process of analyzing the relationships between the first two items, in order to solve an analogy problem, he should be able to solve many problems at this level. However, a heart valve may be unfamiliar to Mr. Jones, and one should question the utility of employing treatment activities that fall outside of his premorbid knowledge base. In other words, there is more to solving verbal analogies than the process of analogical reasoning. To use this type of activity to Mr. Jones's full advantage, the clinician should choose stimulus items that have the greatest relevance to Mr. Jones's personal experience and needs (that is, using carpentry terms if verbal analogies are to be used in treatment). This idea seems straightforward enough, of course, but often it is given little consideration in the course of a busy treatment day. The lack of individualization is one of the major drawbacks to using commercially available treatment materials, and to using a specified curriculum with all "like" patients.

Targeting Executive Functions

For some individuals the difficulties experienced in problem solving may be attributable to poor planning and self-monitoring, or to problems in initiation. The remediation of executive functions, like that of other areas of impairment, requires a systematic approach in which multiple practice opportunities are provided, and reinforcement is applied consistently. Problems in executive control are most readily apparent in natural contexts that lack the organization and structure provided by the clinic setting and the rehabilitation staff. Ylvisaker and Szekeres[21] have indicated that the rehabilitation setting often is a significant obstacle to the daily, natural use and practice of executive skills. "There is a natural tendency of institutions, including schools, to program and structure the affairs of patients or students to such an extent that the individual's executive functioning is taken over by the staff." The intervention for impairments in executive functioning begins with the involvement of individuals in their own program (that is, setting their own goals, planning activities for themselves, and solving their own problems).

Both specific and general treatment strategies for the management of executive control problems have been proposed in the literature, although it must be noted that this is a relatively new treatment arena. The problem-solving models discussed above, and the executive strategy program used by Burke and colleagues,[14] rely on executive functions for success and, at the same time, target executive skills. Awareness and goal setting begin the cycle with the recognition that there is some task to be accomplished (for example, "I want to solve this problem." "I want to remember this information."). Initiation is required to use any strategy effectively and independently. Self-monitoring and regulation of the process, as well as monitoring the results, are indicated in all the models discussed. Although problem solving may be conceptualized as a single process, each of these areas of executive functioning may need to be targeted specifically in treatment.

Initiation, particularly if severely impaired, may be one of the most difficult areas to treat effectively.[21] When severe problems in initiation are observed, environmental restructuring that optimizes natural cues may be the best treatment approach.[21,22,23] Typically, mild to moderate problems in initiation are treated through the use of some type of external cue that serves as a signal to respond or perform some particular activity (for example, a watch alarm or a timer). Sohlberg and colleagues[24] have reported being able to increase the verbal initiation of a patient during group conversations by cuing the individual periodically to ask himself if he was initiating. They did not assess generalization. It is not known if external cues can become internalized over time in this population, but this is an important area to study for functional outcomes. Most clinicians who use external cuing strategies have an optimal goal that internalization of the strategy will occur.

Problems in *planning* can be addressed in a number of ways. Simple sequencing and categorization tasks can provide a starting point, for the purposes of assessment and treatment. Since organization is an important aspect of planning, these activities serve as prerequisites to more complex, multistage organizational tasks. There are many underlying components to organization and planning that should be considered as well. As an example, the successful organization of a complex task, or several simple tasks, requires the ability to divide attention among different aspects, at least momentarily; sustain attention without distraction until certain steps are complete; remember previous steps; monitor strategies for effectiveness, and so on. The completion of tasks within specified times is another aspect of planning that can be systematically addressed by imposing time constraints. Time estimation activities, as well as estimation of ability to accomplish a task, are components of planning, and are useful ways to break down planning as a global process into more manageable components. The estimation of ability is also a technique that can be employed to help individuals in the area of *self-evaluation*. Initially, simple concrete activities should be used to demonstrate the concept.[21] For example, an individual may be asked to estimate how many plastic rings he/she can toss onto a hook. During activities of this nature, *self-monitoring* can be addressed by asking individuals to give an appraisal of how well they think they are doing. If they are not doing well, they can be asked to think of a strategy to improve performance (that is, self-regulation). Individuals may experience personally relevant practice in planning by being given the responsibility for planning a day's treatment or a single session.

At a basic level, self-evaluation and monitoring can be addressed through any number of error detection and error correction activities, with the understanding that the ability to detect errors precedes the ability to make corrections. Simple spelling and arithmetic worksheets can be used for this purpose. Activities of this nature are relatively easy to control for complexity and can be systematically upgraded. They have proven to be particularly useful for students who must check their work for errors of this sort. Similarly, tasks that approximate or simulate an individual's projected work assignments can be used to improve the self-evaluation and monitoring of specific behaviors in the work setting. Many individuals may need to be taught "self-check" strategies through intense, repetitive training and with the use of an external signal (for example, every time the beeper sounds, check work). The charting and graphing of performance variables also can be used to help individuals focus on their responses and behaviors through the evaluation of performance.[21]

The ongoing monitoring of executive functioning in everyday activities is more difficult to address. To be effective, all strategies designed to improve executive functioning must be practiced to the point of habituation. Table 8.1 provides examples of places within a community where problem solving and executive functions can be targeted. As is the case with all skills, generalization must be specifically targeted, and monitored practice outside of the clinic must occur. Family members and significant others need to be carefully trained to cue, monitor, and reinforce any strategies the individual is expected to use beyond the clinical setting. Training cannot occur in a vacuum if it is to be successful.

Table 8.1
Examples of Places Within a Community for
Running Errands.

Bank	Grocery Store
Barber Shop/Hair Salon	Hardware Store
Book Store	Laundromat
Card Shop/Party Goods Store	Library
Discount Department Store	Mall
Dry Cleaners	Medical Clinic
Drug Store	Office Supply Store
Electronics Store	Outdoor Market
Fast Food/Restaurant	Paint Store
Florist/Flower Shop	Picture Framing Shop

COMMUNICATION

Reading and Writing

At this stage of rehabilitation, reading and writing are often the focus of
the speech-language pathologist's treatment, either by direct intervention of
reading and writing skills or by using tasks that require reading and writing.
For example, reasoning skills frequently are addressed with treatment materials that require individuals to draw inferences from a written story or
problem. Clinicians should not assume that intact basic reading and writing
skills (such as, letter and word identification and production, word attack, or
even paragraph comprehension and production) indicate functional reading
and writing for a particular individual. As previously stated, reading and
writing are complex cognitive activities. Good reading comprehension and
written expression at the multiple paragraph level or even complex single
paragraph level require focused attention, the ability to draw upon stored
information, the ability to understand sequences, the ability to retain new
information, the ability to draw inferences, and so on. They also require
vocabulary knowledge and knowledge of the rules of language. Individuals
with traumatic brain injury may experience breakdowns in any of these
abilities and knowledge bases, or in all of them.

As would be expected, students (anyone engaged in educational pursuits)
have the greatest needs for reading and writing. Therefore, it is essential that
clinicians thoroughly investigate high-level (beyond simple paragraphs)
reading and writing skills in this population. In adults who work, job
demands and interests should be evaluated in order to determine an
individual's reading and writing needs.

There are a number of variables regarding reading and writing skills that
clinicians must consider, particularly with adults. Clinicians must establish
the individual's premorbid reading and writing abilities. It is not enough to

determine if the individual could read or write before the injury. Grade levels should be established, as should the frequency with which the person enjoyed and engaged in reading and writing activities. This is not only important for accurate assessment but also for effective treatment planning. Individuals who do not customarily read or write for leisure, and have few reading and writing demands in the work or home environment, should not be engaged in high-level reading and writing treatment activities because we as clinicians think these are worthwhile skills.

Numerous tests and reading materials are available that utilize graded reading materials. (Several have been listed by Nelson and Schwentor.[25]) Many are controlled for important variables such as length, complexity of ideas, vocabulary, and topic and provide measurements of reading rate. In the author's experience, reading rate often is reduced following a traumatic brain injury, and it is important to establish a baseline reading rate through formal assessment. It is often necessary for clinicians to explore commercially available educational materials versus those from the clinical arena to address reading and writing skills in the most effective manner. For those clinicians who work with a large number of patients who have needs for functional reading and writing skills, a library of graded materials that are controlled for the above mentioned variables should be developed. Remember, functional means the expected activity of the individual and should not be limited to the reading and writing demands of simple activities of daily living (that is, signs, menus, phone books, television guides, et cetera) unless indicated.

Discourse

Several scales or inventories have been developed or adapted for the purpose of assessing and monitoring pragmatic behaviors or conversational discourse. A sample of these is provided in Table 8.2. Although variations exist among scales, each is designed to tap similar aspects of communication behaviors. These include: variety of speech acts or language uses; selection, initiation, maintenance, and termination of topic; turn taking and interruptions; repair and revision; lexical selection and syntax; cohesion; intelligibility and fluency; and facial expression, eye gaze, gestures, body posture, and proximity. As with other aspects of an individual's functioning, communication assessment and intervention should not be limited to the treatment session specifically designed to address the problem (for example, communication group) but should be dynamic and should occur in a variety of settings (for example, in other groups, during nontreatment activities such as lunch, outside of the clinical setting in the community and home).

Although there are several studies that have documented the nature of communication impairment following traumatic brain injury, as was indicated in Chapter Five, few studies have been conducted on the effectiveness

Table 8.2
Published scales for rating communication behaviors.

Communication Scale	Source
Communication Performance Scale	Ehrlich J, Sipes A. 1985[26]
Conversational Rating Scale	Ehrlich J, Barry P. 1989[27]
Pragmatic Protocol	Prutting C, Kirchner D. 1987[28]
Pragmatic Inventory for Brain Injury	Kennedy M, DeRuyter F. 1990[29]

of treatment to improve discourse or pragmatic behaviors in this population. In working on communication behaviors, clinicians must avoid the tendency to address too many issues at one time (for example, topic maintenance, turn taking, and proximity). If too many treatment variables are introduced, it becomes difficult to apply reinforcement or shaping techniques (refer to Chapter Six). One solution to this dilemma is to develop subgroups to address particular communication behaviors that a few patients have in common (for example, a topic maintenance group or a turn-taking group). This provides a mechanism for addressing several behaviors during the course of rehabilitation without compromising a clear focus for each session by the introduction of multiple variables. Still, there must be a limit to the number of skills that can be addressed at any one time, and priorities must be established.

Additionally, behavioral strategies are not applied only during a single group or individual session. Rather, to optimize learning, reinforcement should be applied whenever the desired behavior occurs. This necessitates limiting the number of behaviors that can be addressed at any one time by the whole team. For example, if an individual interrupts others whenever engaged in conversation *and* switches topics in midstream, but the interruptions are determined to be the more irritating of the two behaviors, interruptions could be targeted by the entire team, but topic maintenance would be targeted only in specified groups. It is extremely important to establish priorities of "needs" at the postacute stage of rehabilitation. Those behaviors and skills that have the greatest impact on the individual's goals for community re-entry must be placed at the top of the list.[30]

Many of the strategies designed to improve executive functions and problem solving are applicable to communication skills, particularly when communication problems are the result of impaired executive functioning, as they often are. For example, excessive verbalization may be viewed as a problem in the self-monitoring and regulation of verbal output. To improve upon this behavior, there first must be awareness, although, it is possible that the behavior could be extinguished through *carefully applied* behavioral techniques with little awareness from the patient of the extent of the impairment. The awareness of excessive verbalization could be approached through a process similar to error detection using audio or video recordings. Initially all verbalizations of all conversational partners should be tallied, so as to draw comparisons between speakers and to establish a baseline with the patient from which to work. Once the individual understands that his or her verbalization is greater than that of others, a goal can be established for reducing the frequency of utterances within a specified time period (for example, 15 minutes). Initially, the clinician may need to provide an external cue to signal "too much talking." Other communication behaviors that lend themselves to frequency counts can be managed in this manner (for example, interruptions, annoying interjections, idiosyncratic and distracting facial expressions, and excessive questioning).

Because communication is dynamic and interactional, group therapy and the use of video recordings become indispensable means for addressing communication breakdown. Each of these is discussed in the following sections. Video recordings are virtually essential to training individuals to recognize the nonverbal communication signals of others. Although initial training may be done with facial expressions and pictures, the antecedent behavior that elicits the nonverbal response is not available. In conversational discourse, it is the antecedent behavior that often is the true focus of intervention. In other words, the behavior that provokes a nonverbal signal of boredom, confusion, displeasure, or irritation from others is the behavior in need of modification. Often, the identification of the nonverbal behaviors of others merely serves as evidence, or as a way to demonstrate to patients, that something about their communication behavior is offensive to others.

THE USE OF VIDEO RECORDINGS IN TREATMENT

Working with individuals who have traumatic brain injuries frequently gives rise to memory disputes over any number of events. Because many individuals with traumatic brain injury have poor awareness, in addition to faulty memories, the verification of information and of the course of events is often problematic. Video recordings have a distinct advantage over live interactions, in that they provide "evidence" that certain behaviors occurred, and provide a record of how events emerge, unfold, and end. Recordings can be rewound to pinpoint disputed events, and there is less reliance on memories that may be faulty, and that will, in most cases, favor each of the independent participants to the exclusion of the others. For example, John, Marie, and Nancy are having a conversation. A communication breakdown occurs because John does not follow turn-taking rules. Specifically, he is unable to detect nonverbal signals (for example, eye gaze, shoulders raised, hand motions, forward posture) and verbal signals (for example, frank statements such as "Wait, I'm not through yet," and "Don't interrupt," or stallers such as "and . . . ," "I think . . . ," "but . . . ," "well . . . maybe . . .") used by a speaker who wishes to maintain the floor (continue talking). Marie discontinues talking altogether, and Nancy excuses herself from the conversation and leaves. When reviewing this interaction from memory, Nancy may remember that John was rude and cut her off, so she left. Marie may remember that no one ever let her speak, and John will probably remember that no one would let him have a turn unless he interrupted. A video recording of that particular scenario would offer the opportunity for all members to review and critique each other's behaviors *as they occurred.*

Video recordings can offer incredible time savings in the clinical setting. Video cameras that can be mounted in group treatment areas tend to become part of the fixtures and less conspicuous. Hall-mounted cameras or cameras placed in common areas (for example, kitchen/dining, lounge) offer the advantage of capturing "candid" events and natural interactions that can be used to address transfer and generalization. Often, patients do not recognize the relevance of therapy sessions (group or individual) to problems they may face outside of the clinical setting. The step between "this happened in the clinic, so it could happen in the grocery store or on the job" is too large for many individuals to make. A common scenario in working with individuals who wish to return to work is convincing them that inappropriate behaviors and interactions risk their ability to obtain and maintain employment. Candid video recordings of natural interactions can assist in bridging the gap for patients between clinic observations and real world behaviors. Before making any recordings, however, clinicians must take care to ensure that proper releases have been obtained from all concerned. Permission to record for therapeutic purposes only can usually be obtained as part of the admissions paperwork. It should be explained, however, that other staff and patients will view the recordings and comment on them, as part of treatment. The ethical considerations in the use of video recordings are discussed in Chapter Ten. Additionally, many individuals are uncomfortable being recorded or viewed by others on tape. Before group recordings are made or shown, it may be necessary to familiarize individuals with the process and its purpose by using recordings of others (therapists for example), and then recordings of the individual with trusted friends or staff.

Video cameras and recorders have become such popular home equipment items that it is now relatively easy to obtain a library of recordings in addition to those produced in the clinical setting. Recordings from outside the therapy setting, either television recordings or live recordings of non-patient interactions (for example, a therapist's family reunion, wedding ceremony, or birthday party), can serve to motivate patients by using recordings of interest to either an individual or the group. For example, a communication group could choose a particular television show from which they would like to critique conversations and learn conversational rules. This not only increases interest level but also helps patients to understand that the skills they are addressing in therapy *are* important in the real world (not to imply that television necessarily represents the real world).

GROUP THERAPY AND COTREATMENT

Although group therapy can be conducted in the acute phase of rehabilitation, problems in attention and confusion limit the usefulness of this format. In the postacute setting, group therapy is not only a mechanism for providing peer support and feedback, but also a necessary way to address conversational skills. However, when groups are not planned carefully, with clear objectives, or when too many members are included, they can become unruly and time-wasting. Any group or group activity should have the following: criteria for the types of problems to be addressed, specific objectives for the group and for each member, an optimum number of members, a specified leader, and an environment that is without distractions and conducive to the goals of the group. Sohlberg and Mateer[4] and Hartley[31] have reviewed the functions of a group leader; therefore, they will not be reviewed again here.

Although conversational groups may be the most familiar to the speech-language pathologist, any number of groups can be formed, as long as the above conditions have been met. Many facilities primarily conduct therapy in a group format, however, in the author's opinion, the group format should be a supplement to the individual therapy needed by so many individuals with traumatic brain injury. Table 8.3 provides a list of examples of some of the types of groups that can be conducted in a postacute setting, with the community in mind.

The postacute setting affords many opportunities for cotreatment among therapists, not merely for the purpose of having several members focus on one goal, but more importantly, for the purpose of addressing several skills

Table 8.3
Types of Groups for Community Re-entry.

Type: Orientation
Purpose: reinforce the use of compensatory aids for memory and orientation, and facilitate the organization of information needed to perform daily, weekly, or monthly activities.
Focus: reviewing schedules, reviewing previous day's activities for pertinent information, making appointments, organizing memory notebook or organizer

---

Type: Problem Solving
Purpose: develop problem-solving skills for daily activities
Focus: identifying problems, learning and applying a problem-solving model, predicting likely consequences, considering multiple solutions

---

Table 8.3 (continued)
Types of Groups for Community Re-entry.

Type: Psychosocial Adjustment
Purpose: develop skills to improve the adjustment to disability
Focus: understanding nature of brain injury and relationship to current
  functioning, expressing feelings, identifying strengths, identifying coping
  strategies, discussing feelings of others, offering support, acknowledging
  support

Type: Behavior Management
Purpose: develop strategies to identify and manage inappropriate behaviors
Focus: understanding behavioral paradigm (antecedent, behavior, consequence),
  identifying antecedents for individual responses, identifying inappropriate
  behavioral responses, discussing consequences of inappropriate behaviors for the
  individual and others, identifying strategies to improve management of
  inappropriate behaviors

Type: Communication
Purpose: develop conversational skills
Focus: understanding communication intent, introducing topics, taking turns,
  maintaining topic, using and interpreting nonverbal communication, restating
  and rephrasing ideas, summarizing, asking for clarification

---

Type: Career Awareness
Purpose: develop an awareness of employment fields and job requirements
Focus: reading job and career descriptions, making phone inquiries, interviewing
  employed persons, defining strengths and weaknesses relative to employment,
  understanding various job requirements

Type: Job Skills
Purpose: develop skills needed to obtain employment
Focus: writing inquiry letters, resumes, and cover letters, reading advertisements,
  completing job applications, interviewing

Type: Job Communication
Purpose: develop communication skills for the workplace
Focus: following and giving directions in work settings or work-related tasks,
  receiving feedback and criticism, expressing complaints, talking with
  supervisors, talking with coworkers, taking and delivering messages,
  communicating with the public

Type: Leisure Skills
Purpose: develop an awareness of leisure and the skills needed to enjoy leisure
  pursuits
Focus: discussing preinjury leisure lifestyle, identifying benefits of leisure,
  identifying leisure interests, identifying barriers to leisure and strategies to
  overcome them, planning leisure activities

Type: Money Management
Purpose: develop calculation and budgeting skills to manage money

Table 8.3 (continued)
Types of Groups for Community Re-entry.

Focus: calculating money, writing checks, balancing a checkbook, making change, developing a budget, estimating costs of goods and services, evaluating resources, making purchases

---

Type: Meal Planning and Preparation
Purpose: develop skills needed to prepare meals
Focus: reading recipes, planning menus, sequencing steps of meal preparation, identifying nutritionally balanced menus, budgeting and estimating costs, demonstrating equipment safety, making shopping lists, purchasing grocery items

---

needed to complete a complex activity. To be cost effective, cotreatment is usually conducted with more than one patient at a time. Although the type of activity may have several objectives common to all individuals being treated, specific goals should be established for each individual. In addition to many of the groups presented in Table 8.3, the following list offers some examples of cotreatment activities.

Speech-language Pathology and Occupational Therapy

Activity: transportation arrangements
Areas to address: reading schedules; telephoning to obtain or verify schedules, or to make arrangements; sequencing the "trip" with other responsibilities; determining and arranging payment; and evaluating alternatives and backups

Speech-Language Pathology and Physical Therapy

Activity: any physical exercise program or game/sport
Areas to address: following and giving oral directions; learning the steps to a new physical activity; turn taking in a group activity; reading/following an exercise sheet; expressing complaints; and giving praise to others

Speech-Language Pathology and Vocational Rehabilitation

Activity: looking for employment
Areas to address: reading job descriptions and advertisements; job interviewing practice; telephoning to obtain information, schedule an appointment, and answer preliminary interview questions; writing a resume and letters of inquiry or introduction; and on-the-job communication

Speech-Language Pathology and Psychology or Social Work

Activity: group discussion of the treatment day
Areas to address: communication intent; giving and interpreting nonverbal messages; interpreting and expressing feelings; constructive versus destructive criticism; spatial proximity; acknowledging comments; and offering advice

Speech-Language Pathology and Recreation Therapy

Activity: plan a leisure activity to do with a friend
Areas to address: determining interests; listing and evaluating various activities; reading the directions to a game; telephoning to make arrangements; and determining costs or items needed

PSYCHOSOCIAL AND EMOTIONAL ISSUES

It would be a clear error of omission not to address the psychosocial and emotional sequelae of traumatic brain injury as they relate to intervention by all members of the treatment team. Although an exhaustive discussion is not possible, several key issues need to be brought to the reader's attention. One of the greatest impediments to positive long-term outcomes for individuals who have sustained a traumatic brain injury is their apparent lack of awareness of the extent of their cognitive and psychosocial impairments. Prigatano[32] has referred to this as "disturbances of self-awareness of deficit." He describes the problem as follows:

> Although many factors potentially contribute to this phenomenon [poor long-term psychosocial and vocational outcome], clinically it often appears that severely brain-injured patients do not adequately perceive significant changes in their higher cerebral functioning. Consequently, they may choose a level of work that is not appropriate for their abilities, with catastrophic social consequences. The same problem is seen in their interpersonal relationships. They often do not recognize how impulsive, irritable, childish, or demanding they are in certain circumstances. Thus they frequently alienate family and friends, and they appear confused and bewildered in the face of their interpersonal failures. The result is often social isolation. In some instances frank delusional ideation emerges.

The psychotherapist serves a critical role on the team, as a member who can identify the nature and extent of psychosocial needs and recommend the best approaches to helping the individual with these needs. However, a mistake often made in rehabilitation programs is that these problems are referred only to the psychotherapist, who is expected to remediate them in the traditional one or two 1–hour sessions per week. It has now been clearly stated by Prigatano,[33] and others[34] as well, that traditional psychotherapy paradigms are not adequate to facilitate any real change in the traumatic brain injury population. It is not within the scope of this section, however, to discuss the numerous approaches to psychological problems employed by traditional psychotherapy.

Few have postulated how memory impairment affects behavior, but a practical view tells us that it must do so. Obsessive behaviors may develop because of the strong need for order and routine. Patients can become agitated and even hostile when they are unable to remember people's names, the way from one place to another, things they read, or if they ate breakfast. This is not to imply that behavioral disorders are secondary to memory impairment, but only to illustrate the interaction between cognitive abilities and behavioral manifestations. The reader is reminded (see Table 5.1) that behavioral disorders themselves are considered among the most prominent of the neurobehavioral sequelae to traumatic brain injury. Traditionally, great emphasis has been placed on the distinction between behavioral problems that are thought to be organic versus those believed to be pre-existing to the injury. This has caused rehabilitation clinicians to neglect to develop strategies to assist in the management of the psychosocial and behavioral problems that interfere with successful community integration.

The psychosocial problems of individuals with brain injuries must be managed with consistency among all team members. Self-awareness is not merely an awareness of one's feelings about the injury; it also includes awareness about all aspects of functioning. Many of these "aspects" have been addressed in this chapter (for example, awareness of the need to focus attention, to use a memory aid, and to follow a problem-solving guide; awareness of nonverbal communication signals and frequent interruptions of others; and awareness of the tone of voice taken with authority figures). All clinicians have a responsibility to specifically address awareness problems in a systematic and therapeutic manner (in other words, improving awareness is not the steady application of confrontational statements about an individual's deficits). This is not to say that speech-language pathologists should engage in the practice of psychotherapy; they should not, unless they are trained and licensed to do so. Rather, it is to say that awareness is key to successful intervention, and to ignore awareness problems that fall within the domain of one's expertise is to do less for patients than they deserve.

Likewise, concerns about motivation cannot be left to the psychotherapist "to fix." Rehabilitation clinicians who employ or work within a medical model often fall short in their approach to problems in motivation by examining them as either pre-existing personality characteristics—separate from the brain injury—that will be affected little by treatment (for example, "He's always been that way; it's unlikely he can change now with a brain injury."), or by examining them as problems that are the direct result of the brain damage (that is, frontal lobe damage) but not as problems related to the dynamics of having sustained trauma and all that follows. In other words, we fail to appreciate the effects that trauma and the subsequent failure(s) have on motivation. Persons who have sustained brain injuries experience enormous degrees of failure, especially in rehabilitation settings. The repeated process of try/fail, try/fail in and of itself contributes to low motivation, and why would we think otherwise? Few of us have the emotional reserves that would allow us to experience failure over and over and remain completely unaffected by it. The clinical challenge, then, becomes to find things that the patient is motivated towards (that is, personal goals) and to establish a treatment agenda that promotes success and limits failure to the extent possible.

Although charting performance and behaviors can be time consuming for clinicians, it can have immense value in helping individuals "see" improvement, and it has the additional benefit of addressing self-awareness and self-monitoring. Patients can be given the data along with instruction to develop graphs that illustrate their performance, either with paper and pencil or computer programs. As an activity, this may in turn address other skill areas (for example, organization) in a motivating way (for example, "This is my data, and I want to put it in a graph to see what I've done.").

Clinicians are now beginning to recognize that the physical, cognitive, communicative, and psychosocial sequelae to traumatic brain injury are not distinct impairment processes that have little overlap. In an attempt to focus the clinician in this direction, this text has emphasized the importance of viewing the individual with traumatic brain injury from a larger perspective than merely as a study in cognitive-communicative impairment.

SUMMARY

The postacute stage of rehabilitation is challenging to the clinician in that a wide and variable range of impairments may be seen. Postacute rehabilitation may occur in a variety of setting types (for example, outpatient clinic, office building, group home, transitional facility), but at this stage, regardless of setting, rehabilitation efforts should be directed toward helping the individual integrate into the community. Community re-entry programs have a threefold purpose that was listed as: to specifically address skills needed to function as a community member, to help individuals identify and learn to use community resources in the community of residence, and to enhance community acceptance of persons with traumatic brain injury through education, observation, and first-hand experience. To this end, therapy must be directed toward those behaviors that have the greatest impact on the individual's ability to return to the most productive lifestyle possible.

Several approaches to impairments in memory, problem solving and executive functioning, and communication were discussed. The selection and use of memory notebooks were discussed at length, as patients often are given notebooks with little instruction. A number of models of problem solving were presented that can be used to help patients organize their thoughts and approach problems in a systematic manner. Strategies to improve executive functions and communication behaviors were discussed.

Video recordings and group therapy were discussed as important components to rehabilitation, aimed at improving self-awareness and self-monitoring. Several examples of types of groups and activities that can be implemented in a community re-entry program were provided.

Finally, the importance of recognizing the impact of psychosocial sequelae on long-term functioning was stressed. Particular attention was given to the impact of awareness deficits on successful integration into the home and community. The need to address these issues specifically, throughout the rehabilitation program, was emphasized.

REFERENCES

1. Condeluci A, Gretz-Lasky S. Social role valorization: a model for community reentry. *Journal of Head Trauma Rehabilitation*. 1987;2:49–56.
2. Eames P, Wood RL. The structure and content of a head injury rehabilitation service. In Wood RL, Eames PG (eds). *Models of Brain Injury Rehabilitation*. Baltimore, MD: Johns Hopkins University Press; 1989:31–47.
3. Stanczak DE, Hutcherson WL. Acute rehabilitation of the head-injured individual: toward a neuropsychological paradigm of treatment. In Long CJ, Ross LK (eds). *Handbook of Head Trauma: Acute Care to Recovery*. New York, NY: Plenum Press; 1992:125–136.
4. Sohlberg MM, Mateer CA. *Introduction to Cognitive Rehabilitation: Theory and Practice*. New York, NY: Guilford Press; 1989.
5. Parenté R, Anderson-Parenté JK. Vocational memory training. In Kreutzer JS, Wehman P (eds). *Community Integration Following Traumatic Brain Injury*. Baltimore, MD: Paul H Brookes; 1990:157–168.
6. Gianutsos R, Gianutsos J. Rehabilitating the verbal recall of brain-injured patients by mnemonic training: an experimental demonstration using single-case methodology. *Journal of Clinical Neuropsychology*. 1979;2:117–135.
7. Wilson BA. *Rehabilitation of Memory*. New York, NY: Guilford Press; 1987.
8. Little MM. The remediation of everyday memory deficits. In Williams JM, Long CJ (eds). *The Rehabilitation of Cognitive Disabilities*. New York, NY: Plenum Press; 1987:123–138.
9. Crosson B, Buenning W. An individualized memory retraining program after closed-head injury: a single-case study. *Journal of Clinical Neuropsychology*. 1984;6:287–301.
10. Wilson B. Models of cognitive rehabilitation. In Wood RL, Eames PG (eds). *Models of Brain Injury Rehabilitation*. Baltimore, MD: Johns Hopkins University Press; 1989.
11. Lawson MJ, Rice DN. Effects of training in use of executive strategies on a verbal memory problem resulting from closed head injury. *Journal of Clinical and Experimental Neuropsychology*. 1989;11:842–854.

12. Glisky EL, Schacter DL. Extending the limits of complex learning in organic amnesia: computer training in a vocational domain. *Neuropsychologia.* 1989;27:107–120.
13. Mateer CA, Sohlberg MM. A paradigm shift in memory rehabilitation. In Whitaker HA (ed). *Neuropsychological Studies of Non-focal Brain Damage: Dementia and Trauma.* London, England: Springer-Verlag; 1988:202–225.
14. Burke JM et al. A process approach to memory book training for neurological patients. *Brain Injury.* 1994;8:71–81.
15. Fluharty G, Priddy D. Methods of increasing client acceptance of a memory book. *Brain Injury.* 1993;7:85–88.
16. Sohlberg MM, Mateer CA. Training use of compensatory memory books: a three-stage behavioral approach. *Journal of Clinical and Experimental Neuropsychology.* 1989;11:871–891.
17. Ben-Yishay Y. *Working Approaches to Remediation of Cognitive Deficits in Brain Damaged Persons.* New York, NY: New York University Medical Center; 1980:129–174.
18. Ylvisaker M et al. Topics in cognitive rehabilitation therapy. In Ylvisaker M, Gobble EM (eds). *Community Re-entry for Head Injured Adults.* Boston, MA: College-Hill Press; 1987:137–220.
19. Bransford JD, Stein BS *The Ideal Problem Solver: A Guide for Improving Thinking, Learning, and Creativity.* New York, NY: WH Freeman; 1984.
20. Goldstein FL, Levin HS. Disorders of reasoning and problem solving ability. In Meier MJ, Benton AL, Diller L (eds). *Neuropsychological Rehabilitation.* New York, NY: Guilford Press; 1987:327–354.
21. Ylvisaker M, Szekeres SF. Metacognitive and executive impairments in head-injured children and adults. *Topics in Language Disorders.* 1989;9:34–49.
22. Sohlberg MM, Mateer CA, Stuss DT. Contemporary approaches to the management of executive control dysfunction. *Journal of Head Trauma Rehabilitation.* 1993;8:45–58.
23. Stuss DT, Mateer CA, Sohlberg MM. Innovative approaches to frontal lobe deficits. In Finlayson MAJ, Garner SH (eds). *Brain Injury Rehabilitation: Clinical Considerations.* Baltimore, MD: Williams and Wilkins; 1994:212–237.
24. Sohlberg MM, Sprunk H, Metzelaar K. Efficacy of an external cuing system in an individual with severe frontal lobe damage. *Cognitive Rehabilitation.* 1988;6:36–41.
25. Nelson NW, Schwentor BA. Reading and writing disorders. In Beukelman DR, Yorkston KM (eds). *Communication Disorders Following Traumatic Brain Injury: Management of Cognitive, Language, and Motor Impairments.* Austin, TX: Pro-Ed; 1991:191–249.
26. Ehrlich J, Sipes A. Group treatment of communication skills for head trauma patients. *Cognitive Rehabilitation.* 1985;3:32–37.
27. Ehrlich J, Barry P. Rating communication behaviours in the head-injured adult. *Brain Injury.* 1989;3:193–198.
28. Prutting CA, Kirchner DM. A clinical appraisal of the pragmatic aspects of language. *Journal of Speech and Hearing Disorders.* 1987;52:105–119.
29. Kennedy MR, DeRuyter R. Cognitive and language bases for communication disorders. In Beukelman DR, Yorkston KM (eds). *Communication Disorders Following Traumatic Brain Injury: Management of Cognitive, Language and Motor Impairments.* Austin, TX: Pro-Ed; 1990:123–190.

30. Evans RW, Preston BK. Day rehabilitation programming: a theoretical model. In Kreutzer JS, Wehman P (eds). *Community Integration Following Traumatic Brain Injury*. Baltimore, MD: Paul H Brookes; 1990:125–138.

31. Hartley LL. *Cognitive-Communication Abilities Following Brain Injury: A Functional Approach*. San Diego, CA: Singular Publishing; 1995.

32. Prigatano GP. Disturbances of self-awareness of deficit after traumatic brain injury. In Prigatano GP, Schacter DL (eds). *Awareness of Deficit after Brain Injury: Clinical and Theoretical Issues*. New York, NY: Oxford University Press; 1991:111–126.

33. Prigatano GP et al. *Neuropsychological Rehabilitation after Brain Injury*. Baltimore, MD: Johns Hopkins University Press; 1986.

34. Sbordone RJ. A conceptual model of neuropsychologically-based cognitive rehabilitation. In Williams JM, Long CJ (eds). *The Rehabilitation of Cognitive Disabilities*. New York, NY: Plenum Press; 1987:3–25.

9

Motor Speech Disorders

Monica McHenry

Traditional theories expounded by texts on motor speech disorders[1] are inadequate to describe the complexity of motor speech disorders following a traumatic brain injury. The focus of this chapter is primarily on the assessment and treatment of dysarthria, although apraxia of speech is also acknowledged as a motor speech disorder, and is addressed in a separate section. Many components of the various classifications of motor speech disorders may exist, yet they rarely appear in isolation. Because of the diffuse nature of brain damage following a traumatic brain injury, the dysarthria, if present, is usually a mixed type with both upper and lower motor neuron damage.[2] Often, attempting to classify the dysarthria of an individual with traumatic brain injury can cause more confusion than clarity. Further, with today's sophisticated imaging techniques, the differential diagnosis of neurologic disease is no longer as dependent upon the diagnosis of speech disorders as it was thirty years ago. For these reasons, it is advantageous to consider the components involved in speech production and determine the impact of the brain injury on each.

The incidence of dysarthria in individuals with traumatic brain injury has been difficult to determine. Variables precluding a precise estimate include time postinjury, and where and how the data were obtained. Yorkston, Honsinger, Mitsuda, and Hammen[3] conducted a survey of 151 individuals with traumatic brain injury. Patients evidencing mild to moderate dysarthria constituted 65 percent of the acute rehabilitation population, 42 percent of the acute medical population, and 22 percent of the outpatient rehabilitation population. By contrast, patients with severe dysarthria made up 24 percent of the acute care population, 20 percent of the acute rehabilitation population, and only 10 percent of the outpatient rehabilitation population. As with the cognitive-linguistic deficits seen in traumatic brain injury, the severity of motor speech disorders often changes over the course of recovery, as cognitive functions improve.

As acknowledged by Yorkston and Beukelman,[2] apraxia of speech has been reported rarely in published studies of individuals with traumatic brain injury. It is investigated most commonly in people who have sustained damage to the left hemisphere from vascular causes. Clinical experience and occasional case studies,[4] however, suggest that apraxia of speech may be present following traumatic brain injury, varying greatly in severity.

It is not possible to describe a typical patient with motor speech disorders following traumatic brain injury. The potential combination of characteristics is limitless. For example, in addition to severe dysarthria, an individual may present with apraxia of speech and neologisms secondary to receptive aphasia. Components of the speech production mechanism also may be affected differentially. For example, some individuals may evidence an open velopharyngeal port, with intact respiration, voicing, and articulation. Others may have varying degrees of weakness throughout the vocal tract. Because of the cognitive impairment that is a hallmark of traumatic brain injury, assessment and treatment of motor speech disorders can pose a challenge to clinicians. The contributors to reduced intelligibility often cannot be sorted out through traditional evaluation procedures, but must be untangled during "diagnostic therapy."

DYSARTHRIA ASSESSMENT

The depth and complexity of the speech evaluation will depend on the equipment available. The greatest advantage of an instrumentation-based assessment is the objectivity it provides. This facilitates accountability and is invaluable in monitoring progress throughout therapy. Often instrumentation will reveal changes that are not easily perceived, for example in the severity of hypernasality. The author recognizes that many clinicians will not have access to much of the instrumentation described. Nonetheless, it is important to have some understanding of the extent to which instrumentation can provide an objective assessment. Further, knowledge of the assessment options may facilitate the making of appropriate referrals.

It is important to recognize, however, that not all instrumentation-based measures relate well to unstructured conversational speech. Although they can provide information regarding very specific and isolated aspects of speech production, it is an integrated perceptual impression that impacts the listener. Finally, the clinician or researcher must comply with the underlying assumptions on which a measure is based. Without a thorough understanding of the development of a measure, and proper procedures to obtain data, the information may be invalid. Instrumentation-based assessments, as well as normative data, are addressed thoroughly in Baken.[5] Ludlow, Bassich, and Connor[6] proposed an assessment protocol for individuals with dysarthria and also provided normative data.

History and Interview

It is obviously useful to begin a history and interview after having reviewed thoroughly the patient's available medical records. This facilitates prompting and immediate verification of the patient report. Whenever possible, the interview should be recorded on videotape. In this manner, all features of an individual's communication style, such as eye contact, posture, and effortfulness of speech production will be captured. During the history and interview, other aspects of a patient's communication style may be assessed. The clinician should pay particular attention to the following: awareness of errors, reaction to errors, response to requests for repetitions, and self-correction attempts. Useful interview questions include those in Table 9.1.

Behavioral observation should continue throughout the evaluation period. If the patient evidences an unusual behavior, such as looking away when breathing in, or making extraneous noises, the clinician should ask about it to determine the patient's level of awareness and concern. It also is important to probe what the individual is able to change with cuing and modeling.

During the interview, it is essential to determine how the individual feels about his or her speech, and to determine what, if anything, the patient would like to change. It is also of great importance to discuss the patient's expectations. The interview provides a good opportunity to assess an individual's awareness of existing problems, level of motivation to change, and realism regarding outcome. The author has developed an awareness scale adapted from Prigatano, Altman, and O'Brien,[7] and presented in Table 9.2, that is given to both the patient and a family member to complete. A scale such as this provides the clinician with some impression of the patient's and the family's view of speech effectiveness.

Most clinicians also will find it beneficial to discuss the family's expectations regarding speech outcome. Therapy can become very challenging when the patient's and family's expectations differ from one another or from those of the clinician. When this occurs, counseling regarding realistic outcome goals must be initiated.

Table 9.1
Useful interview questions.

Tell me about your injury.
How do you feel about your speech?
How has your speech changed since your injury?
How often do people ask you to repeat yourself?
What do you do when someone asks you to repeat?
What would you like to change about your speech?

Table 9.2
Awareness Scales.

Patient Awareness Scale						
1	I speak clearly	all the time	most of the time	some of the time	not very often	never
2	I speak with appropriate loudness	all the time	most of the time	some of the time	not very often	never
3	I sound natural	all the time	most of the time	some of the time	not very often	never
4	I speak at an appropriate rate	all the time	most of the time	some of the time	not very often	never
5	I speak with an appropriate pitch	all the time	most of the time	some of the time	not very often	never
Family Member Awareness Scale						
1	They speak clearly	all the time	most of the time	some of the time	not very often	never
2	They speak with appropriate loudness	all the time	most of the time	some of the time	not very often	never
3	They sound natural	all the time	most of the time	some of the time	not very often	never
4	They speak at an appropriate rate	all the time	most of the time	some of the time	not very often	never
5	They speak with an appropriate pitch	all the time	most of the time	some of the time	not very often	never

Oral Peripheral Examination

A standard oral peripheral examination is an essential part of the evaluation. Following a traumatic brain injury, the side of weakness may vary according to structure. Often there will be bilateral weakness, with one side somewhat worse than the other. Determining the less affected or "best" side typically has little impact on speech production, but may affect decisions regarding swallowing management.

During the oral peripheral examination, the clinician should note independence of structural movement. For example, can the individual move the tongue independently of the jaw? How much tension in other structures is associated with the movement? Is there evidence of oral apraxia, such as groping behaviors? Are there involuntary movements, and how much control does the patient have over them? These observations will provide further insight into severity and prognosis.

Sensation

The recognition that speech is a sensorimotor process has been highlighted in recent work.[8,9] Although the relationship between sensation and production is not yet clear, the assessment of sensory abilities provides a more complete picture of factors that may contribute to intelligibility.

Oral sensation and stereognosis may be assessed with simple tests such as oral form identification and two-point discrimination, although there are limited normative data available for comparison.[10,11] For oral form identification, three different forms (for example, plastic triangle) are placed in the mouth while the patient's eyes are closed. The patient is allowed to feel the first form for five seconds, and is then asked to report if the next form is the same or different. Each form for comparison is presented three times in random order. Two-point discrimination may be administered with calibrated calipers, available at most drafting supply stores. The distance between the caliper points is adjusted in 5-millimeter increments. The patient reports feeling one or two points. Difference limens, or the thresholds at which the patient feels two points, are determined in ascending and descending trials. Normative data for the procedure are available.[10,12]

Respiration

Noninstrumentation

A number of behavioral observations will provide insight into an individual's speech breathing behaviors. The clinician should observe the patient's breathing at rest. The inspiratory strategy associated with speech breathing should be compared with the resting strategy. Many individuals remain within their tidal volume curve while breathing for speech. Ideally, an inspiration for speech is twice that of rest breathing. During connected speech, the clinician should listen for phrasing strategies. Are phrases in logical breath groups? Does the patient break up words in order to breathe? To what extent does the individual go below resting expiratory level to continue talking? Do the utterances become softer at the end?

Hixon, Hawley, and Wilson[13] designed a useful device to determine the ability to generate adequate subglottal pressure for speech. To perform the procedure, the clinician fills a tall glass with water, to approximately an inch from the top. A millimeter ruler is affixed to the glass, with 0 centimeters aligned with the water line. Held in place with a paper clip, a straw is positioned so that the end is 5 centimeters below the water line. The patient is then requested to blow bubbles for five seconds, wearing nose clips if velopharyngeal valving problems are evident. If the patient can blow bubbles for five seconds, with the straw at the 5 centimeter mark, it can be assumed that subglottal pressure is adequate for conversational speech. By placing the end of the straw at the 10 centimeter mark, the clinician may assess the ability to produce adequate subglottal pressure for loud speech. This method allows one to separate laryngeal valving problems from inadequate respiratory drive.

Instrumentation

The wet spirometer is a basic tool for assessing respiration. The device consists of two open-ended canisters. The lower canister is filled with water. The upper canister, open end down, rests in the lower canister, producing an airtight seal. The canisters are now filled with known volumes of air and water, respectively. The patient breathes into a tube that is in contact with the air within the sealed canisters. When the patient exhales, the upper canister is displaced. The movement is recorded on calibrated chart paper to determine the volume of air exchanged. Wet spirometers are usually available in the pulmonary departments of hospitals. It is useful for individuals with dysarthria to undergo pulmonary function testing, consisting of a few simple maneuvers that provide information regarding lung volumes. Typically the patient will breathe quietly, then inspire maximally, exhale maximally, and immediately repeat the maximal inspiration and expiration. The maneuver will provide information regarding vital capacity (the maximum amount of air that can be exchanged), as well as inspiratory and expiratory volumes. If an individual's vital capacity is reduced, a program of aerobic conditioning may offer improvement. The effect of reduced vital capacity is discussed further under therapeutic intervention.

Although it is possible to assess speech breathing strategies using a spirometer, it is not recommended. Because of both claustrophobic reactions and carbon dioxide rebreathing, individuals alter their breathing strategies with spirometric attachment. Other devices that do not require physical attachment to the airway should be used to assess speech breathing.

One of the more popular devices for clinical use is respiratory inductive plethysmography (commercially available as Respitrace). Elastic bands placed around the patient's ribcage and abdomen produce a voltage output that is related to ribcage and abdominal movement. Chest wall movements must then be correlated to known lung volumes by simultaneously sampling chest wall movements and lung volume. To perform the simplest calibration maneuvers, data are obtained with a mask connected either to a pneumotachograph (to capture airflow) or to a canister containing a known volume of air. It must be recognized that volumes are estimated, and validity will depend on the goodness of fit during the calibration procedure. Using these devices, the clinician is able to obtain valuable information regarding speech breathing strategies. Measures are typically referenced to the person's vital capacity, and may include the points to which the individual inhaled and exhaled during speech, as well as lung volume excursions. Measures may also be referenced to resting end expiratory level. In addition, frequency of paradoxical movements of the rib cage and abdomen may be of interest. These are movements in which the ribcage or abdomen is moving opposite to the expected direction. For example, in abdominal paradoxing, the abdomen moves in during inspiration and out during expiration. Similarly, in ribcage paradoxing, the ribcage moves in during inspiration and out during expiration. Greater variety of movements may reflect respiratory flexibility. For example, patients with severe respiratory impairment may show no variation in strategies across a wide variety of speech and nonspeech tasks. For clinical purposes, speech breathing strategies are interpreted with reference to both muscular effort (that is, the range within the vital capacity curve where the patient speaks) and efficiency (that is, the ratio of inspiratory to expiratory time).

Voicing

Noninstrumentation

It is expected that every clinician will have at least a high quality audio tape recorder. This is an essential piece of equipment for voice and speech production therapy. The battery for noninstrumentation voice assessment should include, at a minimum: pitch range, s/z ratio, sustained /i/ and /a/ for voice quality rating, and conversational speech to determine modal pitch, stability of voice quality, and occurrence of pitch breaks and abrupt phonatory onsets. Titze[14] has proposed standardization of vocal tasks for the purpose of acoustic analysis. His proposed test utterances may provide a useful basis for a comprehensive voice profile. Breathiness, harshness, and hoarseness should be rated separately. The voice quality of individuals with traumatic brain injury may be inconsistent, depending upon their loudness, pitch, affect, and enthusiasm. The clinician should make a point of noting situations that elicit the best voice quality, as well as noting the predominant quality. If the voice quality is dependent on nonphysiologic factors, such as mood, intervention strategies will be drastically different, and voice therapy may not be warranted.

Instrumentation

Many clinicians have access to a Visipitch (Kay Elemetrics). By means of this device, the above phonatory tasks can be analyzed more easily, and a jitter estimation may be obtained, giving a more objective analysis of voice quality. *Jitter* refers to the periodicity of vocal fold vibratory frequency (that is, whether or not one cycle of vibration takes the same amount of time to complete as adjacent cycles), and is a physiologic feature related to the perception of hoarseness.

Aerodynamic assessments also may provide objective information regarding various aspects of voice production. A simple measure proposed by Smitheran and Hixon[15] is the calculation of laryngeal airway resistance. It is based on the assumption that intraoral pressure immediately preceding the release of /p/ is an accurate estimate of subglottal pressure. To obtain data, the patient produces /pi/ syllable trains. Intraoral pressure is sensed with a tube attached to a pressure transducer. The tube is placed in the mouth perpendicular to airflow. Translaryngeal flow is measured with a pneumotachograph attached to the patient with a face mask. Laryngeal airway resistance is calculated as translaryngeal pressure (estimated subglottal pressure minus pharyngeal pressure, assumed to be zero) divided by translaryngeal airflow. Automated computer programs exist to complete the analysis.[16]

Following the original presentation of the theoretical arguments for the method,[15,17] investigations have compared laryngeal airway resistance estimates according to gender,[18,19,20] loudness levels,[21,22,23] pitch,[24] phonation type,[25] and voice disorders.[26,27] Individuals with high and low laryngeal airway resistance estimates have been perceived respectively as producing strained and breathy voices.[26]

Holmberg and colleagues[28] found that the laryngeal airway resistance calculation is limited by large and inconsistent intrasubject variability over time. The authors concluded that the high intrasubject variability also detracted from the usefulness of the estimate's ability to sense subtle change in vocal function. Further, the correspondence between intraoral and subglottal pressure has been questioned in certain conditions,[29,30] and in some disordered populations.[31]

Overviews of instrumentation available for voice analysis may be found in Gould and Korovin.[32] For a comprehensive discussion of voice evaluation, with and without instrumentation, the reader is referred to Colton and Casper.[33] For a review of computer-based speech analysis systems, the work by Read, Buder, and Kent[34] is useful.

Resonance

Noninstrumentation

To assess hypernasality, the clinician should rate the patient's nasality while the patient is reading a non-nasal passage. The clinician should attend particularly to voiceless plosives, in order to determine the presence of nasal air emission. Behaviors that may contribute to the perception of nasality, such as reduced mandibular excursion and low vocal effort, should be observed carefully.

The patient should be asked to read a passage with occasional nasals to determine the presence of assimilative nasality. Since assimilative nasality is often due to poor timing of closure, one should probe the effect of different speaking rates on the perception of nasality.

Denasality (which may be present following a pharyngeal flap procedure, or when wearing a palatal lift), can be assessed by having the patient read a passage loaded with nasals. The inability to nasalize phonemes, following surgical or prosthetic intervention, may often be ameliorated by increasing the duration of the nasals. Therefore, the clinician should probe the effect of reduced speaking rate and prolonged nasal production on the perception of denasality.

Instrumentation

A thorough review of instrumentation used to assess velopharyngeal function is found in McWilliams, Morris, and Shelton.[35] The Nasometer (Kay Elemetrics) is one of the more common tools available to the clinician. It provides an acoustic indication of oral/nasal coupling. Normative data exist for various regional dialects.[36] The advantage of acoustic analyses for nasality is their ability to sample natural connected speech.

The adequacy of velopharyngeal closure may also be determined aerodynamically. Software programs have been developed[16,37] that calculate velopharyngeal resistance and factor out nasal cavity resistance. In addition to a computer, a pressure transducer, to sense intraoral pressure, and a pneumotachograph, to measure nasal airflow, are needed. The patient produces /pi/ syllable trains. Data obtained include mean nasal airflow, peak nasal flow on the plosive release, and intraoral pressure. With minor procedural modifications to the aerodynamic protocol, it is also possible to calculate the size of the velopharyngeal orifice.[38,39] This procedure has also been computer automated in a system called PERCI-PC.[40]

Articulation

Noninstrumentation

Articulation will be considered primarily within the context of intelligibility. Intelligibility testing was dramatically improved with the development of phonetic intelligibility testing. Kent, Weismer, and Rosenbek[41] developed a test based on phonetic contrasts. The patient says carefully chosen single words which are then judged by an unfamiliar listener. The listener selects each perceived word from four choices. Listener confusions are categorized according to the phonetic contrast error they represent. Error categories include, for example, voice/voiceless distinctions, high versus low vowels, place confusions, and final consonant omissions. Phonetic intelligibility testing, therefore, helps focus therapeutic intervention.

It is also useful to obtain an intelligibility score for sentences, using the *Computerized Assessment of the Intelligibility of Dysarthric Speech*, by Yorkston, Beukelman, and Traynor,[42] as well as a subjective rating during a conversational speech sample. If there is a large difference between the patient's intelligibility in single words, compared with intelligibility of sentences, a pacing strategy may be effective. Finally, throughout the evaluation, the clinician should probe the individual's ability to change any observed behaviors that may impact intelligibility.

Instrumentation

Most instrumentation-based assessments of articulation are research oriented and may not be practical or relevant in the majority of clinical settings. The patient's ability to generate and sustain forces produced during speech production may be determined with instrumentation.[43,44,45,46] Spectrographic analysis can provide information regarding the speed of formant transitions and may objectify articulatory imprecision.[47] For therapeutic purposes, however, intelligibility and the factors contributing to it remain the primary concern.

Prosody

A variety of prosodic deficits may be evident following a traumatic brain injury. One of the most common is minimal variation (that is, monopitch and monoloudness). In these cases, it is critical to determine why an individual evidences flat intonation contours. The reduced prosodic variations may be associated with flat affect or with physiologic limitations. It is essential to probe the ability to produce natural stress patterns. This can be done with contrasting stress drills. If the patient is unable to produce the intonation contour spontaneously, the clinician should attempt cuing and modeling to determine physiologic abilities. Rarely would one treat monopitch and monoloudness if it appeared to be the result of flat affect.

Another type of prosodic deficit involves extreme or exaggerated pitch and loudness variations. These features are often associated with a slow speaking rate and imprecise articulation. During the evaluation, the clinician should probe the individual's awareness of these features and the ability to imitate less extreme variations.

Evaluation Summary

At the conclusion of the evaluation, the patient should be provided with information regarding the clinician's immediate observations and recommendations. Ideally the complete evaluation results will be presented in a team meeting, with other disciplines reporting as well. The clinician should assess the patient's level of agreement, and attempt to establish which intervention strategies should have priority. If a patient and clinician disagree regarding the recommendations, a period of trial therapy may provide a neutral basis for exploring goals and determining the appropriateness of intervention.

The Timing of Intervention

The decision to provide motor speech therapy will depend on a number of factors. A frequently encountered problem in traumatic brain injury is lack of awareness. Often a patient's report of how well he or she is able to communicate will be incongruous with the clinician's observations. In these cases, individuals may be encouraged to attempt a period of trial therapy. Often with video and audio feedback, patients will acknowledge that their speech does not sound the way it did before the injury, and they may be more receptive to change. It is also of great value to obtain video and/or audio recordings of the patient's premorbid speech. Viewing these videotapes in conjunction with the evaluation video may highlight the effect of the traumatic brain injury and facilitate the patient's receptiveness to intervention. If some degree of awareness is not present, therapy is unlikely to make an impact. In these cases, it is desirable to periodically reassess a patient's awareness of speech deficits and desire to change.

A second major consideration is the patient's level of cognitive function. This can impact both new learning and generalization of skills. Individuals with poor memory may be required to rely on external cuing, such as "Take a big breath and tell me louder." In other instances, the patient's cognitive deficits may be so severe that certain interventions must be given priority over others. A slight reduction in intelligibility, or a somewhat abnormal voice quality, may be the least of the treatment team's and family's concerns. For patients with reduced cognitive function, key phrases repeated consistently by all conversational partners may facilitate learning. For example, "soft and slow" or "breathe big and talk loud" may make an impact.

A third consideration is patient motivation. Lack of motivation to change may be related to awareness, to attitude, or to premorbid characteristics. Some patients believe that if someone does not understand them, it is the listener's problem, and the listener should try harder. In these cases, it is useful to stress the speaker's role in facilitating successful communication. Other patients will consistently respond to feedback or audiotaped playback with "I always talked that way." Although every effort should be made to motivate the patient in any way possible, it is often necessary for the clinician to acknowledge the patient's right to refuse treatment and to provide the individual with the option of pursuing treatment at a later time.

BASIC THERAPEUTIC CONCEPTS

Determine Premorbid Status

Whenever possible, obtaining a sample of the individual's premorbid speech is beneficial. People with brain injuries and their families often have a difficult time describing how the individual talked before the injury. A premorbid speech sample is useful in assessing speaking style, prosodic patterns, articulation (particularly in populations with heavy accents), and voice characteristics. Fortunately, with the explosion of home videos and even phone answering machines, obtaining a premorbid sample has become more feasible than in the past.

How to Communicate as Intelligibility Improves

Clearly, the goal of any intervention is to facilitate effective communication. When an individual is determined to "learn to talk again," he or she may be reluctant to use any strategies other than oral communication. In the author's clinical practice, the patient is allowed two attempts at oral communication. Then, if the listener has not understood the message, the patient is encouraged to use a backup system, such as an augmentative device, alphabet board, writing, or spelling the word. Clinicians should feel free to stress that to do otherwise is an imposition on the listener. Getting the message across, regardless of the means, is always the paramount goal.

Optimal Positioning

Often, individuals with severe motor speech disorders have other physical limitations. Position is important in facilitating speech production. Clinicians can encourage optimal positioning by asking the patient to sit up straight with shoulders level, relax the face, breathe in with lips apart before speaking, and keep a level chin. Ideally, patients with involuntary movements will wait until they are stable to begin talking. When encouraging correct posture, the clinician should make every effort to model the target behaviors as well.

Work Within the Context of Speech

It is critical to integrate all target features simultaneously. Generalization to spontaneous speech is otherwise extremely unlikely. It is highly probable that, for any given patient, a clinician will be scoring a number of features simultaneously, for example, obvious inspiration, appropriate mouth opening, adequate vowel duration, precise articulation, and eye contact. It is rarely productive to work on a single feature in isolation.

Maintain Naturalness

It is very easy to elicit unnatural utterances in structured spontaneous speech. Many patients stop using contractions because of the formal nature of drills. Others will argue that coarticulation sounds "sloppy" and will insist on overarticulating. Often clinicians will model unnatural productions without realizing it. Making speech practice as natural as possible will facilitate generalization to the real world. Listening to audiotapes of therapy sessions may help both the patient and clinician become aware of this important feature.

Make Practice Functional

Related to the concept of working within speech contexts is practicing functional utterances. Patients will always respond better when drilling on words they are likely to use often, such as a family member's name. It is often useful to ask the patient to write down phrases they say throughout the day and practice these. Focusing on words used in specific hobbies can make practice more enjoyable as well. For example, it is very unlikely that an auto mechanic uses the word "illuminate" for daily communication; although the word may contain all the targeted speech sounds and desired number of syllables, it is more efficient to practice words within the patient's typical vocabulary.

Home Practice

Patients spend relatively little time in structured speech therapy, even in intensive residential treatment programs. Clinicians should help patients find times throughout the day to practice. Depending upon the patient's progress in therapy, practice could involve audiotaping of articulation drills, self-monitoring of a target feature to increase awareness, or conversing while attempting to produce a certain feature. Generalization is more likely with short practice sessions spaced throughout the day than with one long session. Audiotaped stimuli are useful for patients who have difficulty reading. Clinicians can incorporate a self-judging form so the patient is actively monitoring and evaluating productions.

Generalization

The clinician and patient should choose certain features to work on throughout the day. Then, the clinician should involve as many people as possible in the patient's goals. Features that are easy for people to identify and understand, such as adequate loudness, eye contact, pacing, or saliva control, should be chosen for others to reinforce. Therapists in other disciplines can cue and monitor target features. Clinicians should ensure that people involved know how to provide positive reinforcement for success, as opposed to nagging or constantly reminding the patient of what to do, which will yield negative results. It is useful, as training, to videotape the patient using a particular strategy effectively, so that others have a clear picture of the goal.

Encourage Proprioceptive Awareness

If individuals are unable to feel what they are doing in accurate productions, the behaviors are unlikely to generalize. Reliance on external biofeedback or judgments by the clinician does not promote self-monitoring and awareness. When the patient produces target features accurately, the clinician can encourage the patient to focus on what the production felt like and sounded like, and play back the recorded audio sample.

Establish Accurate Self-Monitoring

As soon as possible within the therapy session, clinicians should have the patient judge various features of the productions. It is best to begin with the most obvious and easily assessed features. Initially, audio playback may be required, although many individuals dislike hearing their voice on tape. Ideally, the patient will monitor as he or she speaks, with taped playback used for questionable judgments. Once judgment reliability has been established, self-monitoring can be extended to situations outside of the therapy setting. Clinicians can assist patients in choosing a time of day to monitor their speech, and develop a simple scoring system. It is more effective for the patient to score each utterance than to give an overall impression of success.

Audiotape All Sessions

One never knows when a patient will produce the perfect voice quality, ideal articulation, or balanced resonance. It is very simple to record each session, for the sole purpose of providing audio feedback when the patient does something well. Further, recordings provide reference samples for the clinician, and help to develop realistic speech production goals. Audiotapes are also useful to contrast successive attempts of an utterance, so the clinician can point out the features that improved with each trial.

Specificity of Feedback

The ideal time for the clinician to instruct the patient in physiologic concepts is when providing feedback. Clinicians should never say "try it again" without giving information regarding what the speaker should change to improve the production. Conversely, when the patient produces something accurately, the clinician's feedback should stress the target feature that was produced correctly. This will serve as a cue for the next production. When encouraging self-monitoring skills, clinicians should ask patients what they did during the production, in order to encourage awareness that they are in control, for example, "what did you do on the /n/?" instead of "what happened on the /n/?" Table 9.3 provides examples of specific feedback.

Avoid Jargon

It is very easy for the clinician to use terminology that is unique to the field of speech-language pathology. The goal, however, is effective communication. It is particularly important that clinicians avoid excessive use of professional jargon when reporting progress to the treatment team, patient, and family members. A few examples of jargon are "assistance, cuing,

Table 9.3
Examples of specific feedback.

On the next one, take a bigger breath.
Open your mouth more and stretch out the vowel.
Keep your tongue behind your teeth.
Swallow after you clear your throat.
Keep your lips apart when you say /f/.
Breathe in with your lips apart.
Keep eye contact with me as you breathe in.

---

phoneme, module, moderate, deficit, mobility, subskill, comprehension, evaluation, and assessment." If there is a simpler, more common way to say something, it is best to use it. For example, instead of "You need moderate cuing to produce alveolars accurately," say "You still need some reminders to keep your tongue behind your teeth."

SPECIFIC THERAPEUTIC STRATEGIES

The underlying premise of therapy for individuals with motor speech disorders is compensation. Although it is possible that physiologic functioning may return to premorbid levels, in most cases this is not a realistic assumption. It is essential, therefore, to encourage patients to accept their current level of functioning and develop compensatory strategies to optimize function.

Respiration

Reduced respiratory effort, often coupled with a reduction in vital capacity, is one of the most typical problems encountered in motor speech disorders following traumatic brain injury. This may result in short phrases, reduced loudness, and, in extreme cases, stopping of fricatives to conserve air. The degree of the problem will depend on valving throughout the vocal tract. Clearly, the respiratory strategies will make a greater difference if the patient also evidences poor laryngeal and velopharyngeal valving. Figure 9.1 illustrates the effect of reduced vital capacity on the magnitude of prephonatory inspirations. It is thought that most people breathe in about 20 percent of their vital capacity before speaking.[48] If an individual's vital capacity were reduced to 70 percent of the premorbid level, he or she would need to breathe in about 28 percent of vital capacity to reach the premorbid lung volume. By contrast, if the individual maintained the strategy of inspiring to 20 percent of vital capacity, the lung volume would be markedly reduced. Unfortunately, most individuals with motor speech

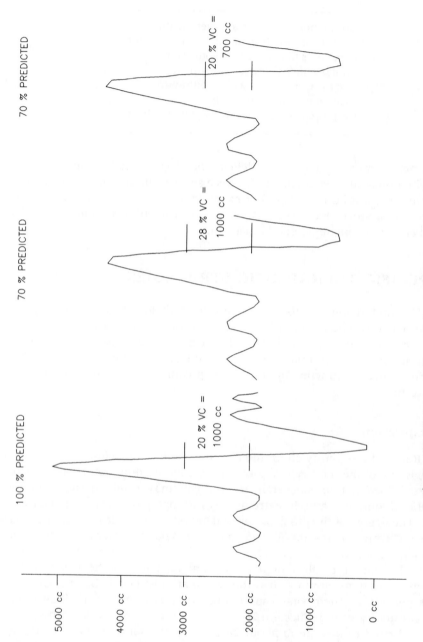

Figure 9.1 Vital capacity/speech breathing range comparisons.

disorders following brain injury have difficulty exerting increased respiratory effort, and typically inspire to much less than 20 percent of vital capacity. In addition to a reduced vital capacity, individuals with closed head injury have also evidenced difficulty coordinating rib cage and abdominal displacements.[49]

The goal of speech breathing intervention is to maximize efficiency and minimize effort. Because airflow is the driving force for phonation and provides the carrying power of the voice, improving inspiratory magnitudes is critical. Many individuals find it more effortful to expire at a level below resting expiratory level than to increase their level of inspiration, so focusing on inspiration is appropriate. Patients can be encouraged to expand their rib cage and abdomen outward, in order to increase inspiration. Mirror feedback is adequate for this. Any tendency to shoulder elevation with increased inspiratory magnitudes should be extinguished immediately. The effort should be exerted below shoulder level. The clinician must also watch for extraneous behaviors such as looking away during inspiration or facial grimaces. Any distracting behaviors must be eliminated before they become a habit. Breathing should be practiced within the context of speech, to avoid hyperventilation. A program of aerobic activity should be initiated concurrently with increasing the awareness of respiratory effort. This will not only improve the individual's vital capacity but will also lessen fatigue, in the long run, making it easier to increase respiratory effort. Consultation and/or cotreatment with a physical therapist is extremely important in developing an effective treatment program of this nature.

It is of obvious importance to keep words and phrases intact. Individuals with severe reductions in respiratory capacity may breathe between syllables, adding to listener confusion. When working with patients who are cognitively able, the clinician should help them plan in advance where to breathe, in order to minimize syntactic disruptions. It is ideal to combine speech breathing with improving loudness, which is addressed in a later section.

Biofeedback can be very useful in settings where the clinician has access to a Respitrace. When using biofeedback, one should obtain several cycles of rest breathing (ideally with the patient's eyes closed for maximum naturalness) to establish a stable baseline and a typical magnitude. The goal for prephonatory inspiration should be set at twice tidal inspiration. Breaths much beyond this point should be avoided. Exaggerated inspiratory magnitudes are harder to control at both the respiratory level (requiring increased checking action) and the laryngeal level (potentially overdriving the vocal folds). The decision to practice expiring at a level below resting end expiratory level must be made on an individual basis. If phonating within expiratory reserve volume elicits excess muscular or vocal tension, it is best to avoid it. Respitrace feedback is illustrated in Figure 9.2. Again, the clinician and patient should work within the context of real speech, moving from short structured phrases to unstructured spontaneous speech. As with any

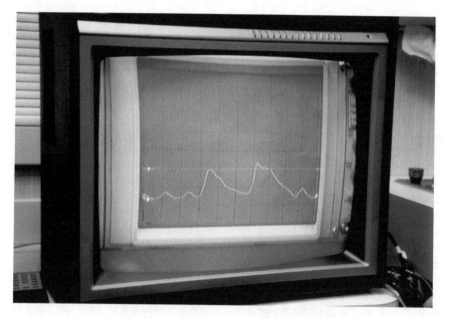

Figure 9.2 Example of Respitrace® feedback.

external biofeedback, it is critical that the patient develop proprioceptive awareness of the ideal strategy. Alternating productions with and without feedback may facilitate generalization. Frequent cues are necessary to help the patient focus on what increased lung volumes feel like, and develop a sense of the effort required.

Voicing

Patients should undergo a laryngeal evaluation by an otolaryngologist before any therapeutic intervention for voicing is initiated. It is essential to know the physiologic status of the vocal folds, in order to plan a therapy program. Laryngeal videostroboscopic evaluation is infinitely preferable to a simple, indirect laryngoscopy. An indirect laryngoscopy will provide only information regarding very gross laryngeal features, such as general appearance of the vocal folds and any signs of paresis. It is also limited by the necessity to evaluate the patient while he or she produces a high vowel at a high pitch, a task which facilitates vocal fold closure. Thus, the patient's performance may not reflect vocal fold activity during typical conversational speech. A videostroboscopic exam, on the other hand, will provide information regarding mucosal wave vibratory patterns. If a flexible endoscope is used, the exam can be performed as the patient performs a wide variety of speech, singing, and nonspeech tasks. A review of videostroboscopic procedures may be found in Karnell.[50]

Several different types of voice problems may be present following a traumatic brain injury. A recent study[51] revealed that 55 percent of males and 75 percent of females with severe head injuries evidenced reduced laryngeal airway resistance, manifested as breathiness. By contrast, subjects with closed head injury and dysarthria, studied by Theodoros and Murdoch,[52] evidenced characteristics associated with laryngeal hyperfunction. It is necessary, therefore, to acknowledge that a wide variety of voice problems may be present following a brain injury. Very often, the patient will evidence reduced loudness. It is ideal to combine work on increased respiratory effort, as described previously, with improving loudness. A sound pressure level meter is useful, but not essential. If one is used, the mouth to microphone distance should be kept constant across sessions. The clinician can establish the target level based on a conversational distance. Many patients report they feel as if they are talking too loudly, when in fact the loudness produced is perfect for conversational speech. Their reported sensation may be attributable to the increased effort required to produce adequate loudness. To help the patient accept the appropriate loudness level, it is useful to elicit feedback from peers, as well as to videotape conversational interactions. Adequate loudness is typically easy for others to judge. It is an ideal goal to establish across disciplines and for eliciting family involvement. All feedback should be positive, such as, "That sounded great. I had no trouble hearing you." Patients will be much more receptive to this than to cuing, which may be perceived as nagging.

Breathiness is characterized by excessive airflow due to inefficient laryngeal valving, and is often associated with reduced loudness. In many cases, increased respiratory effort will result in an improvement of breathiness. If the vocal folds are very weak, however, increased respiratory effort may have the opposite effect. In these cases, the optimum balance of respiratory effort and voicing must be established.

Other traditional approaches to reducing breathiness may be effective. These include beginning phonation with abrupt phonatory onsets (hard glottal attack), a cough, or a throat clearing. If vocal fold paralysis is present, these strategies are not indicated. Rather, the patient should be encouraged to use voice amplification, and be taught voice conservation techniques. If the paralysis has persisted past the period of expected spontaneous recovery (at least one year), the patient may wish to consider surgical intervention. A review of current surgical procedures is found in Colton and Casper.[53] Many patients with traumatic brain injury have no desire to undergo general anesthesia and further surgery. The less extreme intervention strategies will probably be preferred.

Harshness is characterized by aperiodic vocal fold vibration, which may be perceived as tense or pressed phonation. It may be associated with an inappropriately high fundamental frequency due to excessive laryngeal tension. The easiest way to reduce harshness in many patients with brain injury is to reduce loudness. Traditional strategies designed to reduce the force of vocal fold adduction, such as the yawn sigh, may also be appropriate. The difficulty with harshness associated with traumatic brain injury is that often the reduction of effort must occur only at the laryngeal level, and should not be generalized throughout the vocal tract.

Hoarseness is characterized by the presence of both breathiness and harshness. The voices of individuals with traumatic brain injury may be characterized by wet hoarseness. Inefficient swallowing during a meal may lead to residue accumulation in the pyriform sinus. The residue gradually spills onto the vocal folds, causing wet hoarseness. Another cause of wet hoarseness is poor saliva management. With reduced sensation, many individuals may not feel saliva accumulation and recognize the need to swallow. External cuing strategies may be beneficial for individuals who simply need to be reminded to swallow more frequently. (Additional information regarding swallowing was presented in Chapter Seven.)

A patient's pitch may be abnormally high as a result of excess laryngeal muscle tension. This is a difficult problem to address, and often one must rely on spontaneous recovery to facilitate muscle relaxation. Relaxation strategies, including yawn sigh techniques and electromyographic (EMG) biofeedback, may be of benefit. For many patients, pitch increases as utterance length progresses. With these individuals, swallowing often effectively lowers the larynx, restoring optimal laryngeal positioning and lowering pitch.

Abnormal modal pitch is often associated with a restricted pitch range. If the patient was at all musical premorbidly, singing can be a very pleasant and effective intervention strategy. Songs with sections containing small pitch variations, such as "Row, row, row your boat" and "Amazing Grace" are good starting points. The song "Do Re Mi" from *The Sound of Music* is an easy way to track progress in terms of number of semitones produced.

Patients with severe respiratory and laryngeal involvement often have difficulty producing voiceless phonemes. Voiceless phonemes in the final position may be easier to elicit if the patient has adequate respiratory capabilities. To facilitate laryngeal abduction, the clinician can encourage patients "to turn their voice off" and just blow. For some patients, voiceless phoneme establishment in the initial position may be simpler. Again, cues to blow air quietly have been found effective. Following initial voiceless phoneme production, laryngeal adduction is necessary in order to initiate voicing, or the production will be whispered.

Velopharyngeal Valving

Patients with traumatic brain injury present with varying degrees of nasality. In a study by Theodoros and colleagues,[54] listeners perceived nasality in 95 percent of 20 subjects with severe closed head injury. The intervention strategy chosen will depend on the type and severity of the problem, and the patient's ability to use compensatory strategies effectively. An oral peripheral evaluation noting only velar elevation and lateral and posterior pharyngeal wall movement may not adequately describe velopharyngeal function, since much sphincteric activity takes place out of view. Whenever possible, it is ideal to conduct nasal endoscopy to determine the adequacy of closure. Other, less invasive strategies, described previously, also may be used to determine the degree of closure.

A key factor in determining the most appropriate intervention strategy is the patient's ability to compensate. For many patients, increasing vocal effort may result in an increase in velopharyngeal resistance, thereby reducing nasality.[55] Increased mandibular excursion often is associated with louder utterances, but also should be probed in isolation. For patients who evidence excessive effort and appear to "overdrive" the system, a reduction in loudness may be effective. It is also useful to probe the effect of rate variation in case the problem is related to the timing of velopharyngeal closure.

If hypernasality is not affected in any discernible manner by the attempted compensatory strategies, other more invasive interventions may be considered. A palatal lift prosthesis, pictured in Figure 9.3, mechanically impedes airflow through the velopharyngeal port. The extension on the posterior portion of the lift elevates the velum. The effectiveness of the lift may depend on the presence of lateral or posterior pharyngeal wall movement. A lift is useful at the minimum to determine if the patient would be likely to benefit from surgical intervention such as a pharyngeal flap procedure.

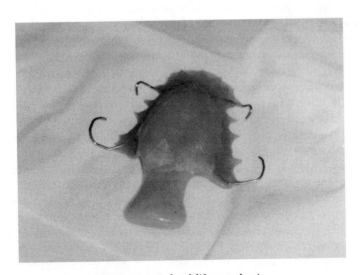

Figure 9.3 Palatal lift prosthesis.

Many individuals have a difficult time tolerating palatal lift prostheses. The two greatest deterrents appear to be the generation of excess saliva and interference with swallowing. Given that many patients with motor speech disorders also have swallowing difficulties, these problems can be serious enough to rule out a lift. Unfortunately, it is typically very difficult to predict who will be able to tolerate a palatal lift. The least likely candidates are individuals with a hyperactive gag reflex. Some patients are able to develop tolerance if the posterior portion is extended gradually over a period of several visits to the prosthodontist. Others may benefit from desensitization procedures, as described by Daniel.[56] The cost/benefit ratio of discomfort to nasality reduction is very obvious to most patients. A patient's decision to tolerate a palatal lift will depend greatly on how its effectiveness is perceived. If the lift is effective, but uncomfortable, the patient may well benefit from a pharyngeal flap or related surgical procedure. Although not yet documented in the literature, some clinicians have become concerned about the effect of pharyngeal flaps on breathing during sleep. It is advised to consult with the patient's surgeon regarding potential problems, and to monitor the patient postsurgically.

Articulation

The relationship between muscle strength and intelligibility is not yet clear. Studies have been conflicting to date.[43,46] No investigation has yet indicated that increasing muscle strength improves intelligibility, and there is considerable doubt that work on nonspeech tasks affects speech production. It is therefore of questionable utility, for example, to drill the patient on tongue strengthening exercises. These procedures may enhance a patient's awareness of articulatory movement and force generation, but they have no proven relation to connected speech. Again, working within the context of connected speech is likely to be the most efficacious way to improve intelligibility.

When working with patients with severe weakness or very poor motor control, the clinician should begin with any movement they are able to make consistently. Functional words are preferable to nonsense words whenever possible. Words such as "bye, no, and hi" are often easy to elicit and can encourage socialization.

Various compensatory strategies may be employed. Bilabial closure, as well as tongue contact, may be enhanced by the patient propping up the chin to reduce mandibular distance. If there is a problem with poor mandibular control, a bite block (as simple as a pen held between the teeth) may help stabilize the jaw. Tucking the chin also facilitates jaw stabilization for some patients.

If an individual is unable to produce /k, g, ng/, elicitation from a high vowel such as /i/ may be successful. The author also has had some success in patients who used a palatal lift by making a "dropped palate," whereby the posterior portion of the lift covering the hard palate is thickened. This modification may facilitate tongue contact, particularly for individuals with posterior lingual weakness.

Some patients produce sounds in a manner that may be perceptually adequate, but visually confusing, (for example, tongue protrusion on alveolars). It is important to explain to the patient that, because of reduced intelligibility, listeners will watch the mouth in order to better understand. Clinicians should convey to their patients the importance of providing accurate visual information to the listener, as another strategy to enhance intelligibility. Mirror feedback can be very useful to develop awareness. Contrasting accurate with inaccurate placement will heighten proprioceptive awareness.

Articulatory imprecision may be due to several factors. Weak movements may respond well to developing more exaggerated articulation. If the imprecision is primarily due to speaking too rapidly, a pacing strategy may be employed. Various options are available for pacing. One of the first decisions to be made is whether the patient will pace once for each syllable or for each word. For people with severe dysarthria, pacing for each syllable seems to enhance precision. More obvious pacing strategies are commercially-available pacing boards, or rulers with large raised numbers. Any device that allows the patient to feel the pacing, rather than to visually monitor it, will facilitate maintenance of eye contact. Strategies that do not involve external devices are tapping with a finger, hand, or foot, and touching each finger to the thumb. Once a strategy has been established, it is important to be consistent. For example, always using the same hand, or always tapping the fingers to the thumb in the same order, will facilitate habituation. Pacing is a difficult strategy to encourage outside of therapy. Most patients are more receptive to the less conspicuous methods than to some type of pacing board. To optimize generalization, it is important that everyone with whom the patient interacts should expect paced speech. Very often, people will tell the patient that they are able to understand without pacing, which undermines the development of the habit. Playback of utterances with and without pacing may help the patient and others become aware of the benefits.

Pacing may be performed accurately with or without audible breaks between the words. The clinician and the patient must determine the best compromise between precision and naturalness. Encouraging the patient to "put breaks between words" is another form of pacing, and may be more effective than asking the patient to "slow down."

Occasionally, imprecise articulation is worsened by excessive saliva accumulation. The simplest solution is for the patient to swallow more frequently. A second, less desirable, option is for the patient to use medication, which dries the mouth. This may have undesirable side effects, and does not encourage the motoric practice of more frequent swallowing.

Prosody

Although the physiologic abilities discussed thus far influence intelligibility, prosodic variations affect the perception of naturalness. There is often a trade-off between intelligibility and naturalness. From a therapeutic standpoint, the author considers intelligibility to be the essential basis for speech production and naturalness to be the fine tuning of the production. In extreme cases, however, prosodic limitations such as excess and equal stress may also detract from intelligibility.

Prosodic variations may be affected with changes in pitch, loudness, and duration. Typically, changes in all three features co-occur to stress a word. Individuals who are limited in their ability to alter these features may stress a word by pausing after it. Finally, rate of change, particularly in pitch, is an important consideration. Both very slow and extremely rapid pitch changes will detract from naturalness.

It must be noted that any stress is relative to the rest of the utterance. Some deviation from the modal pitch and loudness is required. Connected speech practice is therefore critical to the development of naturalness.

As mentioned previously, intervention is typically not warranted if reduced prosody is associated with flat affect, and not related to physiologic limitations. Studies are currently underway in the author's laboratory to determine if an individual's nonspeech dynamic pitch and loudness ranges are related to prosodic variations in connected speech. In the cases of monopitch, the author often uses singing to encourage vocal flexibility and improved pitch range and variation. Singing is a dynamic task requiring good motor control. It may also help the patient develop a sense of being "in tune," a feature critical to naturalness. During singing, the focus should be on pitch, as opposed to loudness variation, because of problems associated with controlling loudness. If an individual attempts to affect stress with an extreme loudness change, he or she often inadvertently sounds angry. The same tasks that can be used for patients with reduced prosody can be effective with individuals who evidence extreme prosodic variations. The therapy goal in the latter case is to minimize variations, often both in the rate and extent of pitch and loudness changes.

A number of tasks, ranging from highly structured to natural conversational speech, may be effective in developing natural prosodic variations. At a basic level, sentence length contrastive stress exercises may be beneficial. Given a standard phrase such as "Mary bought a new dress," the patient responds to questions, emphasizing the word necessary to answer the question. For example, "Who bought a new dress?" should elicit stress on *Mary*, while "Did Mary buy an old dress?" should elicit stress on *new*. Some patients respond best when the standard sentence is personal. For example, "You're wearing a blue cap today" may elicit a more natural response than would be elicited by an impersonal statement.

Common phrases such as "What time is it" and "I don't know" are good practice, because they have fairly standard stress patterns. They can also be practiced immediately in social interactions. Responding to general knowledge questions may be an effective strategy for patients with adequate cognitive abilities. They can be cued to think of the response, and plan the stressed word to effectively answer the question.

If the patient is able to read, acting out simple scripts can be an enjoyable way to practice prosodic variations. Another strategy, effective with some patients, is repetition of the same phrase, such as "I'm going home today," while portraying different emotions. Emotions that tend to elicit very different prosodic patterns include: happiness, sadness, sarcasm, fear, excitement, and boredom.

When working on prosody, both the clinician and patient must have a good ear for naturalness. It is often difficult to determine the ideal balance between flat and extreme variations. Close attention to the natural conversational speech of others will help. In addition, frequent playback of audio or video recordings is essential for developing awareness of appropriate prosody. If the patient produces an unnatural utterance, the clinician should be able to describe the problem as objectively and specifically as possible (for example, "Your pitch went too high on 'I'"), and then model the target pattern. Perception of the appropriateness of prosodic variations is subjective, however. It is difficult for most patients to relate to feedback such as "Your pitch was three semitones too high on 'I.'" Although it is possible to employ visual biofeedback of intonation contours with a Visipitch or comparable equipment, the visual trace often does not correspond with one's perception. The clinician and patient must rely, therefore, on developing good listening skills and realistic judgments of naturalness. Often, unnaturalness will be related to the patient's inability to selectively stress a single word or syllable. Many stress patterns occur in steps, rather than as a gradual increase. Again, specificity of feedback and careful listening enhance therapeutic effectiveness.

AUGMENTATIVE COMMUNICATION

Augmentative and alternative communication has advanced to the extent that it is now an area of subspecialization within the fields of speech-language pathology and special education. Clinicians are well advised to consult with specialists whenever possible. Augmentative communication systems continue to be refined, so details regarding specific systems will soon be outdated. The following is provided as a discussion of some of the issues to address when considering an augmentative system.

The manner by which a patient will access the system will influence decisions. The clinician must determine the individual's most reliable and efficient motor movement. Access options include head movements, sip and blow, touching or pointing, or using switches. Some systems are designed to allow the patient to scan through choices and make selections, minimizing motoric demands. The size of keys the patient can access on a device will be affected by both motor abilities and visual and visuospatial abilities. Additionally, the clinician should determine the patient's best mode of visual comprehension. Can the patient read words, discriminate among pictures, or understand symbols?

The adaptations the individual will need in order to use the system effectively must be considered prior to the final selection of a device. Key guards help an individual access only one key at a time, regardless of motor control. Special mounting can facilitate access through optimal positioning. The patient's physical limitations need to be considered in order to determine if the system will be permanently mounted on the wheelchair, or will be more portable.

Augmentative systems range from the extremely simple, with large picture access, to those with multiple layers using single word prompts. The cognitive abilities of an individual must be carefully considered. Comprehension, memory, and new learning abilities will all impact the decision regarding system complexity.

The clinician must also determine if the patient prefers a synthesized voice or a recorded voice. Recorded voices sound more natural, but obviously limit the patient's output options. Synthesized voices offer more flexibility in output but may be, despite recent advances, unappealing or difficult for some people to understand. The ability to supplement output by means of a printer is helpful in these cases. A printer option also allows the system to be used for written as well as verbal expression.

The clinician and patient should determine to what degree an augmentative system will be the individual's primary means of communication. Utilization may well vary by situation. In familiar settings, listeners may understand the patient in one or two attempts. In unknown contexts or with new listeners, the patient may rely on an augmentative device for effective communication.

Finally, the patient's primary communication partners or discharge environment will affect the selection. If the patient will be discharged to the family home, the device may get little use. Often a patient will be able to communicate with family members because of situational and contextual familiarity. In these cases, family members may inadvertently discourage use of an augmentative system. Similar situations may occur in residential facilities, once staff become familiar with the patient. Many conversational partners find it more convenient to guess the patient's intent rather than allow expression through an augmentative system. Ideally, before the patient's discharge, the clinician should provide training to individuals in the discharge community, in order to improve awareness of the patient's abilities, and to encourage use of the augmentative system.

Because augmentative systems are being refined constantly, it is difficult for a clinician to keep up to date. Again, a good consultant is an invaluable resource. If none is available in the clinician's area, vendors at conferences and workshops will have the latest equipment. The journal *Augmentative and Alternative Communication*[57] is also an excellent resource.

APRAXIA OF SPEECH

Apraxia of speech is a neuromotor programming problem. It can occur in isolation, with the patient evidencing no muscle weakness or linguistic deficit, or in conjunction with dysarthria and aphasia. Apraxia of speech must be distinguished from oral apraxia. The test, *Apraxia Battery for Adults*, by Dabul,[58] is useful in this regard. In oral apraxia, nonspeech oral movements, such as tongue lateralization or licking the lips, may be characterized by searching and groping behaviors. In the author's clinical experience, oral apraxia rarely impacts speech production. Unlike dysarthria, in which phoneme errors will be consistent, apraxia of speech is characterized by inconsistent phoneme substitutions or distortions. Groping or searching behaviors may be evident. In very severe cases, the individual may not be able to initiate speech at all, as the result of inability to coordinate the required movements. It is possible, in these cases, that the individual would benefit from using an augmentative system to communicate.

Apraxia of speech following traumatic brain injury is approached in much the same manner as that resulting from a cerebrovascular accident. A thorough review of treatment for apraxia of speech is found in a chapter by Rosenbek.[59] The basic therapeutic principles cited previously remain relevant. Several therapy protocols may be useful in treatment. As with dysarthria, the consideration of the patient's cognitive abilities is paramount to the choice and implementation of therapy procedures. Because it is difficult to predict which treatment approach will be most beneficial, each is worth a period of trial therapy. The first approach involves an eight-step process designed to facilitate the reorganization of speech. Based largely on imitation, the first step of the process requires that the patient simply watch and listen to the clinician, and then produce an utterance simultaneously. The process progresses through delayed imitation with a visual cue (that is, clinician mimes the utterance), delayed imitation with no visual cue, successive patient productions, written stimuli with simultaneous production, written stimuli and delayed production, utterance elicited by a question, and finally, appropriate response in role playing.

A second approach is *Melodic Intonation Therapy*.[60,61,62,63] Although initially designed to facilitate verbal expression in individuals with severe nonfluent aphasia, it may be useful for some patients in treating apraxia of speech. Also an imitative program, Melodic Intonation Therapy involves the simultaneous verbal production and tapping of phrases, according to an established pattern of pitch, rhythm and stress. A hierarchy, progressing from simultaneous productions to more independent spontaneous utterances, is outlined in Sparks and Holland.[61]

A third approach involves establishing a hierarchy of phonemes from easiest to hardest for the patient to produce. Often, the patient will be able to imitate vowels, liquids, and glides, but will have great difficulty producing more complex sounds, such as affricatives. The clinician can build a repertoire of words based on the sounds easily produced by the patient, gradually adding more difficult sounds, and increasing the length and complexity of the utterances.

As mentioned previously, apraxia of speech rarely occurs in isolation in individuals with traumatic brain injury. Therefore, it is of paramount importance to establish priorities among intervention strategies. It is always useful to determine what will make the biggest difference in the patient's ability to communicate. In this way, the patient and family members will see the benefits of therapy more quickly, and be more likely to maintain motivation.

SPECIAL CASES

There are times when it is very difficult to discern the cause of reduced intelligibility. In these cases, most often a combination of cognitive, linguistic, and physiologic deficits is evident. For example, a patient recently seen by the author presented with severely reduced intelligibility. Only after several weeks of diagnostic therapy was it determined that the contributors to the intelligibility deficit included depression, paraphasic errors, word finding problems, and apraxia of speech, as well as moderate hypernasality and mild articulatory imprecision. Therapy focused on improving language abilities and addressing depression, which in turn enhanced intelligibility.

Even more challenging are those patients who are determined "to learn to talk again," despite severe physiologic and cognitive limitations. The author believes that virtually everyone deserves a period of trial therapy, when funding and time permit. If the patient is truly determined to talk again, the clinician can at least provide basic strategies for independent practice. During this time, however, the clinician must stress the need for effective communication, regardless of modality.

Assessment and treatment of motor speech disorders following traumatic brain injury is demanding, rewarding, and rarely boring. Every patient presents a different combination of cognitive, emotional, and physical strengths and limitations. The challenge for the clinician is to individualize treatment to compensate for deficits and to optimize the patient's strengths.

SUMMARY

Motor speech disorders resulting from traumatic brain injury are complex. Since traditional theories of dysarthria classification are inadequate for traumatic brain injury, a physiologic approach to delineating the characteristics of motor speech disorders in this population was presented. Deficits may occur anywhere along the vocal tract, resulting in disorders of respiration, voicing, resonance, and articulation. Differing degrees of impairment may occur at each level, and the effects are interactive.

The utility of clinical instrumentation for assessment and intervention was reviewed. Instrumentation may be useful to objectify a component of the patient's speech production problem, to provide accountability for therapy, and to serve as biofeedback. Clinicians were cautioned, however, not to rely solely on instrumentation since it is the perception of the integrated processes as a whole that determines an individual's communicative success. Further, biofeedback affords minimal generalization without the patient's proprioceptive awareness of optimal productions.

Since many individuals will not return to premorbid physiologic functioning, therapy emphasizing compensatory strategies was highlighted. In this chapter, the author stressed that the guiding strategy underlying any intervention is to optimize the patient's strengths. Basic therapeutic guidelines were outlined that emphasized functional, contextual speech production practice.

Apraxia of speech was discussed as another type of communication disorder that may occur following traumatic brain injury, although its incidence, like dysarthria, is unknown. Recommendations for assessment and intervention were made. A brief discussion of augmentative communication was presented as it is a necessary alternative for many individuals with severe communication impairments following traumatic brain injury.

REFERENCES

1. Darley FL, Aronson AE, Brown JR. *Motor Speech Disorders*. Philadelphia, PA: WB Saunders; 1975.
2. Beukelman DR, Yorkston KM. *Communication Disorders Following Traumatic Brain Injury: Management of Cognitive, Language, and Motor Impairments*. Austin, TX: Pro-ed; 1991:251–315.
3. Yorkston KM et al. The relationship between speech and swallowing disorders in head injured patients. *Journal of Head Trauma Rehabilitation*. 1989;vol. 1–16.
4. McHenry M, Wilson R. The challenge of unintelligible speech following traumatic brain injury. *Brain Injury*. 1994;8:363–375.
5. Baken RJ. *Clinical Measurement of Speech and Voice*. Boston, MA: Little Brown and Company; 1987.
6. Ludlow CL, Bassich CJ, Connor NP. An objective system for assessment and analysis of dysarthric speech. In Darby JK (ed). *Speech and Language Evaluation in Neurology: Adult Disorders*. New York, NY: Grune & Stratton; 1985:393–425.
7. Prigatano GP, Altman IM, O'Brien KP. Behavioral limitations that traumatic-brain-injured patients tend to underestimate. *The Clinical Neuropsychologist*. 1990;4:163–176.
8. Gracco VL, Abbs JH. Sensorimotor characteristics of speech motor sequences. *Experimental Brain Research*. 1989;75:586–598.

9. Gracco VL. Sensorimotor mechanisms in speech motor control. In Peters, Hulstijm, Starkweather (eds). *Speech Motor Control and Stuttering.* North Holland: Elsevier Science Publishers; 1991:53–76.

10. Rosenbek JC, Wertz RT, Darley FL. Oral sensation and perception in apraxia of speech and aphasia. *Journal of Speech and Hearing Research.* 1973;16:22–36.

11. Ringel RL, Ewanowski SJ. Oral Perception: 1. Two-point discrimination. *Journal of Speech and Hearing Research.* 1965;8:389–398.

12. Maeyama T, Plattig KH. Minimal two-point discrimination in human tongue and palate. *American Journal Of Otolaryngology.* 1989;10:342–344.

13. Hixon T, Hawley J, Wilson J. An around-the-house device for the clinical determination of respiratory driving pressure: a note on making simple even simpler. *Journal of Speech and Hearing Disorders.* 1982;47:413–415.

14. Titze IR. Toward standards in acoustic analysis of voice. *Journal of Voice.* 1994; 8:1–7.

15. Smitheran JR, Hixon T. A clinical method for estimating laryngeal airway resistance during vowel production. *Journal of Speech and Hearing Disorders.* 1981; 46:138–146.

16. Barlow SM, Suing G. Aerospeech: automated digital signal analysis of speech aerodynamics. *Journal for Computer Users in Speech and Hearing.* 1991;7: 211–227.

17. Hixon T, Smitheran J. A reply to Rothenberg. *Journal of Speech and Hearing Disorders.* 1982;47:218–223.

18. Langhans J. Laryngeal airway resistance during vowel production in adult females. *ASHA.* 1981;23:745.

19. Shaughnessy AL, Lotz WK, Netsell R. Laryngeal resistance for syllable series and word productions. *ASHA.* 1981;23:745.

20. Netsell R et al. Vocal tract aerodynamics during syllable productions: normative data and theoretical implications. *Journal of Voice.* 1991;5:1–9.

21. McHenry MA, Reich AR. Effective airway resistance and vocal sound pressure level in cheerleaders with a history of dysphonic episodes. *Folia Phoniatrica.* 1985;37:223–231.

22. Holmberg EB, Hillman RE, Perkell JS. Glottal airflow and transglottal air pressure measurements for male and female speakers in soft, normal, and loud voice. *Journal of the Acoustical Society of America.* 1988;84:511–29.

23. Hillman RE et al. Objective assessment of vocal hyperfunction: an experimental framework and initial results. *Journal of Speech and Hearing Research.* 1989;32: 373–92.

24. Holmberg EB, Hillman RE, Perkell JS. Glottal airflow and transglottal air pressure measurements for male and female speakers in low, normal and high pitch. *Journal of Voice.* 1989;3:294–305.

25. Holmberg EB. Laryngeal airway resistance as a function of phonation type. *Journal of the Acoustical Society of America Supplement.* 1980;68:S101.

26. Netsell R, Lotz WK, Shaughnessy AL. Laryngeal aerodynamics associated with selected voice disorders. *American Journal of Otolaryngology.* 1984;5:397–403.

27. McHenry MA, Wilson RL, Minton JT. Management of multiple physiological system deficits following traumatic brain injury. *Journal of Medical Speech-Language Pathology.* 1994;2:59–74.

28. Holmberg EG, Hillman RE, Perkell JS, Gress C. Relationships between intra-speaker variation in aerodynamic measures of voice production and variation

in SPL across repeated recordings. *Journal of Speech and Hearing Research.* 1994;37:484–495.

29. McHenry MA et al. Comparison of direct and indirect calculations of laryngeal airway resistance in connected speech. *Journal of Voice.* In press.

30. McHenry MA et al. Comparison of direct and indirect measurements of laryngeal airway resistance in various voicing conditions. *European Journal of Communication Disorders.* 1995. In press.

31. Finnegan E et al. Sources of error in estimation of laryngeal airway resistance in patients with spasmodic dysphonia. *National Center for Voice and Speech Status and Progress Report.* 1994;65–75.

32. Gould WJ, Korovin GS. Laboratory advances for voice measurements. *Journal of Voice.* 1994;8,8–17.

33. Colton RH, Casper JK. *Understanding Voice Problems: A Physiological Perspective for Diagnosis and Treatment.* Baltimore, MD: Williams and Wilkins; 1990:165–210.

34. Read C, Buder EH, Kent RD. Speech analysis systems: an evaluation. *Journal of Speech and Hearing Research.* 1992;35:324–332.

35. McWilliams BJ, Morris HL, Shelton RL. *Cleft Palate Speech.* Philadelphia, PA: BC Decker; 1990:163–196.

36. Seaver EJ et al. A study of nasometric values for normal nasal resonance. *Journal of Speech and Hearing Research.* 1991;34:715–721.

37. Barlow SM et al. A high-speed data acquisition and protocol control system for vocal tract physiology. *Journal of Voice.* 1989;3:283–293.

38. Warren DW, DuBois AB. A pressure-flow technique for measuring velopharyngeal orifice area during continuous speech. *Cleft Palate Journal.* 1964;1:52–71.

39. Warren DW et al. A pressure-flow technique for quantifying temporal patterns of palatopharyngeal closure. *Cleft Palate Journal.* 1985;22:11–19.

40. Campbell TF, Linville, RN, Campbell Y. Aerodynamic assessment of speech using the PERCI-PC: evaluation and reliability. *Plastic and Reconstructive Surgery.* 1991;87:365–370.

41. Kent RD et al. Toward phonetic intelligibility testing in dysarthria. *Journal of Speech and Hearing Disorders.* 1989;52:482–499.

42. Yorkston KM, Beukelman DR, Traynor C. *Computerized Assessment of Intelligibility of Dysarthric Speech.* Tigard, OR: CC Publications; 1984.

43. Robin DA, Somodi LB, Luschei ES. Measurement of tongue strength and endurance in normal and articulation disordered subjects. In Moore CA, Yorkston KM, Beukelman DR (eds). *Dysarthria and Apraxia of Speech: Perspectives on Management.* Baltimore, MD: Paul H Brookes Publishing; 1991:3–14.

44. Robin DA et al. Tongue strength and endurance: Relation to highly skilled movements. *Journal of Speech and Hearing Research.* 1992;35:1239–1245.

45. McHenry M, Minton JT, Wilson RL. Increasing the efficiency of articulatory force testing in traumatic brain injury. In Till J, Yorkston KM, Beukelman DR (eds). *Motor Speech Disorders: Advances in Assessment and Treatment.* Baltimore, MD: Paul H Brookes Publishing; 1994:135–146.

46. McHenry MA et al. Intelligibility and nonspeech orofacial strength and force control following traumatic brain injury. *Journal of Speech and Hearing Research.* 1994;37:1271–1283.

47. Weismer G et al. Formant trajectory characteristics of males with amyotrophic lateral sclerosis. *Journal of the Acoustical Society of America.* 1992;2:1085–1098.

48. Hixon TJ, Goldman MD, Mead J. Kinematics of the chest wall during speech production: volume displacements of the rib cage, abdomen, and lung. *Journal of Speech and Hearing Research.* 1973;16:78–115.
49. Murdoch BE et al. Abnormal patterns of speech breathing in dysarthric speakers following severe closed head injury. *Brain Injury.* 1993;7:295–308.
50. Karnell MP. *Videoendoscopy: from Velopharynx to Larynx.* San Diego, CA: Singular Publishing Group; 1994.
51. McHenry MA. Laryngeal airway resistance following traumatic brain injury. In Robin D, Yorkston KM, Beukelman DR (eds). *Disorders of Motor Speech: Recent Advances in Assessment, Treatment, and Clinical Characterization.* Baltimore, MD: Paul H Brookes Publishing; 1995.
52. Theodoros D, Murdoch BE. Laryngeal dysfunction in dysarthric speakers following severe closed head injury. *Brain Injury.* 1994;8:667–684.
53. Colton RH, Casper JK. *Understanding Voice Problems: A Physiological Perspective for Diagnosis and Treatment.* Baltimore, MD: Williams and Wilkins; 1990: 211–234.
54. Theodoros D et al. Hypernasality in dysarthric speakers following severe closed head injury: a perceptual and instrumental analysis. *Brain Injury.* 1993;59–69.
55. McHenry MA. The effect of increased vocal effort on velopharyngeal resistance. Submitted
56. Daniel B. A soft palate desensitization procedure for patients requiring palatal lift prostheses. *Journal of Prosthetic Dentistry.* 1982;48:565–566.
57. *Augmentative and Alternative Communication.* Baltimore, MD: Williams and Wilkins.
58. Dabul B. *Apraxia Battery for Adults.* Tigard, Oregon: CC Publications; 1979.
59. Rosenbek JC. Treating apraxia of speech. In DF Johns (ed). *Clinical Management of Neurogenic Communicative Disorders.* Boston: Little Brown; 1985:267–312.
60. Sparks RW, Helm N, Albert M. Aphasia rehabilitation resulting from melodic intonation therapy. *Cortex.* 1974;10:303–316.
61. Sparks RW, Holland AL. Method: melodic intonation therapy for aphasia. *Journal of Speech and Hearing Disorders.* 1976;41:287–297.
62. Berlin CI. On: melodic intonation therapy for aphasia by RW Sparks, AL Holland. *Journal of Speech and Hearing Disorders.* 1976;41:298–300.
63. Mihailescu, MPL. Melodic intonation in the rehabilitation of Romanian aphasics with bucco-lingual apraxia. *Romanian Journal of Neurology and Psychiatry.* 1992;30:99–113.

10

Ethical and Legal Considerations

Although a number of texts and journals have addressed specific ethical issues in traumatic brain injury rehabilitation, such as competency,[1] autonomy,[2] and allocation of resources,[3] few have included a theoretical framework from which the rehabilitation professional can consider ethical issues. Medical ethicists have only recently begun to analyze the uniqueness of the patient/provider relationships that exists in the field of medical rehabilitation.[4] Most of the moral dilemmas discussed in the literature on medical ethics arise from the acute and emergency care settings. Speech-language pathologists will find little guidance in the literature for confronting ethical dilemmas specific to the discipline.

The majority of schools granting degrees in the health professions do not offer formal courses in medical ethics.[5] According to Dr. L.R. Bristow, the 1995 President of the American Medical Association,[6] at least 25 percent of medical schools have no formal courses in medical ethics. He thinks courses in ethics are greatly needed to help clinicians face the health care challenges of today. It is the opinion of the author, based on clinical experience, that those involved in traumatic brain injury rehabilitation, for even a brief amount of time, will be faced with at least one significant ethical dilemma. Often, ethical challenges and difficult decisions can be managed with greater certainty if options and potential solutions have been previously considered than if one is unprepared and inexperienced concerning the issues. This chapter attempts to prepare the reader to consider some of the ethical dilemmas in rehabilitation, by:

(1) providing a theoretical framework from which to understand medical ethics,
(2) delineating types of ethical issues and dilemmas that occur in traumatic brain injury rehabilitation,
(3) presenting case examples for consideration, and
(4) presenting legal issues that may be encountered.

The case examples presented are not hypothetical, but have been altered for reasons of confidentiality. Possible courses for action are provided to prompt the reader's thinking, but the examples are not intended to limit or dictate the clinician's decision making.

A FRAMEWORK FOR CONSIDERING MEDICAL ETHICS

Robert Veatch, a well-known medical ethicist, defines ethics as "the enterprise of disciplined reflection on the moral intuitions and moral choices that people make."[7] One may ask, rightfully, "What is moral?" Ruth Purtilo,[8] an ethicist and physical therapist, explains to us that morality "is concerned with relations between people and how, ultimately, they can live in peace and harmony." Morality, then, involves the values of society, as well as those of the individual.

A number of ethical theories have been proposed by theologians and philosophers. An additional text would be required to present the numerous interpretations of the different theoretical paradigms used to discuss ethics. Purtilo[8] has outlined two of the categories of theories that have the greatest relevance to health care: deontological and teleological theories. Briefly, those who adhere to *deontological* theories are concerned with duties and rights, and the means by which results are achieved. As an example, if society considers it wrong to lie (it is a duty or responsibility to tell the truth), and an individual member values absolute truth, then it would be wrong for that person to lie, even if doing so would cause a positive result that benefited another member of society. Those who view moral decisions from a *teleological* framework are more concerned with results or consequences than with absolutes (rights and wrongs). The result achieved in the end is more important than the means by which it is achieved. Within this framework, a number of consequences are considered, and thus alternate paths of action are explored. This position is in contrast to a deontological frame of reference, in which the right course (for example, do not lie) is chosen because it is the only course consistent with a given moral principle (for example, always tell the truth). An individual may operate within either framework, depending upon the situation, personal values, and the values of the group at large (for example, a department of a hospital, a rehabilitation team, a religious organization, or a family). These theories are presented as a means by which clinicians can evaluate their own behaviors and modes of operation when making difficult decisions.

There are a number of components to ethics, as well as a number of theoris. Duties and rights are the two concepts considered in this chapter. Included under *duties,* or *obligations,* are bringing about good (benevolence), doing no harm (nonmaleficence), telling the truth, with the implication of not being deceitful (veracity), keeping promises (fidelity), and justice.[8] Justice is perhaps the most complex of these, and is concerned with fairness and impartiality. It concerns the fair allocation of benefits among all members of a society. Needs, resources, equity, and deservedness are all factors that must be considered when justice is an issue. The practicing clinician will quickly recognize justice as an area that often presents great ethical conflict.

Rights are defined by Purtilo[8] as "stringent claims a person or group makes on society in general or on a specific individual or group."[7] Some of the rights protected in our Western society include the right to life, the right to privacy, the right to autonomy, and the right to equal opportunity for education and employment. In a society that values equality among its members, all members should have not only equal protection of their rights but also equal access to the goods of the society at large. Much of the difficulty in the political debate over health care costs arises from a lack of consensus among consumers, providers, and policy makers regarding the status of health care as a right. On the surface, it would seem logical to assume that health care providers (professionals) have a consensus; yet, providers are also consumers and may be competing for the same goods as other members of society (for example, rehabilitation services for a loved one). Rehabilitation services, as a form of health care, clearly are not considered the right of all individuals, as evidenced by the frequent use of admission criteria designed to limit the access to these services to a select few. These services are in contrast to emergency medical care, which is available to all, but struggling against financial cutbacks. Rights are important issues for clinicians to consider, from both personal and professional perspectives.

Not all uncomfortable situations that arise in the rehabilitation setting are true ethical dilemmas.[4,8] Purtilo[8] uses the term *ethical distress* to refer to situations in which the morally correct choice is obvious, but a barrier (such as an institutional policy) prevents one from acting upon that choice. An *ethical dilemma* exists when there are two or more morally correct paths of action, but only one can be followed. In a pluralistic society, it is to be expected that individual values will be tolerated, perhaps even encouraged, and will certainly be self-promoted. Because of the sheer number of professionals involved in the treatment of a single individual, rehabilitation is an extremely value-laden enterprise.[5] Clinicians bring to the treatment setting not only the values of their professional organization, but also their own religious values, family values, educational values, and social values. It is imperative that rehabilitation professionals, often vying for a place of representation on the team, be aware of their own values and the influence these have upon the decision-making process.

MEDICAL ETHICS AND REHABILITATION

Much of the way in which we practice our profession in the rehabilitation setting is based on the medical model[7,9] with its roots in the Hippocratic Oath, which dates to the fourth or fifth century B.C. The Hippocratic Oath is the foundation of the codes of ethics of many of the organizations of the allied health professions as well.[7] The place of the Hippocratic Oath in modern medicine (and that of the medical model it fosters) has come under a great deal of criticism from medical ethicists, and even physicians, in the last 20 years. The medical model is considered to be paternalistic, with the physician in the sole authoritative role, empowered to act on behalf of and in the best interests of the patient. The physician is placed in this role because of the special skills and knowledge he or she possesses. In all health care, when the provider (physician or other professional) acts as the authority and sole decision maker, the model of service delivery is labeled the medical model. Speech-language pathologists and other rehabilitation professionals can be said to deliver care under the medical model, and it appears to be the model most often practiced in hospital settings.

Under the guidelines of the Hippocratic Oath, nonmaleficence and beneficence are paramount. As stated by Sanders[10] "Nonmaleficence is the duty to avoid doing harm" (primum, non nocere: first, do no harm) and "beneficence is the duty to prevent harm, to remove evil, and to promote or do good." Some consider nonmaleficence and beneficence to be separate truths to follow, and others may view the two on a continuum.[8]

Adhering to the guiding principle of "do no harm," many nonphysician health care providers have followed in physicians' footsteps by interpreting that principle to include withholding information, particularly if it is thought that revealing information about a poor prognosis could further harm the patient and impede progress. A health care professional can take the idea of withholding bad news that might impede progress (not doing harm) and rationalize it to mean promoting a more positive outcome than would be likely if negative information were given out (that is, promoting good). The intentional withholding of information is not acceptable practice today, in large part because of the need for informed consent (discussed later), but also because this is the new age of consumerism. Today, patients are encouraged to take an active role in their health care and to assume responsibility for their health. Additionally, the increasing competition among health care providers has, to some extent, forced providers to better meet the particular needs of the individuals seeking services today than was the case in the past. To meet this challenge, health care professionals must communicate with their patients on equal ground.

Rehabilitation, unlike other fields of medicine, is not primarily concerned with providing a cure. In almost all other fields of medicine, with the possible exception being psychiatry, the expectation of both patient and provider is that the treatment rendered is intended as a cure.[5,9] Seldom in rehabilitation is the goal to cure; it is rather to restore as much function as is possible, and to teach the patient to compensate for that which cannot be restored. Rehabilitation works best when the patient assumes an active, participatory role. In most instances of traumatic brain injury, patients and their families have entered the health care system first through the emergency and acute care settings. Often, the expectation of cure is still present. Patients and their families may not be ready to assume a participatory form of care when first entering the rehabilitation setting. Additionally, many persons who have a traumatic brain injury do not have the cognitive capacity to choose to take an active role. All of these factors contribute to the ethical conflicts that arise in the rehabilitation setting, as opposed to the critical care setting.

INFORMED CONSENT

In contrast to the development of professional codes of ethics, written to guide professional behavior, informed consent is relatively new, first appearing in the literature in 1957.[11,12] There is actually little written information in the general field of rehabilitation medicine that addresses *informed consent*, and even less in the specific allied health fields. As with other aspects of medical ethics, many of the established precedents for issues concerning informed consent come from cases in the critical care setting. Most health care professionals and lay persons think of informed consent as the written contract that patients sign prior to entering the hospital. The written consent document used in hospitals is a means of obtaining consent to administer care in a very general sense. When specific procedures are indicated, patients are requested to sign additional documents to indicate their consent to the specific intervention, and to acknowledge an understanding of any potential risks associated with the procedure or intervention. The legal system has focused largely on informed consent in this context, and in the context of disclosure of information.[11] As indicated earlier in the chapter, disclosure may be best viewed in regard to the practice of withholding information about a condition (benefits/risks of treatment, prognosis, and so on), as an act of beneficence.

Informed consent is both ethically and legally binding. In concept, informed consent is much more than the process of disclosing information. The basic principle underlying informed consent is an individual's right to autonomy or self-determination.[5,7,9] Informed consent is viewed by some as a commitment to democracy, an indication of mutual participation[13] and a process of shared decision making between the patient and professional.[11] Caplan[9] describes it as the guarantee to patient self-determination. If one's right to self-determination is respected, then the right to determine what will or will not be done to one's body is protected.[14] Informed consent must include the right to refuse treatment.

Brody[15] has stated that "legitimate nondisclosure or deception can occur only when an autonomous patient requests this of the physician." If informed consent is honored absolutely, the only way a provider can withhold full disclosure is with the patient's permission. Fundamental to the concept of informed consent is the belief that knowing a patient's preferences will positively affect the patient-provider relationship and foster trust.[8]

In order to be autonomous, one must have the information needed to make informed decisions. Some of the information that must be made available to patients, in order to have informed consent, includes an explanation of the nature and purpose of treatment, the expected outcome and anticipated success, an explanation of risks, a discussion of alternative treatment(s) available for the same conditions, and the potential effects (or risks) of withholding or not providing treatment.[16] According to Beauchamp[11] "the mere act of signing a form cannot qualify as an informed consent." One cannot really know if informed consent has been given unless the circumstances under which it was obtained are known. Informed consent must be given freely and without coercion.[9] Although it is not necessary to have a signed document in order to have informed consent, the clinician should document carefully the circumstances under which information was revealed, and include: the patient's level of understanding; other persons present; adaptive means used to facilitate comprehension and indication of the patient's agreement/disagreement; questions asked; and the date, time, and length of discussions.[16]

A number of criticisms of medical rehabilitation have suggested that rehabilitation professionals have defended the practice of not obtaining informed consent, citing a number of reasons.[9,16] The reasons suggested have included the fact that rehabilitation is not finite, and that care is delivered by a team of professionals rather than by a single physician.[13] Should consent be obtained for each physical or occupational therapy session before treatment is rendered? Other arguments have posited that it is unreasonable to expect patients to make decisions that will affect their future during the initial stages of adjustment to a disabling condition.[9,16] These are legitimate issues in rehabilitation; they do not facilitate the process of informed consent, but neither do they prohibit it.

Although the writings of those outside of the rehabilitation field[7,9,17] have not suggested that the rehabilitation team treatment plan, or plan of care, functions as a document of informed consent, those in the field might very well argue that it is an exemplary model of informed consent. Because of the requirements set forth by the Commission for the Accreditation of Rehabilitation Facilities,[18] which aim to ensure patient and family participation in rehabilitation planning, rehabilitation facilities that have certification (and adhere to the requirements) are informing patients and their families on a regular basis. It is the author's contention that when used to its fullest extent, the treatment plan does, and should, function as the document of informed consent. Because of the complexity of most comprehensive treatment plans and the abundance of medical jargon typically present, the rehabilitation team does have an obligation to ensure that the information contained in the document is understood. Each member of the rehabilitation team has an obligation to inform the patient of treatment procedures in such a manner that an informed choice can be made. Clinicians should use treatment plans to their full advantage to inform their patients and families about proposed treatment. To use the treatment plan to its full power, as an instrument of informed consent, requires that the team as a whole, or a team member, meet with the patient and/or family members *prior* to the establishment of goals, in order to truly consider patient preferences. In order to honor the patient's right to autonomy, he or she must always be given the option of deleting specific aspects of the program, if portions of the treatment plan are unacceptable. Accordingly, the aspect of care that is perhaps most difficult is ascertaining the patient's level of comprehension as it relates to competence and autonomy.

In traumatic brain injury rehabilitation, a patient's autonomy can pose unique dilemmas in and of itself. How autonomous is the patient who has loss of insight, poor memory, and poor reasoning? How morally correct is it to expect the patient to answer questions requiring reasoning? Should one trust the answers to be an accurate indication of the person's preinjury or current wishes? The issues surrounding the capacity to give informed consent are discussed in the following section. In the competitive market of rehabilitation services, time constraints have been the predominant defense offered for failure to ensure the patient's complete understanding of the rehabilitation plan. This problem is real and is not likely to diminish, since clinicians are expected to be highly accountable for treatment hours rendered. There is great incentive to limit the amount of time spent with patients and their families if that time cannot be billed as a reimbursable service, or if time spent in education seriously limits a therapist's ability to deliver treatment to other patients. Additionally, at the point rehabilitation enters into the continuum of care for a brain-injured patient, family members will frequently have resumed work and other daily routines, making it difficult for team members to consult with them when treatment plans are changed. The coordination of rehabilitation efforts is no doubt a significant task; yet, if patient autonomy is determined to be the priority for the entire rehabilitation team, time and resources must be made available.

COMPETENCY

The relationship between *competence* and *informed consent*, as presented in the literature, appears ridiculously circular. The competent person is one who is able to give informed consent, and as such, one from whom consent should be obtained. Competence is therefore a necessary condition of informed consent. Conversely, the incompetent person is one from whom consent need not or should not be solicited. Competence may be based on factual information or may be presumed categorically.[11] Adults are legally assumed to be competent,[16] while minors are presumed not to be. There are no precise definitions of competence as a legal or medical construct. To add further to the imprecision, *autonomy* is also closely tied to competence. Sanders[10] states that "autonomy is a concept which requires the presence of adequate intellectual capacities to make an informed decision."

In brain injury rehabilitation, questions of competence arise frequently. Being mentally competent to make medical decisions implies an ability to deliberate about the risks and benefits of a proposed treatment, and to understand the consequences of a decision to choose no treatment.[9,16,17] When an individual is thought to be incompetent, consent to treatment should be obtained by proxy. Rehabilitation providers might assume that reasonable persons would always desire rehabilitation immediately following an injury. Therefore, an admission to a facility before a patient is truly competent to make decisions would be an act in the patient's best interest (benevolence). Nonetheless, Banja[19] offers a strong argument against such reasoning in the following:

> The only legally safe course to pursue when contemplating the admission of an incompetent patient is to ensure that a legally authorized proxy consenter has been identified and is available for making treatment decisions. Relying on a next-of-kin who is not empowered by a court or named in a state statute or law to make decisions for the patient is tantamount to providing unauthorized treatment.

The person(s) qualified to give consent on behalf of an individual varies from state to state, depending upon the way the laws are written. It is best for rehabilitation providers to be aware of the laws in their state governing proxy consent.

Rehabilitation is filled with case examples where patients do not wish to pursue the goals clinicians find most appropriate, and they often wish to pursue goals we consider unrealistic and unattainable.[20] It is under these circumstances that we must use extreme caution, so as not to usurp patients' autonomy on the grounds of incompetence. As a clinician, one may choose not to render a particular treatment requested by a patient, if the treatment is considered to be clinically unsound or not in the patient's best interest, provided that the patient is informed and given the option to seek treatment in an alternative manner (for example, at another facility, with another clinician) or to obtain no treatment. However, a clinician may not force a preferred treatment on a patient on the grounds that the patient is incompetent to choose, because the patient has not made the "correct" treatment decision. It is important for clinicians to understand that declaring an individual incompetent is a legal act. Clinicians, other than physicians and occasionally psychologists, do not have the recognized authority to provide information to the court regarding a patient's competence. Nevertheless, in a rehabilitation setting, the professional opinions of other clinicians will be considered, and in most cases they will influence the physician's recommendation. Thus, it is important that clinicians' opinions be based on factual information that is supported by documentation. To have an individual declared incompetent is to take away that person's autonomy, and in a society that values individualism and choice, loss of autonomy is extremely devaluing. Assisting individuals with brain injury in their struggle to regain autonomy is a primary objective of rehabilitation. Yet, at the same time, the care and "safeguarding" of a patient is entrusted to the health care professional. Concerns over liability are justified in our litigious environment. Autonomy is not an all or none proposition, and great clinical judgment must be exercised as to how much self-determination can be encouraged without endangering the patient or other members of society.

Current views of competence suggest that there can be specific areas in which an individual can be competent to make decisions, and that competence is not necessarily an all or none matter.[1] An individual may be competent to decide a preferred treatment but not competent to manage personal finances. This relative scale of competence requires that during rehabilitation all efforts be made to provide patients with the opportunity to make decisions regarding their own care. It is important that incompetence not be assumed on the basis of a diagnosis or a limited sampling of behavior, that all patients be afforded every opportunity to act autonomously, and that their decisions be honored when competence has been demonstrated.

Case Example 1:   Keith was a 20-year-old high school graduate who worked part-time for his father in an automotive repair shop. His mother and father were divorced and resided in different states. Keith had been living with his father for an indefinite period when he was involved in a motorcycle accident resulting in a severe traumatic brain injury with severe apraxia of speech and right-sided hemiparesis. He was in a coma for several months and initially treated in an acute care hospital. He was later treated for six months in a rehabilitation hospital in the state where he lived with his father. Upon his discharge from the rehabilitation hospital, his mother admitted him to a transitional residential facility approximately 30 miles from her home. Following three months of further comprehensive rehabilitation, he returned to his mother's home and continued therapy in a day treatment facility. He was enrolled in an intensive program of speech and language therapy, two to four hours daily, with an additional hour each of physical and occupational therapy. At the end of a two-month period, he was able to walk with a cane and had some isolated finger movement in his right hand. His speech was limited to a few words, typically spontaneous greetings, and was virtually unchanged in comparison to initial reports from the transitional facility. Reading and spelling remained severely impaired; however, he was able to recognize letters on a keyboard and could type some simple words. Other cognitive skills, such as attention, memory, and reasoning, were impaired, but Keith was considered competent by the rehabilitation team. Accordingly, the team made all attempts to act upon his treatment preferences and to assist him in making his wishes known to others. He and the speech-language pathologist, together, decided that an augmentative communication device with synthesized voice would best enable him to communicate his needs to others. Funding was available for the device and for an additional month of therapy, after which all funding would end. Numerous family conferences had been conducted, during which the speech-language pathologist's plan was discussed with Keith's mother, who had indicated agreement with Keith's wishes. Knowing that it would be several weeks before an augmentative system would be available to use with Keith, the speech-language pathologist focused most of the remaining treatment sessions on teaching Keith to use a computer keyboard in preparation for using an augmentative system. Keith's mother asked to attend one of the speech-language pathologist's therapy sessions and, with Keith's permission, observed one of the sessions. Following the session, she met with the speech-language pathologist and requested that the therapist resume working with Keith exclusively on speech production. The speech-language pathologist consulted with Keith and his mother about the limited amount of therapy time available to learn all of the information he would need to use an augmentative system. Keith's mother insisted that treatment primarily be focused on speech production, and in her presence Keith acquiesced.

Possible Courses of Action:
  (1) Change the treatment plan according to Keith's mother's wishes.
  (2) Meet with Keith privately to clarify his preferences, then insist that his mother follow them.
  (3) Ask to consult with Keith's father, with whom he still has contact.
  (4) Refer them to another facility to receive the desired services.
  (5) Ask the insurance carrier to intervene.

Considerations: Legally, Keith is considered competent until factual information proves otherwise, in which case a surrogate would need to act on his behalf. Keith does not need a surrogate according to professional opinions. Therefore, he is "free" to accept his mother's recommendation, although the speech-language pathologist does not consider the decision to be in his best interest. This case is a good example of the way in which disability interferes with or limits an individual's freedom, and hence autonomy, even if the individual is competent. Because of financial constraints, as well as physical and cognitive-communicative limitations, Keith is dependent on his mother and will be so for many years. The value the speech-language pathologist places on communication must be weighed by Keith against the value he places on his mother's ongoing financial and emotional support. Is Keith truly free to choose?

CONFIDENTIALITY

Many ethicists argue that the potential for violation of an individual's right to privacy is great in the rehabilitation setting because of the number of professionals involved in providing services.[4,8] Although it is considered acceptable practice to share information among professionals treating a particular individual, caution must be exercised so as not to overextend the limits of that practice by sharing information with persons marginally associated with the care of a patient. Further, because of the number of persons who have access to medical records and the increased ease of accessibility due to computerized record keeping, caution should be exercised regarding what is documented in the medical chart. The only information that should be documented in the medical record is that which is true and pertinent to the condition for which the patient is seeking treatment.[8] Extreme discretion should be used when documenting information about the behavioral problems often exhibited by persons with severe brain injuries. Information regarding sexual preference, desires, and activities should not be entered into the medical record unless it falls within the realm of treatment offered, which would not apply in the case of treatment by a speech-language pathologist. This is not to state that information about aspects of the patient's care other than cognitive-communicative impairment cannot be discussed with other members of the team, only that the medical record is not the mechanism by which sensitive information should be conveyed. This advice may appear to be common sense; nevertheless, the records of persons with traumatic brain injuries are filled with scenarios of past and present behaviors that have little to do with the therapy being provided. In the rehabilitation setting, where team members often have differences of opinion, clinicians are sometimes tempted to substantiate one opinion over another through the documentation process. The medical record is not the appropriate means for settling such differences.

In traumatic brain injury rehabilitation, it is not an unusual practice for facilities to pass information from one setting to the other when patients are trying to qualify for services, or the parties involved are trying to determine if there is a "good fit" between patient profile and facility profile. This seems to be a reasonable practice, because the shared information can be vital to the provision of cost effective treatment, reducing duplication of services and rehabilitation efforts. Because of the high costs of duplicating materials, conservative organizations may maintain records of persons not receiving services from the organization for some time after the records have been reviewed, under the assumption that individuals may seek services again at a later date. Many small organizations are without a department of medical records, and do not have procedures in place for the management of these types of records; yet, it is essential that clinicians take precautions to safeguard the information in these records as scrupulously as if the patients were being treated.

Although the field of head injury rehabilitation has grown immensely, it remains a closely connected network of both patients and professionals, particularly within a given locale. Regardless of the familiarity one may seem to have with a particular patient, through medical records or through colleagues, it is a violation of confidentiality and the patient's right to privacy to discuss information, obtained from either written clinical reports or verbal reports, with individuals not involved in the direct care of that patient. One only need place himself or herself in the role of the patient to understand the implications of this type of violation. Professionals often form unjustified impressions of patients based on old medical reports or on the opinions of professionals offered in casual conversations. As a consequence, an additional level of discrimination is leveled against the patient with an unfavorable report.

Another variable affecting the confidentiality of patients in the rehabilitation setting, aside from the large number of professionals involved in the brain injury program, is the number of relatives and friends. In virtually all rehabilitation settings, family members are encouraged to be active participants in treatment along with the patient. This is particularly true of those family members with whom the patient is most likely to reside upon completion of rehabilitation. Although the professional team seeks to involve family members, it should not assume that the patient always wants information shared with the family. Yet, seldom do we ask our adult patients if we have permission to discuss their condition and progress with family members, or who is to be included in the family group. It is often assumed that the family who accompanies the patient to the rehabilitation setting has a close association with the individual and should therefore have access to confidential information, but in fact the patient may not want information shared with certain family members.

Because of the nature of the treatment speech-language pathologists provide, with its focus on promoting communication, the speech-language pathologist is in a privileged position. Patients often confide in their speech-language pathologists. Sometimes secrets are revealed because the speech-language pathologist is able to communicate with the patient when others cannot, and at other times, confidences are shared because of a close, trusting relationship that has evolved over the course of treatment.

When severe communication disability exists, the speech-language pathologist may be called upon to speak on behalf of the patient or to serve as a translator. These instances usually have implied consent, with the patient present during communication exchanges. Difficulties arise in keeping confidences when patients communicate to a therapist injustices or abuses that they have experienced but have been unable, or unwilling, to report, because of the communication impairment, or out of fear of worsening the unpleasant situation. If unable to obtain the patient's consent to address the abuses with the proper authorities, or even with the persons accused, the therapist is faced with a true ethical dilemma: the good of the patient versus the confidence of the patient. Brody[15] has offered the following three guidelines for when confidentiality may be overridden:

(1) Revealing the information would produce some considerable public good.

(2) Revealing the information would prevent some possible risk of harm to someone, but we cannot identify with certainty who that would be.

(3) Revealing the information would prevent some very likely harm to specific and identifiable individuals.

Additional precautions need to be taken by speech-language pathologists who frequently use video recordings, either for communication purposes or dysphagia evaluations. These must be treated with utmost confidentiality because of the manner in which they represent the patient (that is, a readily identifiable representation of the individual as opposed to a written report that is interpretive). Banja and Higgins[21] have suggested that written informed consent be obtained for all video recordings. The consent should provide a clear indication of the purpose of the recording, including delineation of persons who may have access to the video (for example, other patients or family members), and it should specify the period for which the consent is valid. The greater the specificity of the consent, the better it serves as an indication of the patient's knowledge of the procedure (that is, informed consent).

A final "warning" regarding confidentiality in all settings, but again particularly in brain injury rehabilitation, is to ensure that consent has been obtained from either the patient or a representative before information is disclosed to third parties: these include attorneys, insurance case managers, current and former employers, and representatives of other agencies such as the Department of Human Services, Vocational Rehabilitation, or Workers' Compensation. It is not sufficient that a person identify himself or herself as knowing the patient or as representing an agency attempting to assist the patient in some manner. Some form of written or verbal consent should be obtained prior to even acknowledging that a patient is receiving, or has received, treatment.

Case Example 2:   Albert was a 55-year-old man who fell from a ladder while working on the roof of his daughter's home. When he fell, the left side of his head struck a brick ledge, and he suffered left frontal lobe damage, as well as diffuse damage, resulting in apraxia of speech and right hemiparesis as the predominant impairments. He received acute medical care and six months of inpatient and outpatient rehabilitation in the city where his daughter lived, so that she could help provide for his care. Albert's wife was not employed outside of the home and was able to stay with him at their daughter's home.

Following the six months of rehabilitation, Albert and his wife returned to their home, and he continued to receive physical therapy and speech and language therapy, as an outpatient at their local rehabilitation center. He made good progress with the speech-language pathologist and developed a trusting relationship with her. Although he was able to communicate most of his needs to the majority of listeners, this required patience on the part of the listener. Albert was extremely sensitive to this and did not want to "bother" people with his slow communication. As a result, he confided almost exclusively in the speech-language pathologist. Over the course of several weeks, he informed the speech-language pathologist of at least three occasions on which he had fallen to the floor, and his wife had either beaten him with a broom or kicked him, before he was able to rise. Albert was a tall man and required the assistance of a stable object or a person to pull himself up from the floor. He showed the speech-language pathologist large bruises on his leg and back, that could have been caused by blows or possibly by a fall alone. Albert admitted that he was afraid of his wife and of what she might do to him (both physically and financially) if he tried to report her. But he admonished the speech-language pathologist not to speak to anyone about this, and threatened to discontinue therapy if she revealed his secret.

Possible Courses of Action:
   (1)   Use all methods of influence to persuade Albert that the proper authorities must be informed.
   (2)   Report Albert's wife to the Department of Adult Protective Services.
   (3)   Meet with the facility's social worker to obtain a professional opinion about the course of action to take.
   (4)   Call Albert's daughter without his permission.
   (5)   Talk to Albert's wife without his permission.

Considerations: The speech-language pathologist has a special relationship with Albert and probably could lead him, by phrasing questions skillfully, into giving consent to reveal his secret. This type of interaction could very easily become coercive instead of persuasive; coercion, in and of itself, is unethical. It is possible that Albert is blaming his wife for the falls he has had. Without additional information, it is impossible to know with certainty. If the suspected abuse concerned a child, would the answers be more readily apparent? If the relationship between Albert and his wife is worsened by the actions of the speech-language pathologist, what will happen to him? If the speech-language pathologist violates Albert's trust and he discontinues therapy, who will serve as his advocate?

Case Example 3:   Mr. Brown was a 73-year-old man. Until his wife's death from cancer, he had enjoyed working in the interior decorating business they owned. For six months following her death he was quite depressed, but he finally began to resume his business activities and engage in activities with his three daughters. Mr. Brown was always very independent and drove himself wherever he chose. Not long after resuming activities, he was involved in a motor vehicle accident that resulted in a traumatic brain injury. He was unconscious for an undetermined amount of time following the accident, but regained consciousness in the emergency room and remained in the hospital for less than a week.

Following discharge from the hospital, Mr. Brown received services as an outpatient. He saw a speech-language pathologist for mild cognitive deficits and an occupational therapist for mild visual-perceptual deficits. Mr. Brown discussed with the speech-language pathologist and the occupational therapist his intense desire to drive again, and the thought of driving really seemed to brighten his outlook on his future. Following two weeks of daily treatment, the two therapists were discussing Mr. Brown in the weekly staff conference, and concurred that he should be referred to the hospital for a driving evaluation. The occupational therapist discussed this with Mr. Brown and informed him that she would make the referral. He was delighted.

When two of Mr. Brown's daughters came to the clinic later that day to drive him home, the speech-language pathologist took the opportunity to bring them up to date on Mr. Brown's progress and to discuss the driving evaluation. They informed the therapist that it was forbidden for Mr. Brown to drive because he probably had lost consciousness while driving, which was the suspected cause of the accident. Further, his car had hit another automobile, killing the driver, and there were possible legal charges pending. The speech-language pathologist explained that Mr. Brown had never mentioned this, and that if he had done so, the occupational therapist would not have recommended the evaluation. The daughters informed the therapist that Mr. Brown did not know a person had been killed, or even involved, in the accident. They had not told him because of his previous depression.

Mr. Brown is not incompetent, nor is any if his daughters his legal guardian. They asked the speech-language pathologist for a professional opinion about whether or not Mr. Brown should be told the truth, and actually urged the therapist to tell him during the next day's therapy. The clinicians' dilemmas were what to tell Mr. Brown about the driving evaluation, given his recent depression, and how to proceed with documentation that already contained information about the driving evaluation.

Possible Courses of Action:
   (1)   Insist that the family tell Mr. Brown, before he returns for therapy the next day, that they do not want him to have a driving evaluation. The reasons offered for not having the evaluation will be up to the daughters.
   (2)   Briefly meet with the occupational therapist to relay the new information, and ask her to tell Mr. Brown that the evaluation will be canceled because he lost consciousness while driving.
   (3)   Conduct a family conference as soon as everyone can meet, and, with all persons involved present, explain to Mr. Brown that he

cannot drive until the reason for his loss of consciousness is known.

(4) Tell the daughters that Mr. Brown has a right to know *all* information, and that they must tell him themselves.

(5) Recommend that the family seek a psychological consultation to better determine Mr. Brown's psychological status and ability to manage the tragic information.

(6) Document the results of all conversations, including the reason for canceling the driving evaluation referral.

(7) Document none of the conversations, except the fact that the daughters were given a progress update, and do not mention the driving evaluation again.

(8) Document that the driving evaluation has been discussed with family members, who are not in agreement with the recommendation; therefore, it has been placed "on hold."

Considerations: The clinicians possess confidential information about the patient that was not released to them by the patient. The probability of a legal investigation into this case is high. What should the clinicians document about the information they possess, about the reason for the decision not to refer the patient for a driving evaluation, and about the consultation with the family? What are their obligations to the patient with regard to self-determination and autonomy? Are there larger obligations to society that should be considered?

THE REHABILITATION TEAM AS A UNIQUE ETHICAL CHALLENGE

One of the most rewarding aspects of being a professional working in a rehabilitation setting with a traumatic brain injury program is the opportunity to share in a common goal with a group of peers. The rehabilitation team offers clinicians the opportunity to expand their knowledge through association and collaboration with other disciplines. Ideally, the rehabilitation team provides a method of checks and balances for the professional competence of the individual team members. Yet, in reality, there are numerous accounts of professionals protecting their incompetent colleagues out of a sense of loyalty.[22] Although most of the rehabilitation disciplines have licensure requirements and written codes of ethics, they are primarily self-governing. The assurance of conformity and adherence to regulations rests largely with peers.

Through shared joys and frustrations, the rehabilitation team can offer its members support, encouragement, and a sense of belonging.[8] It can also provoke great moral conflict when individual members are in disagreement, not only with the patient but with each other, regarding what is "best" for the patient. Additionally, patients divulge different information to individual team members according to what they think each professional wants to hear. It is not an uncommon scenario for a patient to tell the speech-language pathologist on the team that the most important goal is to "speak clearer," and to tell the physical therapist that the most important goal is to "walk without a cane." Although both goals are important, conflict may arise because of time constraints and/or financial limitations. The speech-language pathologist and the physical therapist each may think that two hours of therapy daily is needed to adequately address the patient's goal, when only three hours are available. Placing the patient in the role of decision maker takes the responsibility away from the team and gives it to the person to whom it rightfully belongs: the patient. Yet, to make these types of decisions (two hours of physical therapy or two hours of speech-language therapy), patients and their families must be knowledgeable about the benefits and the expected outcomes of each therapy. At present, we are unable to provide our patients with the quantitative information needed to make these decisions, so we leave them with little choice but to defer to the experts' opinion. For reasons such as these, it is important to have a team leader who functions as an arbitrator, or as patient advocate. In most settings, the team leader will come from one of the disciplines treating the patient. Speech-language pathologists often function in the role of team leader or program director. The hazard inherent to this approach to team leadership is the tendency for the team leader to have stronger allegiance to his or her discipline than to the patient and the team as a unit. Only in poorly functioning teams would this misplaced loyalty be accepted for any length of time.

Conflict can also arise as a result of team dynamics. Team members may leave the facility and be replaced, but even when this is not the case, the team composition is not necessarily stable. Sometimes it changes with each new patient. Team functioning almost always changes when there is an increase in perceived stress. Old grudges among members, once put to bed, may resurface under stressful situations.[23] Although the practice is unacceptable, labeling of professionals (as well as patients) does occur in the rehabilitation setting, even within departments. "Susie, speech-language pathologist, never gets her hands dirty. Mary, social worker, always sides with the family, and Bob, physical therapist, is such an idealist." Labeling does little to promote the well-being of the team or the patient, and should be avoided at all times.

The administrative pressures placed on health care teams by policy restraints and financial limitations create additional stresses beyond the day-to-day care of the patients. Administrative stresses can divide team member loyalty between the institution, for which they work, and the patient. Clinicians may experience conflict when departmental demands interfere with the needs of the team, and vice versa.[24] In a pluralistic society such as ours, there will necessarily be differences in values, belief systems, and duties, which must all be weighed against each other. Team membership requires great tolerance and flexibility. Self-awareness and the ability to accept constructive criticism are two important traits of effective team members.

ALLOCATION OF RESOURCES

Buchanan[25] states that "to allocate is to distribute resources among alternative uses." In the context of this chapter, *resources* refer to rehabilitation services, and *uses* refer to the population of persons with traumatic brain injuries in need of those services. However, any discussion of the allocation of rehabilitation resources must necessarily be put in the larger context of health care resources. It is virtually impossible to discuss health care without considering societal views on *quality of life*. However, it is not within the scope of this text to represent the many competing views on quality of life and meaning of life. A brief presentation of two major views should give the reader a sense of how one's views on quality of life issues affect subsequent views on the allocation of health care resources, and in particular rehabilitation.

The *physical* or *vitality* view considers that life in and of itself (regardless of perceived quality) is precious and should be preserved at all costs.[3] This view has dominated in critical care medicine and dictated the manner in which emergency medical care is rendered in the United States. The implied societal goal of preservation of life, above all else, is one of the reasons it is unnecessary to obtain informed consent in emergency situations. This sanctity-of-life view considers that all physical existence, regardless of limitations or capacity, warrants all measures needed to maintain that existence. Issues of resource allocation and quality of life really do not enter into the equation for weighing benefits, once the physical existence is assured.[3] One can assume that, from this perspective, rehabilitation will be on a low priority list, given that its primary goal is one of life enhancement, not life preservation.

In contrast, the *utilitarian* view maintains that the worth of each life (in terms of resource allocation) must be considered in relation to the benefits to, and burdens on, society at large. The utilitarian principle, in operation, has to be based on some predetermined formula to weigh the benefits and burdens, such as the amount of financial contribution a brain-injured person can make to society, offset by the costs of rehabilitation. Other views of quality of life consider a person's ability to be self-determining (autonomous), and hold that if that goal is achievable, all necessary interventions are justifiable.[3]

In the United States, we do not have a unified perspective of what constitutes life, and certainly not of what constitutes quality of life. For professionals involved in rehabilitation in general, and in traumatic brain injury rehabilitation in particular, it is the concern over the quality of life of the individuals we treat that drives us. It is the decisions that we have to make, or that are made for us by policy and payers, regarding the allocation of resources, that frustrate us.

Unlike acute care medicine, the field of rehabilitation has always been concerned with the issue of allocation of resources. Although much has been said and written about systems of justice and models for the allocation of resources, today, in many aspects of health care, it appears that services are distributed on the basis of ability to pay. Frequently, one of the primary criteria for acceptance into a rehabilitation program is the ability to pay for the services delivered or to be delivered.[26] This also has become a condition for a number of other services in recent years (for example, organ transplants and noncritical surgeries). Most institutions concerned with the fair distribution of services implement policies to guide the process of determining who will receive services that are in high demand and low supply. Pressures to contain costs are not merely evident at the institutional level, but are encountered at the level of individual service providers as well. Speech-language pathologists, as well as other providers (clinicians), may be called upon to write or implement policies to manage the distribution of their own services, or to decide who, among a group of select patients, will receive grant funds or funds from private donors.

Clinicians trained in a model of "to serve, to serve, to serve" can become disillusioned quickly in the rehabilitation arena, particularly in the for-profit arena, where goals are often to save (use the limited resources of an individual with great discrimination, or even withhold them) or to make a profit. It is unreasonable to expect rehabilitation centers to provide quality care and not be financially solvent. However, there have been gross abuses in the field of traumatic brain injury rehabilitation,[27] and it is often clinicians who have felt the most abused.

Dr. Purtillo[8] and Dr. G.F. Krieger,[28] a physician, have each raised the following question: To whom is the professional accountable? Likely choices in the past would have been the patient or the patient's family, of course, or perhaps even the organization of employment or professional membership. In today's business-minded market, with its increasing demands for both outcome accountability and financial accountability, the answer is not simple, and we must add to those choices the state and federal government, the case manager, and the insurance company or health maintenance organization (HMO). Dr. Krieger further asks: To whom is Congress accountable? To whom is the insurance company accountable? The tone implied in Dr. Krieger's questions reflects the frustration many professionals are experiencing in today's health care arena. The question of accountability, particularly with regard to financial accountability, may present the greatest number of ethical dilemmas facing the health care professional. Years of education and professional training do not prepare the clinician adequately to address the ethical dilemmas surrounding the allocation of health care resources.

PROFESSIONAL COMPETENCE AND ACCOUNTABILITY

All health professionals in fields with licensure requirements have minimal standards of practice and qualifications they are expected to follow. Most standards state the scope of practice for the profession. It should be noted that not all rehabilitation professionals are required to obtain a license in order to provide services (for example, Therapeutic Recreation Specialists and Vocational Counselors). The *American Speech, Language and Hearing Association (ASHA)* and individual state licensing boards are the governing bodies for speech-language pathologists. Most state requirements for licensure have followed the guidelines initially set forth by the American Speech, Language and Hearing Association for the Certificate of Clinical Competence. A point of clarification may be in order; the American Speech, Language and Hearing Association is a professional organization to which one pays dues for membership on a *voluntary* basis. The certificate of clinical competence is not required to practice, by law, although many organizations of employment require certification as a minimal standard of entrance. Possessing and maintaining a current state license is a legal requirement if one is to practice outside of a state- or federally-funded institution (for example, the public school system) in most states.

Because of the comprehensive nature of traumatic brain injury, with multiple specialties and multiple stages at which the clinician can become involved, there is a lack of standardization of practice. For example, a particular treatment method that would be considered acceptable in an intensive care unit may be completely inappropriate in a state- and federally-funded work re-entry program, from both a clinical perspective and a financial one. In the field of traumatic brain injury rehabilitation, the expertise needed is not uniform from setting to setting. The skills required to work with patients in the intensive care unit have overlapping characteristics with, but in practice are quite different from, those needed to work in a community reintegration program. This is not to say that a clinician coming from one type of rehabilitation setting is unqualified to work in another setting, but it should be noted that different skills are needed in each setting in order to maximize its benefits for the patient. It is the responsibility of the clinician, as well as the supervisor, to recognize when skills different from those possessed are needed, and to obtain additional education. With regard to working as a member of an interdisciplinary team, where roles sometimes overlap, Malec[29] offers strong advice in his statement that "ethical practice in a transdisciplinary model requires individual team members to recognize their own limitations and refrain from assuming provider roles that, even with consultation from other team members, are beyond their competencies."

We all must become more accountable for outcome. A simple review of the most recent literature in brain injury rehabilitation alone would seem to support this statement.[30,31,32,33] Traumatic brain injury rehabilitation has moved beyond its infancy. Although still representing an underserved population, traumatic brain injury is not unrecognized, as it was twenty years ago. During the last two decades, professionals interested in traumatic brain injury have enjoyed relative freedom to delineate sequelae (exhaustively and redundantly) and to experiment with unproven treatment techniques. It has been a path of discovery not unlike that encountered with other diagnoses. (A quick review of the literature on focal lesions and the aphasias elucidates this point.) Rehabilitation therapies are too expensive, as are most aspects of health care, for the clinician not to know the effectiveness of a specific intervention. Cost consciousness alone, however, should not be the primary force that pushes us to increase our accountability. Patient benefit and time (that is, efficiency) should be the guiding forces.

Large institutions have departments of medical records and quality assurance capable of analyzing significant amounts of information, such as that collected from functional assessment measures (for example, the Functional Independence Measure). The details needed to prove the effectiveness of a cognitive-communicative intervention are often not available from such global scales because they lack sufficient sensitivity to measure small increments of change.

Developing scales of functional communication that can measure small amounts of change is a time-consuming process, and such instruments often lack the rigor of statistical testing needed to be accepted by groups unfamiliar with the scale, such as insurance companies. While there continues to be a need for rigorous research in the field, specifically with regard to remediation of cognitive deficits, there is also a great need for particular institutions and programs to validate their effectiveness. Performance data need to be analyzed in such a manner that outcomes can be attributed to specific types of intervention. It is imperative that clinicians take responsibility for accountability within their own setting and be able to demonstrate results, if referrals and funding for services are desired.

Case Example 4:   Mr. Jones was a 34-year-old truck loader for a major restaurant chain. Following a severe traumatic brain injury from an automobile accident, he had a moderately severe dysarthria and a severe impairment in reading comprehension. His speech was intelligible to the familiar listener, particularly if limited to short phrases. Although reading comprehension was severely affected, he was able to recognize some single words of high imagery value. Mr. Jones had worked for the same company for ten years, and his employer was supportive of his rehabilitation program and wanted Mr. Jones to return to work if at all possible.

The most important goal to Mr. Jones was to improve his speech. His wife supported this goal, but also was eager for him to return to work as soon as possible because they were expecting their second child. The physical therapist thought that Mr. Jones would be able to perform the manual (physical) tasks of his previous job. The limiting factor to his return to employment was the reading disability, which was a handicap because of the job requirement that he be able to read an inventory list and then load the necessary boxes. His job required very little oral communication.

The speech-language pathologist had previously treated a patient with a similar reading disability, but of a lesser severity than Mr. Jones's. The treatment approach used had the goal of being able to match a core set of printed words from one list to another list, and had proven to be 80 percent effective with the similar patient. As an additional gain, single word sight recognition also improved. The treatment period had been four 1 to 2-hour sessions per week, for ten weeks, with a highly motivated individual. The speech-language pathologist had worked also with similar cases of dysarthria, and thought, with approximately 75 percent certainty, that Mr. Jones's speech intelligibility could improve by 10 percent in four weeks with aggressive treatment (a minimum of five 2-hour sessions per week). Additionally, the speech-language pathologist preferred treatment of dysarthria to that of reading disorders.

Mr. Jones's insurance company required that all services be approved before therapy was initiated. The company agreed to reimburse for five 1-hour sessions per week, for eight weeks maximum, with a positive progress report every two weeks. Further, the insurance company noted that this was an "extension" in coverage at the request of Mr. Jones's employer. Mr. Jones was informed of all these circumstances, but remained adamant that if his speech improved, he would be able to return to work. He agreed to work on reading "some."

Possible Courses of Action:
  (1) Treat the reading disability for 30 minutes and the dysarthria for 30 minutes each day.
  (2) Treat the reading disability two times per week and the dysarthria three times per week.
  (3) Ask another clinician, who has greater expertise in treating reading impairments, to work with Mr. Jones.
  (4) Treat only the dysarthria, to honor Mr. Jones' desire.
  (5) Design a rigorous home program for the dysarthria, or the alexia, and train his wife.
  (6) Work after hours and do not bill for the service beyond the approved amount.

(7) Explore alternative funding with the family, to be used when insurance will no longer reimburse.

(8) Ask Mr. Jones to consult with his employer in hopes that the employer can persuade him to address the skill most needed to perform his job.

Considerations: If the clinician is working in a setting with high productivity standards, requiring seven hours of billable service, when will there be time to design the home program, unless it is during Mr. Jones's treatment session? Should a precious treatment hour be used to design a program and then another one or two used to train his wife? What is the wife's level of motivation to carry out the program? In order to design the most efficient reading program, the work site should be observed and words chosen from that setting. This will require additional time from the clinician and may not be a billable service, yet it seems an essential step to providing effective treatment. Both speech and reading therapy are indicated. How much should the speech-pathologist's decisions be affected by Mr. Jones's employment situation? How are limited resources allocated best?

LIFE-SUSTAINING TREATMENT

The speech-language pathologist will most likely not be involved in decisions regarding the discontinuation of life-sustaining interventions, with the possible exception of providing consultation regarding swallowing and nonoral feeding. However, it is highly probable that the speech-language pathologist will be asked to give a professional opinion or personal advice to families regarding the termination of ventilation, particularly if a professional relationship has been established while training the family in coma stimulation techniques and providing educational information. In times of crisis, one must understand how desperately family members or friends want to know which decision will be the right one. If a relationship of trust has been established between the clinician and family, and information has been shared previously, it is not unreasonable to expect that the clinician's professional opinion will be sought. In all cases of this nature, it is best to qualify any statements with a preface that even a professional opinion is not conclusive, because of the individual variability of each case, and unknown factors. The clinician should always reiterate that decisions have to be based on one's personal values. In some cases, when asked for one's own personal opinion, it may be appropriate to provide it; however, it must be stated as a personal opinion, and not as a professional one. If the clinician is knowledgeable about current, well-documented statistics on outcome relevant to the matter in question, he or she may offer this information, if appropriate. Because medical settings are service industries, people are the predominant concern. Many opinions are shared among professionals in both formal and informal discussions. One should never give information to a family (or patient, for that matter) obtained from a colleague without his or her permission; rather, refer the family to the original source. In an attempt to comfort family members, there may be a temptation to offer information that is beyond one's area of expertise, particularly if one is unprepared for the situation. This temptation should be resisted. It is best for the clinician to be prepared for the above situations, in order to give the family the most thoughtful response.

Case Example 5:   Mr. and Mrs. Smith have been married for 40 years, and Mrs. Smith has recently retired. They have two children, Brenda and Tommy. Brenda has graduated from college and works in another state. Tommy is 22 years old and has recently been accepted into medical school for the upcoming semester. He was walking from the university to his apartment, in his home town, when he was assaulted and robbed. His head was beaten severely with a baseball bat, and he sustained massive brain damage with brain stem involvement. He has been on a ventilator in the intensive care unit for six days. The speech-language pathologist, who is the member of the rehabilitation team responsible for providing consultation to the acute hospital for rehabilitation candidates, has been assessing Tommy's responsiveness over the last three days and has met with his parents during each visit to provide educational information. They have developed a trusting relationship with the therapist. During each visit they have optimistically asked the speech-language pathologist if Tommy's responsiveness has changed, and it has not. The trauma surgeon and neurosurgeon have discussed with them the possibility of discontinuing the ventilator. The Smiths have asked the speech-language pathologist: "Don't you think he's shown some signs of responding? We can't even consider turning it off as long as he's showing some signs. Could you?"

Possible Courses of Action:
  (1)   Answer the first question in accordance with professional observations.
  (2)   Avoid answering the first question definitively, because it is possible that the family may have observed a response, since Mrs. Smith has not left the intensive care unit.
  (3)   Talk with all of the nursing staff and other professionals or family who have observed Tommy to discuss their observations, before talking with the Smiths.
  (4)   Defer to the attending physician.
  (5)   Discuss with the Smiths their observations and the fact that Tommy is still severely brain damaged, explaining the long-term implications.

(6) Answer the first question as a professional and the second question from a personal framework.

(7) Arrange for the Smiths to meet with members of other families who have been faced with a similar situation.

Considerations: The trauma surgeon may be unfamiliar with the role of the speech-language pathologist. Providing the family with encouragement contradictory to the recommendations already suggested could endanger the relationship between the physician and the family. The family trusts the speech-language pathologist, implicit in that trust is truth telling. Should the speech-language pathologist answer if unable to separate his or her personal values from the professional observations, if these are in conflict? If members of other families are available to speak with the Smiths, should they be chosen on the basis of the outcomes of their relative with a traumatic brain injury (that is, should one family be chosen who terminated ventilator support and one who did not)?

LEGAL CONSIDERATIONS

Liability Issues

Many of the issues presented up to this point are legal as well as ethical issues, such as informed consent and competency, and they will not be discussed further here. Physicians and other health care providers can be involved directly in legal issues in a number of ways, two of which are discussed below. The following information is not intended in any way to provide legal advice to the clinician, but only to serve as an introduction to certain important issues with which one might be faced personally or through association with colleagues. In the face of litigation, ignorance will not serve the clinician well as a justifiable defense, and in today's litigious environment, clinicians should be aware of areas of potential legal involvement.

Within the legal system, two different areas of legal theory have been invoked and have served as the underlying basis in liability cases. This is not to say that other areas of legal theory have not been applied to liability cases. Under the theory of *battery*, a clinician could be held liable for intended physical contact (in health care, a medical procedure) that occurred without the permission of the patient, or for any consequences resulting from a procedure of which the patient had not been fully informed.[11] The operational condition necessary for battery to be the basis of a legal investigation is that the procedure was *intended*. Under the legal construct of *negligence*, a clinician who failed to exercise proper skill and care in performing a procedure or delivering treatment (was careless) could be held liable for any negative consequences of the treatment.[11] Charges of battery would result in a *criminal* suit, whereas negligence would result in a *civil* suit.[1]

In the author's opinion, the area with the greatest potential legal liability for the speech-language pathologist is dysphagia treatment, for two reasons. It is one of the most invasive treatments we provide, and it has the greatest degree of associated risks as compared to other types of treatment. The risks associated with dysphagia treatment vary considerably from setting to setting, and it is important to recognize some of the differences. In the acute hospital setting, numerous physicians, nurses, and support personnel are available for consultation and follow-through of the speech-language pathologist's recommendations, as well as for monitoring the patient. This provides not only for a potentially higher level of care than in some other settings, but also for additional documentation substantiating the speech-language pathologist's findings. In long-term care facilities, as an example, the level of medical care provided by physicians, nurses, and other therapists is less intense, and support personnel are less well trained. The costs of providing services in long-term care facilities are typically considerably lower than those of hospitals, in part because of the staffing patterns. It is not unusual to find persons with traumatic brain injuries, some of whom have dysphagia, in long-term care facilities. Speech-language pathologists marginally qualified to provide dysphagia treatment (that is, in a learning phase) would be well advised to insist upon adequate supervision, regardless of the practice setting. Speech-language pathologists who have not been trained to treat swallowing disorders should refrain from doing so in all types of settings.

Expert Testimony

Traumatic brain injuries frequently occur as a result of motor vehicle accidents, sports- or work-related injuries, or assaults, incidents for which compensation for personal injury may be sought from persons who are considered responsible or legally liable.[34] The purpose of expert testimony is to provide the court (judge and jurors) with a more precise picture of the extent of injury sustained by an individual than would otherwise be available. Sidley[35] states that two conditions must be present to warrant legal counsel's use of expert testimony:

(1) The subject of the inference to be drawn must be so distinctively related to some science, profession, business, or occupation as to be beyond the ken of the average or "nonexpert" layman.
(2) The witness must have sufficient skill, knowledge, or experience in the field, such that his opinion or inference will probably aid the trier of the case in his search for the truth.

It is important that any expert be careful not to veer from his or her area of expertise. The speech-language pathologist is not qualified in the role of expert witness to establish the presence or absence of psychiatric illness (for example, depression, psychosis, personality disorders) and should not attempt to do so, even if psychiatric behaviors are thought to contribute to cognitive-communicative impairments. Cognitive impairments should be characterized in relation to communication abilities (that is, speech, written and verbal expression, reading and auditory comprehension, nonverbal symbolism, and pragmatics). One needs to be completely knowledgeable of the information available from documentation produced during the delivery of any speech-language pathology services to the patient, in order to definitively address the needs and abilities of the patient. The legal firm representing the patient should have copies of all records involving the patient's medical care. Terminology should be explained in language that can be understood by the lay person.

The role the speech-language pathologist will be expected to fill as an expert witness will depend considerably upon the setting in which he or she practices, as well as the community. If the speech-language pathologist practices in a setting where all cognitive interventions are provided by that discipline, and neuropsychology services are unavailable, he or she may be expected to comment on the full range of treatment services being provided. In cases where large settlements are being sought, it is not unusual for patients to travel great distances to be evaluated by experts, or for experts to travel to patients. In such cases, someone in the field other than the therapist treating the patient may be asked to give testimony, or may give testimony for the opposing side. In either case, legal counsel will instruct the expert in the manner of the proceedings and will provide useful advice that should help put the clinician at ease. Many cases are settled out of court, especially in the presence of strong evidence. If a case is taken before a court, the clinician's display of confidence is particularly important. Unlike the role of defendant in a liability case, the role of expert witness is one that the speech-language pathologist can be called upon to fulfill with confidence. However, it is imperative that expertise be the basis for serving in the role.

SUMMARY

Most rehabilitation professionals have not been trained in the theoretical or practical application of medical ethics. In fact, studies of ethical principles as applied in rehabilitation are limited. This chapter has presented a theoretical framework from which to consider ethical dilemmas that may, and do, arise in the traumatic brain injury rehabilitation setting, along with some specific case examples.

A number of components of ethics were discussed, including benevolence (bringing about good), nonmaleficence (doing no harm), veracity (truth telling), fidelity (keeping promises), and justice (being fair and impartial). These broad ethical constructs are translated into clinical issues that include complex topics such as informed consent, confidentiality, competency, autonomy and self-determination, and the allocation of health care resources.

Each of these was discussed in relation to clinical practice and the clinician's duties. The unique ethical challenges of working with a team, answering questions about termination of life supports, and being an expert witness were also discussed.

It is not unusual to find ethical conflicts in the rehabilitation setting. In traumatic brain injury rehabilitation, a major concern for providers is obtaining informed consent, particularly in view of variable degrees of competence. The fine line between protecting individuals from undue harm and promoting their self-determinism and autonomy is most challenging to clinicians. Confidentiality is a significant issue because of the sheer numbers of clinicians involved in the delivery of treatment. However, it is perhaps the fair and just allocation of resources that poses the greatest ethical dilemma to clinicians. Rehabilitation, as a field of medicine, has been criticized by medical ethicists for having the luxury of choosing who will be admitted to a facility for service, and who will not. Few in rehabilitation would consider it a luxury to have to refuse services to those in need of them.

REFERENCES

1. Haffey WJ. The assessment of clinical competency to consent to medical rehabilitative interventions. *Journal of Head Trauma Rehabilitation*. 1989;4:43–56.
2. Banja J. Ethical issues in staff development. In Durgin CJ, Schmidt ND, Fryor LJ (eds). *Staff Development and Clinical Intervention in Brain Injury Rehabilitation*. Gaithersburg, MD: Aspen Publishers; 1993:23–41.
3. DeJong G, Batavia AI. Societal duty and resource allocation for persons with severe traumatic brain injury. *Journal of Head Trauma Rehabilitation*. 1989; 4:1–12.
4. Haas J, MacKenzie CA. The role of ethics in rehabilitation medicine. *American Journal of Physical Medicine Rehabilitation*. 1995;74(suppl):3–6.
5. Caplan AL, Callahan D, Haas J. *Ethical and Policy Issues in Rehabilitation Medicine*. Briarcliff Manor, NY: The Hastings Center; 1987:1–20.
6. McCormick B. AMA President seeks unity, increased emphasis on ethics. *American Medical News*. 1995;June 5:5.
7. Veatch RM. Medical ethics: an introduction. In Veatch RM (ed). *Medical Ethics*. Boston, MA: Jones and Bartlett Publishers; 1989:1–26.
8. Purtilo RB. *Ethical Dimensions in the Health Professions, 2nd ed*. Philadelphia, PA: WB Saunders; 1993:3–48.
9. Caplan AL. Informed consent and provider-patient relationships in rehabilitation medicine. *Archives of Physical Medicine and Rehabilitation*. 1988;69:312–317.
10. Sanders JM. Ethical implications of disablement. In Greenwood R, Barnes MP, McMillan TM, Ward CD (eds). *Neurological Rehabilitation*. Edinburgh, Scotland: Churchill Livingstone; 1993:59–63.
11. Beauchamp TL. Informed consent. In Veatch RM (ed). *Medical Ethics*. Boston, MA: Jones and Bartlett Publishers; 1989:173–200.
12. Piper A. Truce on the battlefield: a proposal for a different approach to medical informed consent. *Journal of Law, Medicine and Ethics*. 1994;22:301–313.

13. Scofield G. Ethical considerations in rehabilitation medicine. *Archives of Physical Medicine and Rehabilitation.* 1993;74:341–346.
14. Wier RF, Gostin JD. Decisions to abate life-sustaining treatment for non-autonomous patients; ethical standards and legal liability for physicians after Cruzan. *Journal of the American Medical Association.* 1990;264:1846–1853.
15. Brody H. The physician/patient relationship. In Veatch RM (ed). *Medical Ethics.* Boston, MA: Jones and Bartlett Publishers; 1989:65–91.
16. Venesy BA. A clinician's guide to decision making capacity and ethically sound medical decisions. *American Journal of Physical Medicine and Rehabilitation.* 1995; 74(suppl):41–48.
17. Ho V. Marginal capacity: the dilemmas faced in assessment and declaration. *Canadian Medical Association Journal.* 1995;152:259–263.
18. Commission on Accreditation of Rehabilitation Facilities. *Standards Manual and Interpretative Guidelines for Medical Rehabilitation.* Tucson, AZ: Commission on Accreditation of Rehabilitation Facilities; 1995.
19. Banja J. Proxy consent to medical treatment: implications for rehabilitation. *Archives of Physical Medicine and Rehabilitation.* 1986;67:790–792.
20. Haas J. Ethical considerations of goal setting for patient care in rehabilitation medicine. *American Journal of Physical Medicine and Rehabilitation.* 1995;74:16–20.
21. Banja JD, Higgins P. Videotaping therapeutic sessions and the right of privacy. *Journal of Head Trauma Rehabilitation.* 1989;4:65–74.
22. Purtilo RB. Ethical issues in teamwork: the context of rehabilitation. *Archives of Physical Medicine and Rehabilitation.* 1988;69:318–322.
23. Purtilo RB, Meier RH. Team challenges: regulatory constraints and patient empowerment. *American Journal of Physical Medicine and Rehabilitation.* 1995; 74(suppl):21–24.
24. Wood R. The rehabilitation team. In Greenwood R, Barnes MP, McMillan TM, Ward CD (eds). *Neurological Rehabilitation.* Edinburgh, Scotland: Churchill Livingstone; 1993:41–49.
25. Buchanan A. Health-care delivery. In Veatch RM (ed). *Medical Ethics.* Boston, MA: Jones and Bartlett Publishers; 1989:291–327.
26. Haas JF. Admission to rehabilitation centers: selection of patients. *Archives of Physical Medicine and Rehabilitation.* 1988;69:329–332.
27. Kerr P. Centers for head injury accused of earning millions for neglect. *New York Times.* March 16, 1992:(sec)D4:1.
28. Krieger GF. Accountability must be restored to health care system. *American Medical News.* May 22/29, 1995:18–19.
29. Malec JF. Ethics in brain injury rehabilitation: existential choices among western cultural beliefs. *Brain Injury.* 1993;7:383–400.
30. Bryant ET et al. Managing costs and outcome of patients with traumatic brain injury in an HMO setting. *Journal of Head Trauma Rehabilitation.* 1993;8:15–29.
31. Evans RW, Ruff RM. Outcome and value: a perspective on rehabilitation outcomes achieved in acquired brain injury. *Journal of Head Trauma Rehabilitation.* 1992;7:24–363.
32. Cope DN et al. Brain injury: analysis of outcome in a post-acute rehabilitation system Part 1. General analysis. *Brain Injury.* 1991;5:111–125.
33. Cook L, Smith DS, Truman G. Using functional independence measure profiles as an index of outcome in the rehabilitation of brain-injured patients. *Archives of Physical Medicine and Rehabilitation.* 1994;75:390–393.

34. Rosenthal M, Koplan KI. Head injury rehabilitation: psycholegal issues and roles for the rehabilitation psychologist. *Rehabilitation Psychology.* 1986;1:37–46.
35. Sidley N, Petrila J. On being involved personally in lawsuit, as a plaintiff, expert witness, or defendant. In Sidley N (ed). *Law and Ethics: A Guide for the Health Professional.* New York, NY: Human Sciences Press; 1985:355–378.

11

Family Issues

Rosenthal and Hutchins[1] have stated that "the most valuable asset a person with head injury can have is a supportive family." Clinicians who have practiced in the field of traumatic brain injury rehabilitation for very long know this to be true. Romano[2] reminds us that although the person with a traumatic brain injury becomes a part of the health care or medical system, the person was first, and remains, a member of other systems. The family system, perhaps the most important, is the one addressed in this chapter.

There are several thorough reviews covering much of the literature to date that have addressed family issues in traumatic brain injury.[3,4,5,6] An additional review is not undertaken in this chapter, but an introduction to the literature is indicated. Initially, the emphasis of study relating to family members of persons with traumatic brain injury was not on studying the family members themselves. Instead, the reports of families regarding the observed characteristics and behaviors of their relative with a brain injury were used during a period of investigation (the early 1970s) when the delineation of deficits was the primary concern.[4] The information that family members provided to investigators was valuable because of the questionable reliability of self-reporting from persons with brain injuries, who often have problems in the area of self-awareness. In the 1970s and early 1980s, studies that addressed some of the impact of traumatic brain injury on specific family members began to appear in the literature.[7,8,9] Much of the research during this period obtained information from families in an anecdotal manner (that is, reporting information that families shared, without, in some cases, conducting research designed to objectively measure burdens experienced). As an example, the financial burden that a traumatic brain injury places upon families has been reported frequently,[3] but with little documented evidence of the actual costs and financial losses experienced, and the kind of hard evidence needed to impact political and social policy. Current research has as its focus the impact of traumatic brain injury on family functioning, viewing the family as a whole unit or system.[4] This line of inquiry has as its basis the family systems theory common to the training of social workers and psychologists involved in family counseling. Investigations that take this approach should help clinicians better understand the needs of family members as they are directly related to, and affected by, the needs of the person with the traumatic brain injury. In future years, we can hope to understand more fully the skills on the part of the whole family that are needed for a positive *family* outcome. As rehabilitation professionals, we need to ask ourselves: Have we really obtained a successful outcome for society if, in the process of returning one person with a traumatic brain injury to work, two additional family members have become disengaged, lost employment, depleted all financial resources, or become health impaired?

EARLY NEEDS OF FAMILIES

With rare exceptions, families of persons who have sustained a traumatic brain injury enter the medical system through the emergency or trauma center of a hospital. This immediately casts them in the role of passive recipients, sometimes waiting hours for information regarding the status of their loved one. Often, family members have been awakened in the middle of the night and summoned to appear at the hospital as quickly as possible, sometimes after being given the information that their loved one may die at any moment, and at other times, little more than the information that their loved one has been involved in a serious accident, the details of which are still unclear. Regardless of the conditions, few are prepared to face the realities that lie ahead.[10] For some families, the last occasion they had to be in the hospital was none other than the birth of the individual now on the brink of death. Their feelings of disbelief that this person may now be taken from them are understandable.

Although television dramas make attempts to emulate the hospital environment, the fact remains that most people are quite unfamiliar with the workings of a real medical setting. Popular conceptions, fostered by the media, may give families a false idea of the realities of a severe injury, especially a brain injury. Given the widespread misrepresentations of coma, it is quite often impossible for families and friends to believe that the patient, their loved one lying in the intensive care unit, will not wake up in a few hours, even as those hours stretch into days. In the initial stages of a traumatic brain injury, families are in crisis—not in the overused, popular sense, but in the true psychiatric model of crisis. Cope and Wolfson[11] describe the situation as follows:

> A crisis may be thought of as a stressful, novel situation, suffused with the perception of danger, for which the participant has no adequate frame of reference. There are not understood or clear rules of how to behave or what to expect. There is not a sense of when it will be 'over' or what the outcome may be.

Two important concepts are presented in the above description: there is *no frame of reference* for the family to draw upon, and there are *no rules to help guide their behavior*. Intervention with the family at this stage should be focused on helping the family to use their resources (time and energy) wisely, and in a way that helps them feel useful. Providing consistency for family members is as important as providing consistency for the patient. A single member of the professional staff should serve as a liaison to help guide the family through the system and to provide support.[11] This member is typically a social worker, but other staff can serve in this role, if specified, and if skilled in the management of stressful situations.

Depending upon the hospital setting, the speech-language pathologist may be a member of the acute care rehabilitation team or, in some cases, the trauma team. In all stages of a traumatic brain injury, family education is important, and the speech-language pathologist will be involved in providing education. In the early stages, education may involve dysphagia and/or coma stimulation. In some cases, the speech-language pathologist may be the member of the acute care consult team designated as the contact person for rehabilitation services. In this role, more comprehensive education about rehabilitation services and outcome will be expected. Families need to be provided with concrete information and to have technical terms clearly explained. It is equally important, however, that they not be overloaded in single sessions with too much information. All verbally presented information should be supplemented with written information that can be accessed easily at a later time. There are several published family guides that can be given to families as reference material.[12,13,14,15] Although the information presented may be highly familiar to the clinician, it is foreign to the family. The family in crisis is in a confused state, often having gone without sleep for extended periods. They will not be able to grasp fully all of the information presented at this stage.[16] Families need *to be made comfortable* with asking for clarification or repetition of information. The intensive and acute care stages of recovery present a unique opportunity, and sometimes the only opportunity, for clinicians to talk with families and to establish a relationship. At this stage, families are desperate for information, anxious to learn about their loved one's condition, and not yet disillusioned by the professionals who have made "failed" predictions of outcome.[11,17] Cope and Wolfson[11] refer to this as a *window of opportunity* when families will be receptive to the information professionals have to share.

Given this caveat, clinicians need to gradually introduce families to the prospects that lie ahead. The timing and the manner of presentation of information to families, as intimated, are crucial.[18] Some of the most common stories clinicians hear in rehabilitation settings (at all stages) are that "the neurosurgeon or trauma surgeon told us he'd be a vegetable if he lived," or "they told us in the hospital he'd never walk, and look at him now." Most stories are stories of hope proved true, hope that the individual would live. It is within this context that clinicians must present prognostic information. Families should be told that progress will be a series of ups and downs, with great individual variability. They should be told of the unknowns, and they should be given the facts. And, although realistic information regarding prognosis should be presented, families need to be permitted their own opinions.[11] Clinicians do not need to agree, only to listen attentively and acknowledge the family's right to an opinion. If families are alienated in the beginning, they will tend to distrust professional advice later[2,19] (for example, "the doctor told us she wouldn't live, but she did, so why should we believe you when you say she will probably not be able to return to the university this year?").

Clinicians who work in intensive care units or in acute care are prone to great emotional stress over the loss of life, as are families. Nonetheless, it is imperative that clinicians respond differently than family members do. JoAnn Kramer,[19] the parent of a daughter with a traumatic brain injury, wisely advises the clinician as follows:

> Family members get tired and in time may address some of their latent anger for the situation . . . with the . . . health professionals. If professionals are aware of the possibility of prolonged stress on a family and its manifestations, they can attempt to help the family rather than take the criticism personally.

Staff are a logical target for the family's anger and frustrations.[3] Brooks[3] states that "failure to identify the underlying processes driving the reactions of family members can have a profound effect upon the ability and competence of staff members, and can destroy the therapeutic alliance built up between staff, family and patient." The feelings of underappreciation staff sometimes experience as a result of family frustrations can be placed in proper perspective if *team members support each other while supporting the family.*

As stated earlier, families need to feel useful. Purposeful activity can occupy the mind, thus relieving some of the anxiety, and can assuage some of the feelings of helplessness experienced by families in the intensive care unit. The technological assistance provided to some patients in the intensive care unit can be intimidating to families. The education provided to families at this stage should include a number of "how to's": how to touch the patient, how to talk with the patient, how to perform oral hygiene and other tolerated grooming, how to provide range of motion exercises, how to personalize the environment, and so on. This is not to suggest that family members should be expected to "take over" the care of the patient, only that they be given permission and shown how to interact with the patient in a way that can be ultimately beneficial. To the extent that they are able, families should be involved in the care of the patient as soon as possible.[11] It is too often the case that one day families are limited to 15-minute intervals of interaction with the patient, then two days later are expected to take their family member home and provide all aspects of care. At the very least, clinicians have an obligation to recognize the possibility of early discharge and to prepare families as best, and as early, as possible.

The needs of family members, as much as those of the person with a traumatic brain injury, change over the course of recovery. Throughout the literature the need that is cited most often is the need for information.[1,20] As the patient and the family progress, the type of information needed by families changes. In the early stages, basic information is needed, as discussed above. As would be expected, families want to know about the day-to-day medical status of their loved one, and they need emotional support to help them through the crisis. Once the question of survival is no longer the foremost concern, family needs change to wanting to know how to help the patient "get well fastest." With experience, clinicians become familiar with the type of information most often requested in their particular work setting. In the author's experience, it is not acquiring the information that is difficult for clinicians, but rather learning how to interact with families in a therapeutic way. The next section is presented to help clinicians view families as persons with needs that are not completely distinct from those of the patient, needs that must be addressed in order to have an effective rehabilitation program.

VIEWING THE FAMILY AS A SYSTEM

In "Understanding Families from a Systems Perspective" (from *Head Injury: A Family Matter*), Turnbull and Turnbull[21] help professionals view families within a basic framework that is applicable to any family structure, which is exactly the point of reference they wish us to adopt. The family who suddenly find themselves with a member with a traumatic brain injury is a family first. And, although their lives have been completely disrupted by this unwanted and unexpected event, they remain a family. The basic structure of the family does not change, unless additional members are added or subtracted through birth, marriage, and/or death. Family systems theory places the family, as opposed to the individual, as the unit of emphasis for analysis and intervention.[22] From a systems perspective, as characterized by Turnbull and Turnbull,[21] the family should be viewed as having components, which are summarized in the following discussion. Families have *characteristics* such as the number of members, the ages, the cultural background, and the "idiosyncratic personal characteristics of each family member."[21] Within each family system are communication groups or *subsystems* such as husband and wife, parent and child, brother and sister, and extended family subgroups. Each subsystem has its own relationship or manner of interacting. The authors state as an essential point to remember "that any change or major need in one subsystem [group] will have an effect on all other subsystems in the family." Family *functions* are another component, identified by the authors as "the tasks that families carry out to meet their needs," such as financial, work and education, daily living, and leisure needs. Lastly, they describe the life cycle of the family, a model of family progression that has been applied to the family dealing with traumatic brain injury by several other authors as well.[22,23,24] The life cycle of a family, or the developmental cycle, is an extremely useful framework for helping the clinician to conceptualize the major disruption a traumatic brain injury has on the family system. The developmental stages presented are predictable, but vary somewhat from author to author. The stages, also referred to as transitions, include being a couple, having young children (births), who move into adolescence, followed by young adulthood, and then leave the home. At this point parents often reunite, focusing on their relationship, then on preparing for and moving into their later, aging years. These developmental transitions are expected in families and are often eagerly anticipated. Families are prepared for these transitions, for the most part. It is the nondevelopmental transitions that can occur at any time, without being anticipated, that cause disruption to the family cycle. Traumatic brain injury is a nondevelopmental transition. The point at which it occurs in the family cycle has an effect on the family's reaction and coping abilities, as well as on the coping skills of the member with an injury.[23] The family whose only child has a traumatic brain injury after entering college experiences extreme loss because their dream of a great physicist, artist, or teacher is gone (possibly along with the prospect of grandchildren), and because their own opportunity to reunite has to be put off indefinitely.

In addition to the components of a family described above, within each family, members have specific roles. The equilibrium of a family is maintained when different members fulfill their roles, and it is disrupted when roles are not fulfilled.[22] Sometimes these roles are not immediately apparent to the outsider. When the family structure has been disrupted, as it has with traumatic brain injury, families experience a loss of control, in part because of a loss of identity and role definition.[25] Although all members of a family have significant roles, at different times in the family cycle one person's role may have greater significance than another's. If the role of a father in a family is that of primary financial provider, the wife or oldest child may be expected to fill, and in reality have to fill, that role in the case of the father's sustaining a brain injury—and it may be a role neither is prepared to fill. The role of the wife as primary caretaker becomes stretched beyond its previously established boundaries. Role strain is a term used by Maitz[22] to refer to the "stress that is generated within an individual when he or she experiences difficulty meeting the demands of a particular role." The preceding example illustrates obvious role loss and role strain. Not all roles within a family are as obvious. The son who is the last of three, expected to be the only one to finish college, whose role in the family has been to help his father maintain sobriety, and who becomes brain injured while driving under the influence of alcohol, demonstrates a role less visible to the outsider, but one of extreme importance to the family.

According to Stambrook and colleagues,[23] the child who experiences a traumatic brain injury probably creates the least degree of role change for families. Parents are already in a caretaker role; however, when parents are young, they may not have the financial or community resources available to them to sustain future goals (for example, purchasing a home, having additional children, taking family vacations). Parents who have a child with a disability may be unable to experience the "empty nest" if the child is unable to live independently at adulthood. Siblings who have a brother or sister with a traumatic brain injury may have to assume a larger role than normally expected, often with less support and attention than they received previously. When a parent is the member with an injury, the financial strain upon the family and the strain of single parenting can be tremendous, especially if there are young children in the home. It is doubtful that, as clinicians, we can fully understand the significance of role change for family members, or the disruption in the family cycle caused by a traumatic brain injury. We can, however, have an appreciation that role changes occur in a family, ask families to discuss previous roles,[24] and utilize this information when working with family systems.

Although formal family assessment is often the responsibility of the social worker or psychologist, all clinicians are involved with families.[26] In some settings where speech-language pathologists may work, there will be no social worker or professional with a similar role. It is imperative that clinicians recognize the unique characteristics, functions, relationships, and roles of the families with whom they interface. Understanding the dynamic nature of the family system, and the interrelatedness of its members, should help clinicians in their evaluation of both the patient and the family. This framework should also help clinicians realize that a one-time assessment of a family will be completely inadequate to provide a thorough indication of the family's strengths and resources.[27] It is strengths and resources that must be identified to understand how to best work with families and patients. Therefore, a thorough, multidimensional family assessment (input from all therapists, input from all family members, and assessment in different settings) is crucial to the rehabilitation process.

FAMILIES AND REHABILITATION

Families enter the rehabilitation setting at various points in the recovery process. Few therapists will work in a setting that encompasses a full continuum of services. Even if an organization provides an extensive range of services, a single clinician typically does not provide service throughout the continuum. A more typical staffing pattern is to have one team of therapists dedicated to the acute hospital setting, another team to inpatient rehabilitation, and another to outpatient services. Family reactions to a traumatic brain injury, and their needs, vary from setting to setting. Few patients will have access to a full, uninterrupted continuum of rehabilitation. Therefore, clinicians must be sensitive to the expectations of families at these different points of entry into the rehabilitative process.

In the early stages of rehabilitation, families are often full of hope and anticipation for what rehabilitation can offer. They are no longer in the initial period of shock, and often have new-found hope because their loved one has survived a sometimes lengthy period of intensive care and crisis.[28] Families may feel that clinicians who limit potential have given up hope or do not understand the incredible obstacles already overcome. Although clinicians understand the permanence of disability, families may not be familiar with this concept, or may be unable to understand and assimilate it. Families often come to the rehabilitation setting under the impression that their injured relative has an illness, and with the expectation that, like illness, the injury is time limited.[17]

The work ethic in America signifies that there is a positive correlation between hard work, what one deserves, and the respect one receives.[29] Many families enter the rehabilitation setting with the expectation that with enough hard work (therapy), the patient will obtain what is deserved (a cure). Clinicians encourage hard work, but often they only imply what the results might be (for example, "you have to work really hard if you expect to get better"). It is important that clinicians present family members with concrete information about what to expect, to the best of their knowledge. This is not the same thing as confronting family members with all the deficits of their loved one, and what will never be accomplished. Nor is it the same as being evasive about known limitations, and goals that are highly unlikely to be achieved. Rather, clinicians have an obligation to help families understand what are reasonable expectations, while validating their sense of loss and supporting their need for hope.

Clinicians, like patients and families, have their own needs, one of which may be the need to be successful and not fail. If a clinician agrees to a goal that is overly optimistic, and then is unable to accomplish the goal with the patient, the clinician may experience a fear of being blamed or being held liable in some way, not to mention a personal sense of failure. This level of concern is more understandable in the critical care setting, where the liability risks are much greater than in the rehabilitation setting. Supporting a family's need for hope by acknowledging it, and even hoping with them, is not the same as promising miracles or unrealistic outcomes. It is this distinction that rehabilitation professionals perhaps fail to make, when presenting overly negative and pessimistic information in the interests of not wanting to create "false hope."

In the acute care medical setting, families learn to rely on professionals and their opinions. When families move into the rehabilitation arena, and are presented with options and encouraged to make decisions, they may perceive professionals as not being knowledgeable about their loved one's condition. They may be uncomfortable with this new, more active role, and be unclear of what is expected of them. Professionals may see families as being resistant or indecisive when they do not readily switch roles.[26] Although family members are *expected to participate* in the rehabilitation program in most centers, their specific *roles are generally undefined*.[25] Therapists often vary considerably in terms of their own level of comfort with families, and the degree to which they desire family involvement. This degree of variation can make it difficult for families to understand the role they have in rehabilitation. The words of Beth O'Brien,[17] the mother of a young man with a traumatic brain injury, can help clinicians understand the immense struggle family members experience in trying to find a role and purpose in the rehabilitation program.

> A struggle for control may occur initially among all the parties involved in the rehabilitation of the individual with head injury. The family may seek control by being highly critical of staff in those areas that would normally fall within the purview of parents: personal care, food service, . . . They are asserting themselves as caregivers in an attempt to rebuild confidence and establish new role identities.

It is important that rehabilitation teams and programs identify a role for families that will allow them to expend their energy in a constructive and beneficial way.[25]

All too often, as rehabilitationists, we see the family as a resource or adjunct to therapy, when in fact it is they who need help and resources.[30] We mistakenly value a family's worth by how effective they are in helping the patient in the rehabilitation program. Family members can be a great addition to the therapy program when utilized to motivate, and in many cases they provide effective intervention. Clinicians should not assume, however, that all families have the ability to provide supplemental intervention. As Brooks[3] states "it may simply be asking too much of already overloaded family members to be friends, partners, supporters *and* therapists or behavior managers."

As discussed in Chapter Two, a primary goal of rehabilitation is education of the patient and the family. Education must not be limited to 45-minute inservices or family conferences.[31] To assume that family members are able to comprehend, in one sitting, all the information presented by a group of professionals or even one professional, is unrealistic. Clinicians do not obtain their knowledge in one course. It is also incorrect to assume that, because families do not grasp all the details of the information presented, they are in denial or unrealistic,[25] something clinicians often do assume. Chad Pierro,[32] a person with a disability, advises that "learning about a disability or a chronic illness does not happen in a single session; rather, it is a process that continues over time."

Because professionals deal with numerous persons over time, often relaying similar details over and over, *our passage of time is quite different from that of the family* or the individual with an injury. Clinicians often feel as if they have delivered the message over and over, when in fact they have not. Whether a clinician has or has not repeated information should have little to do with ensuring that families have the opportunity to ask questions until they feel satisfied. Families have different learning styles, just as our patients do. Some families understand written information, and others do better in a question and answer format. Some prefer one-on-one sessions and others may be perfectly comfortable in a large group, such as in a meeting with the rehabilitation team. It is important that consideration be given to identifying different learning styles by observation and by asking. Although large family and team meetings are necessary, especially during the initial goal-setting period, family members should be given the opportunity to meet with individual team members. They should also have a contact person to whom they can go for additional information and clarification. The team leader or case manager is the logical choice for this role, but may not be able to establish the rapport with the family that is necessary for open communication. If the family gravitates to a particular team member who does have rapport with them, the team should take advantage of the therapeutic relationship to facilitate communication and relay information. This could be accomplished by relieving that member of some other responsibility in order that time can be made available for communication.

One of the roles of clinicians in rehabilitation is to help families move beyond "what was," in order to set goals based on the new self of the person with a traumatic brain injury. This can be a difficult task to accomplish for two reasons. First, persons with traumatic brain injury often do not have adequate judgment, insight, and flexibility to develop an emotional acceptance of the disability.[30] Second, *clinicians use the word acceptance to mean an awareness of the strengths and limitations* of the new person, while *families take this to mean giving up*. Some families are afraid to change their focus from preinjury to postinjury goals, for fear that merely doing so will limit the individual's progress. It is important for clinicians to establish a common vocabulary with families before basing goals on an assumption of acceptance. Acceptance should be defined and discussed. As professionals, we are often torn between the needs of the individual with a brain injury, to whom we feel our allegiance is owed, and the needs of the family. When these are in conflict, as they often are, clinicians might do better to obtain consensus between the family and the patient, than to act solely upon professional goals, the goals of the patient, or the goals of the family. Without this consensus, therapeutic efforts are surely doomed to fail, regardless of the appropriateness of the goals and the clinicians' good intentions.

Williams[18] reminds us that for individuals with traumatic brain injury and for their families, *loss is episodic*. It can occur again and again, perhaps *with the passage of each memorable event or missed opportunity*, such as the occurrence of the high school prom or college graduation. Some families fear that with each missed opportunity the loved one slips further and further away from what should have been. Therefore, many families make great sacrifices, of themselves as well as the patient, to ensure that these events do not go by without participation. Clinicians can help families by viewing these events as the source of a great sense of loss, and focusing their efforts on helping families to find new passages (cycles) for their loved one, instead of focusing on the reasons why it would be inappropriate for the person to attend such and such an event. A number of rehabilitation programs have graduation ceremonies or other types of ceremonies to recognize the efforts and achievements of the individuals who have completed the rehabilitation program. These types of events can help create the new passages needed to replace the missed developmental milestones, and in some cases they can serve as a source of inspiration for other individuals with traumatic brain injury and their families.

Although most rehabilitation programs offer family counseling services, families may be reluctant to focus on their own needs, or to assume a "patient" role, because of the belief that attention will be focused away from their injured family member.[25] In many family cultures, any form of psychological support or counseling is still considered quite taboo. Understanding the family culture and preconceptions can save considerable time and financial resources. Therapy cannot be forced on families any more than it can be forced upon a person with a traumatic brain injury. It is important that clinicians not "wash their hands of" family members who refuse offers of formal counseling; instead, the professional should investigate other avenues for support. Families often find support from other families who have had similar experiences. Providing a common space, where family members can talk while waiting for their loved ones in treatment, often can facilitate the development of an informal support network. Sometimes, these informal exchanges can later be structured into a formal support group that incorporates professional involvement.

The rehabilitation professional's presence is temporary in the lives of persons with traumatic brain injury and their families.[4] Although clinicians know, in theory, that a supportive family is the most valuable asset for a person with a traumatic brain injury, they often fail in practice to value the contributions of the family and validate their needs. It is often too easy for clinicians to assume that patients might be "better off" without involving their families, but it is wrong to assume that families have a limited role in rehabilitation.[33] It is better to recognize that it is families, not we, who will ultimately have to care for the person with a traumatic brain injury and to do everything possible to prevent the disintegration of the family unit.

FAMILIES AS CONSUMERS

As previously indicated in this chapter, families of persons who have sustained a traumatic brain injury enter the medical system through the hospital's trauma or emergency center, even in the case of mild brain injuries. In the United States, the emergency and intensive care stage will perhaps be the last time families will be provided with access to seemingly unlimited medical resources without financial qualification. With increasing frequency, families are expected, early on, to be educated consumers of the medical resources needed for the care of their loved one. In some instances, families will be expected to assume an active role that requires negotiating and bargaining for services, while they are still in the midst of anguish over loss, guilt, fears of the unknown, and exhaustion from days and nights of vigil. It should be of little surprise to clinicians that some families have difficulty adjusting to the long-term, often grueling, and costly course of rehabilitation.

Regardless of the current state of health care, which proffers health care services as if they were any other commodity, to be purchased as one would purchase a pair of shoes, most families are ill prepared to make such crucial decisions. Families are often expected to be active consumers at a time when they are least able to make informed choices. Many are emotionally fragile and financially vulnerable. Few of the variables about the appropriate rehabilitation program are known to families, and only in rare, exceptional cases do they actually have the buying power to purchase the needed goods and services.

Therefore, clinicians may find themselves in the unfamiliar role of trying to help families be good consumers, often with the realization that the family may choose services other than their own. It is, however, ethically unacceptable for clinicians to promise a family services that cannot be delivered or that are not indicated. Clinicians *do have an obligation* to maximize the effects of their treatment by helping families identify additional services as needed.

In the case of traumatic brain injury, long-term rehabilitation and support services are almost always needed but are in short supply.[2] Although discharge placement is often a function of the social services department in inpatient facilities, many settings in which the speech-language pathologist may work will not have a designated department responsible for discharge placement. In either case, the speech-language pathologist will probably have the most knowledge of the cognitive-communicative needs of the patient and will need to make specific recommendations for continued service and integration into the work, community, and/or school setting. Some families develop a quite sophisticated understanding of the services needed and the services available, but many do not, and these need the help of professionals. It is wise for clinicians in this position to develop files of resources that can be shared with families, and to become familiar with other agencies in the community in order to network and to facilitate transitions.[17]

Speech-language pathologists are often involved in helping families find appropriate educational services for the student who sustains a traumatic brain injury. It is a worthwhile effort for clinicians to know the structure of the public school system in their particular locale, as these vary considerably from state to state and city to city. A file of private schools and contact persons should also be maintained to share with families. Additionally, clinicians should be knowledgeable about advocacy groups for persons with other types of disabilities. If the speech-language pathologist is not involved in an area support group for traumatic brain injury, a list of current officers and contact persons should be obtained from the organization and made available to families, as should information from the Brain Injury Association in Washington, D.C. For persons living in small communities with limited resources, clinicians will need to expand their region of networking in order to help families obtain services and support.

Although case management services are available from some third party funding sources, case managers often operate from a cost-savings perspective. Additionally, in this author's experience, case managers are poorly informed about the long-term needs of persons with traumatic brain injuries. Networking with other agencies to find appropriate services is time consuming. Clinicians are sometimes tempted to think "it's not my job," but in order to truly be an advocate for this population, a working knowledge of local resources is essential.

SOME SUGGESTIONS FOR WORKING WITH FAMILIES

- Family adjustment is not an end, resulting in acceptance, but an ongoing process.[22]
- Denial is a coping mechanism that should not necessarily be viewed as pathological, particularly in the early stages of recovery.[3,11]
- Families need hope to get through the crisis of traumatic brain injury; clinicians should work with families to find a balance between hope and reality.[26]
- A formal assessment that includes a family systems analysis should be done with the family, including the individual with a traumatic brain injury whenever possible.[27] Measures of psychosocial adjustment also should be administered to determine baseline functioning and note progress or deterioration.
- A key family member should be identified as the person "in charge" or spokesperson, to reduce confusion and facilitate the flow of information back and forth. This should be an agreed upon role by the family, patient, and team. However, all family members and significant others should be given the opportunity to voice concerns, and joys, through regular meetings.
- The family should be considered a member of the rehabilitation team, not merely an affiliate.
- If a family cannot be present for a team meeting, a member of the rehabilitation team should be designated to represent the family's position.[26]

- Written educational material should provide concrete information, and include graphics to enhance understanding.[1,17]
- Information should be presented in different formats to accommodate the various learning styles of families.[17,25]
- Clinicians need to teach families (by demonstration) how to be effective communicators with the person with a traumatic brain injury, beyond merely understanding the utterances of the patient.[21]
- Clinicians need to be open and honest about the uncertainty of outcome.[2]
- Families need consistency.
- Families should be encouraged to ask their questions, and their opinions should be heard.

SUMMARY

As clinicians, we sometimes forget that the person with a brain injury, who has become a member of the rehabilitation system, was once a member of several other systems, the family system being one of the most important. In this system, all individuals have roles; the individual with a brain injury filled a unique role that now must change in some way. Clinicians must learn about the roles in each family system to know how to capitalize upon each member's strengths in a way that supports the entire family system. It is also important to understand the developmental nature of the family system and to appreciate how a traumatic brain injury alters this progression. For example, when the last child of a family becomes disabled in the last year of college and must return to the parents' home to live, the injury presents a disruption not only to the individual's cycle of college, job, family, and so on, but also to the parents' transition into a time of reunion for themselves.

Like the patients going through rehabilitation, families have needs that change over the course of recovery. The literature indicates, however, that the need for information remains basic. The initial informational needs are for medical knowledge and an understanding of the technology as it relates to survival. Once the critical concerns for survival have passed, the needs turn more to "how to" and "what next" information. The needs of family members are met better when the family is incorporated into the rehabilitation team as a member, not as an adjunct. It is sometimes difficult for clinicians to accept that family members do know their loved one better than the professionals who are temporarily part of their lives. Because families are the ones who provide long-term assistance and support, they must be included in all aspects of rehabilitation, and valued for their contributions. It is also important to recognize that families are a variable group, just like the patient population. Individualized approaches must be developed for them as well. These approaches should accommodate different learning styles, different communication styles, and different priorities. Emotional support from all staff is indicated throughout rehabilitation, as families come to the gradual realization of the permanence of disability, and struggle to replace lost dreams with new goals.

REFERENCES

1. Rosenthal M, Hutchins B. Interdisciplinary family education in head injury rehabilitation. In Williams JM, Kay T (eds). *Head Injury: A Family Matter*. Baltimore, MD: Paul H Brookes Publishing; 1991:273–282.
2. Romano MD. Family issues in head trauma. In Horn LJ, Cope DN (eds). *Traumatic Brain Injury: Physical Medicine and Rehabilitation State of the Art Reviews*. Philadelphia, PA: Hanley and Belfus; 1989:3(1),157–167.
3. Brooks DN. The head-injured family. *Journal of Clinical and Experimental Neuropsychology*. 1991;13:155–188.
4. Kay T, Cavallo MM. Evolutions: research and clinical perspectives. In Williams JM, Kay T (eds). *Head Injury: A Family Matter*. Baltimore, MD: Paul H Brookes Publishing; 1991:121–150.
5. Livingston MG. Effects on the family system. In Rosenthal M, Griffith ER, Bond MR, Miller JD (eds). *Rehabilitation of the Adult and Child with Traumatic Brain Injury, 2nd ed*. Philadelphia, PA: FA Davis; 1990:225–235.
6. Livingston MG, Brooks DN. The burden on families of the brain injured: a review. *Journal of Head Trauma Rehabilitation*. 1988;4:6–15.
7. Thompsen IV. The patient with severe head injury and his family. *Scandinavian Journal of Rehabilitation Medicine*. 1974;6:180–183.
8. Rosenbaum M, Najenson T. Changes in life patterns and symptoms of low mood as reported by wives of severely brain injured soldiers. *Journal of Consulting and Clinical Psychology*. 1976;44:881–888.
9. Oddy M, Humphrey M, Uttley D. Stresses upon relatives of head-injured patients. *British Journal of Psychiatry*. 1978;133:507–510.
10. Talbott R. The brain-injured person and the family. In Wood RL, Eames P (eds). *Models of Brain Injury Rehabilitation*. Baltimore, MD: Johns Hopkins University Press; 1989:3–16.
11. Cope DN, Wolfson B. Crisis intervention with the family in the trauma setting. *Journal of Head Trauma Rehabilitation*. 1994;9:67–81.
12. Marshall LF, Sadler GR, Bowers SA. *Head Injury*. San Diego, CA: Central Nervous System Foundation; 1985.
13. Hawley LA. *A Family Guide to the Rehabilitation of the Severely Head-Injured Patient*. Austin, TX: Healthcare Rehabilitation Center; 1987.
14. Gronwall D, Wrightson P, Waddell P. *Head Injury the Facts: A Guide for Families and Care-givers*. New York, NY: Oxford University Press; 1990.
15. Deboskey DS, Hecht JS, Calub CJ. *Educating Families of the Head Injured: A Guide to Medical, Cognitive and Social Issues*. Gaithersburg, MD: Aspen Publications; 1991.
16. Graheme L. The family system in acute care and acute rehabilitation. In Williams JM, Kay T (eds). *Head Injury: A Family Matter*. Baltimore, MD: Paul H Brookes Publishing; 1991:153–164.

17. O'Brien BB, Fralish KB. A family perspective on participation in rehabilitation. In Deutsch PM, Fralish KB (eds). *Innovations in Head Injury Rehabilitation*. New York, NY: Mathews Bender; 1994:2A.01–2A.10.

18. Williams JM. Family reaction to head injury. In Williams JM, Kay T (eds). *Head Injury: A Family Matter*. Baltimore, MD: Paul H Brookes Publishing; 1991:81–99.

19. Kramer J. Special issues from a parent. In Williams JM, Kay T (eds). *Head Injury: A Family Matter*. Baltimore, MD: Paul H Brookes Publishing; 1991:9–17.

20. Kreutzer JS, Gervasio AH, Camplair PS. Patient correlates of caregivers' distress and family functioning after traumatic brain injury. *Brain Injury*. 1994;8: 211–230.

21. Turnbull AP, Turnbull HJR. Understanding families from a systems perspective. In Williams JM, Kay T (eds). *Head Injury: A Family Matter*. Baltimore, MD: Paul H Brookes Publishing; 1991:37–63.

22. Maitz E. Family systems theory applied to head injury. In Williams JM, Kay T (eds). *Head Injury: A Family Matter*. Baltimore, MD: Paul H Brookes Publishing; 1991:65–79.

23. Stambrook M et al. Family adjustment following traumatic brain injury: a systems-based, life cycle approach. In Finlayson MAJ, Garner SH (eds). *Brain Injury Rehabilitation: Clinical Considerations*. Baltimore, MD: Williams & Wilkins; 1994:332–351.

24. DePompei R, Zarski JJ, Hall DE. A systems approach to understanding CHI family functioning. *Cognitive Rehabilitation*. 1987;5:6–9.

25. Novack TA, Bergquist TF, Bennett G. Family involvement in cognitive recovery following traumatic brain injury. In Long CJ, Ross LK (eds). *Head Trauma: Acute Care to Recovery*. New York, NY: Plenum Press; 1992:329–355.

26. Williams J. Training staff for family-centered rehabilitation. In Durgin CJ, Schmidt, ND, Fryer LJ (eds). *Staff Development and Clinical Intervention in Brain Injury Rehabilitation*. Gaithersburg, MD: Aspen Publishers; 1993:45–56.

27. DePompei R, Zarski J. Assessment of the family. In Williams JM, Kay T (eds). *Head Injury: A Family Matter*. Baltimore, MD: Paul H Brookes Publishing; 1991: 111–120.

28. Spanbock PD. Understanding head injury from the families' perspective. *Cognitive Rehabilitation*. 1987;5:12–14.

29. Silver SM, Price P, Barrett A. Family and return to work. In Williams JM, Kay T (eds). *Head Injury: A Family Matter*. Baltimore, MD: Paul H Brookes Publishing; 1991:179–201.

30. Florian V, Shlomo K, Lahav V. Impact of traumatic brain damage on family dynamics and functioning: a review. *Brain Injury*. 1984;3:219–233.

31. Ylvisaker M, Feeney TJ, Urbanczyk B. Developing a positive communication culture for rehabilitation: communication training for staff and family members. In Durgin CJ, Schmidt ND, Fryer LJ (eds). *Staff Development and Clinical Intervention in Brain Injury Rehabilitation*. Gaithersburg, MD: Aspen Publishers; 1993:57–85.

32. Pierro C. Talking with your child about disabilities. *Exceptional Parent*. 1995;25(6):92.

33. Gleckman AD, Brill S. The impact of brain injury on family functioning: implications for subacute rehabilitation programs. *Brain Injury*. 1995;9:385–393.

Appendix A

Glossary of Acronyms

AAC: augmentative and alternative communication

ABR: auditory brain stem response

ABER: auditory brain stem evoked response

ACPM: American Congress of Physical Medicine

ADA: Americans with Disabilities Act

ADD: attention deficit disorder

ADH: antidiuretic hormone

ADL: activities of daily living

AIDS: acquired immune deficiency syndrome

AEP: auditory evoked potential

AFO: ankle foot orthosis

AOTA: American Occupational Therapy Association

APA: American Psychological Association

APTA: American Physical Therapy Association

ASHA: American Speech, Language and Hearing Association

BAER: brain stem auditory evoked response

BIA: Brain Injury Association

BS: breath sounds

CACR: computer assisted cognitive rehabilitation/retraining

CARF: Commission on Accreditation of Rehabilitation Facilities

CHI: closed head injury

CN: cranial nerve (followed by number, e.g., CN3)

CNS: central nervous system

COBRA: Consolidated Omnibus Budget Reconciliation Act

COTA: certified occupational therapist assistant

CPAP: continuous positive airway pressure

CPT: current procedural terminology

CQI: continuous quality improvement

CR: cognitive rehabilitation/retraining

CRC: certified rehabilitation counselor

CRRN: certified rehabilitation registered nurse

CRT: cognitive rehabilitation therapy or cathode ray tube

CSF: cerebrospinal fluid

CT: computerized tomography

CTRS: certified therapeutic recreation specialist

DAI: diffuse axonal injury

DHHS: Department of Health and Human Services

DHI: diffuse hypoxic injury

DI: diabetes insipidus

DRG: diagnosis-related group

DRS: Disability Rating Scale

DTR: deep tendon reflex

ECG: electrocardiogram

EDH: epidural hematoma

EEG: electroencephalogram

EMG: electromyogram

EOM: extra-occular motion

ER: emergency room

ERP: event-related potentials

ET: endotracheal

ETT: endotracheal tube

EVP or EP: evoked potential

FAS: Functional Assessment Scale

FC: Foley catheter

FFS: fee for service

FH: family history

FIM: Functional Independence Measure

FMP: functional maintenance program

FNP: family nurse practitioner

FUO: fever of unknown origin

GABA: gamma-aminobutyric acid

GCS: Glasgow Coma Scale

GOAT: Galveston Orientation and Amnesia Test

GOS: Glasgow Outcome Scale

GSW: gunshot wound

GT: gastrostomy tube

H & P: history and physical

HCFA: Health Care Finance Administration (Medicare)

HO: heterotopic ossification

HMO: health maintenance organization

ICD: International Classification of Diseases

ICIDH: International Classification of Impairments, Disabilities, and Handicaps

ICP: intracranial pressure

ICU: intensive care unit

IDEA: Individuals with Disabilities Education Act

IM: intramuscular

IV: intravenous

JCAHO: Joint Commission on the Accreditation of Healthcare Organizations

KAFO: knee ankle foot orthosis

KAS-R: Katz Adjustment Scale-Relative's Form

LOC: loss of consciousness or level of consciousness

LOCF: levels of cognitive functioning

LOS: length of stay

MBS: modified barium swallow

MCA: motorcycle accident

MEP: multisensory evoked potentials

MHI: mild head injury

MMPI: Minnesota Multiphasic Personality Inventory

MRI or MR: magnetic resonance imaging

MVA: motor vehicle accident

NARF: National Association of Rehabilitation Facilities

NC: nasal cannula

NG: nasogastric

NHIF: National Head Injury Foundation (now Brain Injury Association)

NICU: neurosurgical intensive care unit

NIDRR: National Institute on Disability and Rehabilitation Research

NOS: not otherwise specified

NPH: normal pressure hydrocephalus

NSAID: nonsteroidal anti-inflammatory drugs

OBRA: Omnibus Budget Reconciliation Act

OBS: organic brain syndrome

OR: operating room

OTR: occupational therapist registered

PA-C: physician assistant certified

PASAT: Paced Auditory Serial Addition Task

PDR: Physicians' Desk Reference

PE: physical exam or pulmonary embolus

PEEP: positive end-expiratory pressure

PEG: percutaneous endoscopic gastrostomy

PERRL: pupils equal, round, and reactive to light

PERRLA: pupils equal, round, and reactive to light, accommodation

PET: positron emission tomography

PFT: pulmonary function test

PHI: penetrating head injury

PMH: past medical history

PNS: peripheral nervous system

POC: plan of care

POMR: problem oriented medical record

PPO: preferred provider organization

PPS: prospective payment system

PRO: peer review organization

PROM: passive range of motion

PT: physical therapist

PTA: physical therapist assistant

PTA: post-traumatic amnesia

PTE: post-traumatic epilepsy

PTH: post-traumatic hydrocephalus

PVS: persistent vegetative state

QA: quality assurance

RIPA: Ross Information Processing Assessment

RLA: Rancho Los Amigos

ROM: range of motion

SAH: subarachnoid hemorrhage

SCI: spinal cord injury

SDH: subdural hematoma

SH: social history

SOC: start of care

SPECT: single photon emission computed tomography

SSDI: Social Security disability insurance

SSI: supplemental security income

SSN: Social Security number

TBI: traumatic brain injury

TEF: tracheoesophageal fistula

TEP: tracheoesophageal puncture

TLC: transitional living center

TPN: total parenteral nutrition

TQM: total quality management

UR: utilization review

URI: upper respiratory infection

UTI: urinary tract infection

VAMC: Veterans Affairs Medical Center

VC: vital capacity

V/F: videofluoroscopy

VR: vocational rehabilitation

WAIS: Weschler Adult Intelligence Scale

WC: Workers' Compensation

WFL: within functional limits

WHO: World Health Organization

WMS: Wechsler Memory Scale

WNL: within normal limits

Appendix B

Selected Readings by Topic

ACUTE REHABILITATION

See Rehabilitation

ATTENTION

Auerbach SH. Neuroanatomical correlates of attention and memory disorders in traumatic brain injury: an application of neurobehavioral subtypes. *Journal of Head Trauma Rehabilitation.* 1986;1:1–12.

Mack JL. Clinical assessment of disorders of attention and memory. *Journal of Head Trauma Rehabilitation.* 1986;1:22–33.

McCaffrey RJ, Gansler DA. The efficacy of attention-remediation programs for traumatically brain-injured survivors. In Long CJ, Ross LK (eds). *Handbook of Head Trauma: Acute Care to Recovery.* New York, NY: Plenum Press; 1992:203–217.

Mesulam MM. Attention, confusional states, and neglect. In Mesulam MM (ed). *Principles of Behavioral Neurology.* Philadelphia, PA: FA Davis; 1985:125–168.

Nissen MJ. Neuropsychology of attention and memory. *Journal of Head Trauma Rehabilitation.* 1986;1:13–21.

Sohlberg MM, Mateer CA. Effectiveness of an attention-training program. *Journal of Clinical and Experimental Neuropsychology.* 1987;9:117–130.

von Zomeren AH, Brouwer WH, Deelman BG. Attentional deficits: the riddles of selectivity, speed, and alertness. In Brooks, DN (ed). *Closed Head Injury: Psychological, Social, and Family Consequences.* Oxford, England: Oxford University Press; 1984:74–107.

Weber AM. A practical clinical approach to understanding and treating attentional problems. *Journal of Head Trauma Rehabilitation.* 1990;5:73–85.

Whyte J, Rosenthal M. Rehabilitation of the patient with head injury. In DeLisa J (ed). *Rehabilitation Medicine: Principles and Practices.* Philadelphia, PA: JB Lippincott; 1988;585–611.

Whyte J. Attention and arousal: basic science aspects. *Archives of Physical Medicine and Rehabilitation.* 1992;73:940–949.

Wood RL. Rehabilitation of patients with disorders of attention. *Journal of Head Trauma Rehabilitation.* 1986;1:43–53.

COGNITIVE DEFECTS

Assessment

Baxter R, Cohen S, Ylvisaker M. Comprehensive cognitive assessment. In Ylvisaker M (ed). *Head Injury Rehabilitation: Children and Adolescents.* San Diego, CA: College-Hill Press; 1985:247–274.

Lezak MD. *Neuropsychological Assessment, 2nd ed.* New York, NY: Oxford University Press; 1983.

Sohlberg MM, Mateer CA. *Introduction to Cognitive Rehabilitation: Theory and Practice.* New York, NY: Guilford Press; 1989:63–89.

Tupper DE, Cicerone K (eds). *The Neuropsychology of Everyday Life: Assessment and Basic Competencies.* Boston, MA: Kluwer Academic Publishers; 1990:125–168.

Comprehensive Overviews

Ben-Yishay Y, Diller L. Cognitive deficits. In Rosenthal M, Griffith ER, Bond MR, Miller JD (eds). *Rehabilitation of the Head Injured Adult.* Philadelphia, PA: FA Davis; 1983:167–183.

Brooks DN. Cognitive deficits. In Rosenthal M, Griffith ER, Bond MR, Miller JD (eds). *Rehabilitation of the Adult and Child with Traumatic Brain Injury, 2nd ed.* Philadelphia, PA: FA Davis; 1990:163–178.

Brooks DN. Cognitive deficits after head injury. In Brooks DN (ed). *Closed Head Injury: Psychological, Social, and Family Consequences.* Oxford, England: Oxford University Press; 1984:44–73.

Levin HS. Neurobehavioral sequelae of head injury. In Cooper PR (ed). *Head Injury, 2nd ed.* Baltimore, MD: Williams and Wilkins; 1987:442–463.

Levin HS. Part II: Neurobehavioral recovery. In Becker D, Povlischock (eds). *Central Nervous System Trauma Status Report.* Bethesda, MD: National Institute of Neurological and Communicative Disorders and Stroke; 1985:281–299.

Prigtano GP. Cognitive dysfuntion and psychosocial adjustment. In Prigatano G (ed). *Neuropsychological Rehabilitation after Brain Injury.* Baltimore, MD: Johns Hopkins University Press; 1986:2–17.

Attention, Memory, Executive Functions

Refer to each heading

COGNITIVE REHABILITATION

Comprehensive Overviews

Adamovich BB, Henderson JA, Auerbach S. *Cognitive Rehabilitation of Closed Head Injured Patients: A Dynamic Approach.* San Diego, CA: College-Hill Press; 1985.

Benedict RH. The effectiveness of cognitive remediation strategies for victims of traumatic head-injury: a review of the literature. *Clinical Psychology Review.* 1989;9:650–626.

Ben-Yishay Y. Working Approaches to Remediation of Cognitive Deficits in Brain Damage. *Monograph 61.* New York, NY: New York University Medical Center; 1980.

Ben-Yishay Y, Diller L. Cognitive remediation. In Rosenthal M, Griffith ER, Bond MR, Miller JD (eds). *Rehabilitation of the Head Injured Adult.* Philadelphia, PA: FA Davis; 1983:367–380.

Duke LW et al. Cognitive rehabilitation after head trauma. In Long CJ, Ross LK (eds). *Handbook of Head Trauma: Acute Care to Recovery.* New York, NY: Plenum Press; 1992:165–190.

Ellis DW, Christensen AL (eds). *Neuropsychological Treatment after Brain Injury.* Boston, MA: Kluwer Academic Publishers; 1989:1–11.

Kreutzer J, Wehman P (eds). *Cognitive Rehabilitation for Persons with Traumatic Brain Injury: A Functional Approach*. Baltimore, MD: Paul H Brookes; 1991.

Meier MJ, Benton AL, Diller L (eds). *Neuropsychological Rehabilitation*. New York, NY: Guilford Press; 1987.

Moehle KA, Rasmussen JL, Fitzhugh-Bell KB. Neuropsychological theories and cognitive rehabilitation. In Williams JM, Long CJ (eds). *The Rehabilitation of Cognitive Disabilities*. New York, NY: Plenum Press; 1987:57–76.

Prigatano G et al. *Neuropsychological Rehabilitation after Brain Injury*. Baltimore, MD: Johns Hopkins University Press; 1986.

Sbordone RJ. A conceptual model of neuropsychologically-based cognitive rehabilitation. In Williams JM, Long CJ (eds). *The Rehabilitation of Cognitive Disabilities*. New York, NY: Plenum Press; 1987:3–25.

Sohlberg MM, Mateer CA. *Introduction to Cognitive Rehabilitation: Theory and Practice*. New York, NY: Guilford Press; 1989.

Szekers SF, Ylvisaker M, Cohen SB. A framework for cognitive rehabilitation therapy. In Ylvisaker M, Gobble EM (eds). *Community Re-entry for Head Injured Adults*. Boston, MA: College-Hill Press; 1987:87–136.

Trexler L (ed). *Cognitive Rehabilitation: Conceptualization and Intervention*. New York, NY: Plenum Press; 1982.

Uzzell BP, Gross Y (eds). *Clinical Neuropsychology of Intervention*. Boston, MA: Martinus Nijhoff; 1986.

Wood RL, Fussey I (eds). *Cognitive Rehabilitation in Perspective*. London, England: Taylor and Francis; 1988.

Ylvisaker M et al. Topics in cognitive rehabilitation therapy. In Ylvisaker M, Gobble EM (eds). *Community Re-entry for Head Injured Adults*. Boston, MA: College-Hill Press; 1987:137–220.

Computer Assisted

Bracy OL. *Psychological Software Services*. Indianapolis: Neuroscience Publishers.

Levin, W. Computer applications in cognitive rehabilitation. In Kreutzer J, Wehman P (eds). *Cognitive Rehabilitation for Persons with Traumatic Brain Injury. A Functional Approach*. Baltimore, MD: Paul H Brookes; 1991:163–178.

COGNITIVE-COMMUNICATIVE

Aphasia

Groher M. Language and memory disorders following closed head trauma. *Journal of Speech and Hearing Research*. 1977;20:212–223.

Hartley LL, Levin HS. Linguistic deficits after closed head injury: a current appraisal. *Aphasiology*. 1990;4:353–370.

Arseni C et al. Considerations on posttraumatic aphasia in peace time. *Psychiatria, Neurologia, Neurochirurgia*. 1970;73:105–112.

Heilman K, Safran A, Geschwind N. Closed head trauma and aphasia. *Journal of Neurology, Neurosurgery, and Psychiatry*. 1971;34:265–269.

Kriendler A et al. Aphasia following non-missile injury of the brain. *Reviews in Romanian Medicine, Neurology and Psychiatry*. 1975;13:247–254.

Levin HS. Aphasia in closed head injury. In Sarno MT (ed). *Acquired Aphasia*. New York, NY: Academic Press; 1981:427–463.

Levin HS et al. Linguistic recovery after closed head injury. *Brain and Language*. 1981;12:360–374.

Levin HS, Grossman RG, Kelly PJ. Aphasic disorder in patients with closed head injury. *Journal of Neurology, Neurosurgery, and Psychiatry*. 1976;39:1062–1070.

Luria AR. *Traumatic Aphasia: Its Syndromes, Psychology and Treatment*. Bowden D (trans). The Hague, The Netherlands: Mouton; 1970.

Najenson T et al. Recovery of communicative functions after prolonged traumatic coma. *Scandinavian Journal of Rehabilitation Medicine*. 1978;10:15–21.

Sarno MT. The nature of verbal impairment after closed head injury. *Journal of Nervous and Mental Disease*. 1980;168:685–692.

Sarno MT, Buonaguar A, Levita E. Characteristics of verbal impairment in closed head injured patients. *Archives of Physical Medicine and Rehabilitation*. 1986;67: 400–405.

Stone JL, Lopes JR, Moody RA. Fluent aphasia after closed head injury. *Surgical Neurology*. 1978;9:27–29.

Russell WR, Espir MLE. *Traumatic Aphasia: A Study of Aphasia in War Wounds of the Brain*. London, England: Oxford University Press; 1961.

Thompsen IV. Neuropsychological treatment and longtime follow up in an aphasic patient with very severe head trauma. *Journal of Clinical Neuropsychology*. 1981;3:43–51.

Thompsen IV. Verbal learning in aphasic and non-aphasic patients with severe head injuries. *Scandinavian Journal of Rehabilitation Medicine*. 1977;9:73–77.

Thompsen IV. Evaluation and outcome of traumatic aphasia in patients with severe verified focal lesions. *Folia Phoniatrica*. 1976;28:362–377.

Thompsen IV. Evaluation and outcome of aphasia in patients with severe closed head trauma. *Journal of Neurology, Neurosurgery, and Psychiatry*. 1975;38:713–718.

Comprehensive Overviews

Beukelman DR, Yorkston KM (eds). *Communicative Disorders Following Traumatic Brain Injury: Management of Cognitive, Language and Motor Impairments*. Austin, TX: Pro-Ed; 1991.

Halper AS, Cherney LR, Miller TK. *Clinical Management of Communication Problems in Adults with Traumatic Brain Injury*. Gaithersburg, MD: Aspen Publications; 1991.

Hartley LL. *Cognitive-Communicative Abilities Following Brain Injury: A Functional Approach*. San Diego, CA: Singular Publishing; 1995.

Ylvisaker M, Urbanczyk B. Assessment and treatment of speech, swallowing, and communication disorders following traumatic brain injury. In Finlayson MAJ, Garner SH (eds). *Brain Injury Rehabilitation: Clinical Considerations*. Baltimore, MD: Williams and Wilkins; 1994:157–186.

Ylvisaker MS, Holland AL. Coaching, self-coaching, and rehabilitation of head injury. In Johns DF (ed). *Clinical Management of Neurogenic Communicative Disorders, 2nd ed.* Boston, MA: Little Brown and Company; 1985:243–257.

Language and Discourse

Chapman SB, Levin HS, Culhane KA. Language impairment in closed head injury. In Kirshner H (ed). *Handbook of Neurologic Speech and Language Disorders*. New York, NY: Marcel Dekker; 1995:387–414.

Coelho CA, Liles BZ, Duffy RJ. Discourse analyses with closed head injured adults: evidence for differing patterns of deficits. *Archives of Physical Medicine and Rehabilitation.* 1991;72:465–468.

Ehrlich JS. Selective characteristics of narrative discourse in head-injured and normal adults. *Journal of Communication Disorders.* 1988;21:1–9.

Hagen C. Language disorders secondary to closed head injury: diagnosis and treatment. *Topics in Language Disorders.* 1981;1:73–87.

Hartley LL, Jensen PJ. Three discourse profiles of closed-head-injury speakers: theoretical and clinical implications. *Brain Injury.* 1992;6:271–282.

Mentis M, Prutting C. Cohesion in the discourse of normal and head-injured adults. *Journal of Speech and Hearing Research.* 1987;30:88–98.

Milton SB, Prutting CA, Binder GM. Appraisal of communicative competence in head injured adults. In Brookshire RH (ed). *Clinical Aphasiology Conference Proceedings.* Minneapolis, MN: BRK Publishers; 1984:114–123.

Wiig EH, Alexander EW, Secord W. Linguistic competence and level of cognitive functioning in adults with traumatic closed head injury. In Whitaker HA (ed). *Neuropsychological Studies of Nonfocal Brain Damage: Dementia and Trauma.* London, England: Springer-Verlag; 1988:186–210.

Reading and Writing

Nelson NW, Schwentor BA. Reading and writing disorders. In Beukelman DR, Yorkston KM (eds). *Communication Disorders Following Traumatic Brain Injury: Management of Cognitive, Language, and Motor Impairments.* Austin, TX: Pro-Ed; 1991:191–249.

Speech

See Motor Speech

COMA

See Medical Management

COMMUNITY RE-ENTRY

See Rehabilitation, Community Integration

DYSPHAGIA

Cherney LR, Halper AS. Recovery of oral nutrition after head injury in adults. *Journal of Head Trauma Rehabilitation.* 1989;4:42–50.

Goher ME (ed). *Dysphagia: Diagnosis and Management, 2nd ed.* Stoneham, MA: Butterworth-Heinemann; 1992.

Hutchins BF. Establishing a dysphagia family intervention program for head-injured patients. *Journal of Head Trauma Rehabilitation.* 1989;4:64–72.

Lazurus CL. Diagnosis and management of swallowing disorders in TBI. In Beukelman DR, Yorkston KM (eds). *Communicative Disorders Following Traumatic Brain Injury: Management of Cognitive, Language and Motor Impairments.* Austin, TX: Pro-Ed; 1991:367–417.

Lazarus C, Logemann J. Swallowing disorders in closed head trauma patients. *Archives of Physical Medicine and Rehabilitation.* 1987;68:79–84.

Logemann JA. Evaluation and treatment planning for the head-injured patient with oral intake disorders. *Journal of Head Trauma Rehabilitation*. 1989;4:24–33.

Logemann JA, Pepe J, Mackay LE. Disorders of nutrition and swallowing: intervention strategies in the trauma center. *Journal of Head Trauma Rehabilitation*. 1994;9:43–56.

Yorkston KM et al. The relationship between speech and swallowing disorders. *Journal of Head Trauma Rehabilitation*. 1989;4:1–16.

EPIDEMIOLOGY

Frankowski RF, Annegers JF, Whitman S. Epidemiological and descriptive studies part I: epidemiology of head trauma in the United States. In Becker DP, Povlishock JT (eds). *Central Nervous System Trauma Status Report*. Bethesda, MD: National Institute of Neurologic and Communicative Disorders and Sciences; 1985:33–43.

Kalsbeek WD et al. The national head and spinal cord injury survey: major findings. *Journal of Neurosurgery*. 1980;53:S19–S31.

Willer B, Abosch S, Dahmer E. Epidemiology of disability from traumatic brain injury. In Wood RL (ed). *Neurobehavioural Sequelae of Traumatic Brain Injury*. New York, NY: Taylor and Francis; 1989:18–33.

ETHICS

Agich GJ. *Responsibility in Health Care*. Dodrecht, Holland: D Riedel Publishing, 1982.

Banja J. Ethical issues in staff development. In Durgin CJ, Schmidt ND, Fryer LJ (eds). *Staff Development and Clinical Intervention in Brain Injury Rehabilitation*. Gaithersburg, MD: Aspen Publishers; 1993:23–41.

Banja JD, Higgins P. Videotaping therapeutic sessions and the right of privacy. *Journal of Head Trauma Rehabilitation*. 1989;4:65–74.

Calman KC. The ethics of allocation of scarce health care resources: a view from the centre. *Journal of Medical Ethics*. 1994;20:71–74.

Caplan AL. Informed consent and provider-patient relationships in rehabilitation medicine. *Archives of Physical Medicine and Rehabilitation*. 1988;69:312–317.

Caplan AL, Callahan D, Haas J. *Ethical and Policy Issues in Rehabilitation Medicine*. Briarcliff Manor, New York, NY: The Hastings Center; 1987:1–20.

DeJong G, Batavia AI. Societal duty and resource allocation for persons with severe traumatic brain injury. *Journal of Head Trauma Rehabilitation*. 1989;4:1–12.

Garrett TM, Baillie HW, Garrett RM. *Health Care Ethics: Principles and Problems, 2nd ed.* Englewood Cliffs, NJ: Prentice Hall; 1993.

Haas J, MacKenzie CA. The role of ethics in rehabilitation medicine. *American Journal of Physical Medicine Rehabilitation*. 1995;74(suppl):3–6.

Malec JF. Ethics in brain injury rehabilitation: existential choices among western cultural beliefs. *Brain Injury*. 1993;7:383–400.

Purtilo RB. *Ethical Dimensions in the Health Professions, 2nd ed.* Philadelphia, PA: WB Saunders; 1993.

Purtilo RB. Ethical issues in teamwork: the context of rehabilitation. *Archives of Physical Medicine and Rehabilitation.* 1988;69:318–322.

Purtilo RB, Meier RH. Team challenges: regulatory constraints and patient empowerment. *American Journal of Physical Medicine and Rehabilitation.* 1995:74(suppl):21–24.

Romano MD. Ethical issues and families of brain-injured persons. *Journal of Head Trauma Rehabilitation.* 1989;4:33–41.

Sanders JM. Ethical implications of disablement. In Greenwood R, Barnes MP, McMillan TM, Ward CD (eds). *Neurological Rehabilitation.* Edinburgh, Scotland: Churchhill Livingstone; 1993:59–63.

Veatch RM. *The Patient-Physician Relationship.* Bloomington, IN: University Press; 1991.

Veatch RM. *Medical Ethics.* Boston, MA: Jones and Bartlett Publishers; 1989.

Venesy BA. A clinician's guide to decision making capacity and ethically sound medical decisions. *American Journal of Physical Medicine and Rehabilitation.* 1995;74(suppl):41–48.

EXECUTIVE/FRONTAL LOBE FUNCTIONS

Levin HS, Eisenberg HM, Benton AL (eds). *Frontal Lobe Function and Dysfunction.* New York, NY: Oxford University Press; 1991:173–195.

Lezak MD. Newer contributions to the neuropsychological assessment of executive functions. *Journal of Head Trauma Rehabilitation.* 1993;8:24–31.

Prigatano GP. The relationship of frontal lobe damage to diminished awareness: studies in rehabilitation. In Levin HS, Eisenberg HM, Benton AL (eds). *Frontal Lobe Function and Dysfunction.* New York, NY: Oxford University Press; 1991:381–397.

Sohlberg MM, Mateer CA, Stuss DT. Contemporary approaches to the management of executive control dysfunction. *Journal of Head Trauma Rehabilitation.* 1993;8:45–58.

Stuss DT. Contribution of frontal lobe injury to cognitive impairment after closed head injury: methods of assessment and recent findings. In Levin HS, Grafman J, Eisenberg HM (eds). *Neurobehavioral Recovery from Closed Head Injury.* New York, NY: Oxford University Press; 1987.

Stuss DT, Benson DF. *The Frontal Lobes.* New York, NY: Raven Press; 1986.

Stuss DT, Benson DF. Neuropsychological studies of the frontal lobes. *Psychological Bulletin.* 1984;95:3–28.

Stuss DT, Mateer CA, Sohlberg MM. Innovative approaches to frontal lobe deficits. In Finlayson MAJ, Garner SH (eds). *Brain Injury Rehabilitation: Clinical Considerations.* Baltimore, MD: Williams and Wilkins; 1994:212–237.

Ylvisaker M, Szekers SF. Metacognitive and executive impairments in head-injured children and adults. *Topics in Language Disorders.* 1989:9:34–49.

FAMILY

Bond MR. Effects on the family system. In Rosenthal M, Griffith E, Bond M, Miller JD (eds). *Rehabilitation of the Head Injured Adult.* Philadelphia, PA: FA Davis; 1983:209–217.

Brooks DN. The head-injured family. *Journal of Clinical and Experimental Neuropsychology.* 1991;13:155–188.

Brooks DN. Head injury and the family. In Brooks DN (ed). *Closed Head Injury: Psychological, Social, and Family Consequences.* Oxford, England: Oxford University Press; 1984:123–147.

Cope DN, Wolfson B. Crisis intervention with the family in the trauma setting. *Journal of Head Trauma Rehabilitation.* 1994;9:67–81.

DePompei R, Zarski JJ. Families, head injury, and cognitive-communicative impairments: issues for family counseling. *Topics in Language Disorders.* 1989; 9:78–89.

Florian V, Shlomo K, Lahav V. Impact of traumatic brain damage on family dynamics and functioning: a review. *Brain Injury.* 1989;3:219–233.

Lezak MD. Brain damage is a family affair. *Journal of Clinical and Experimental Neuropsychology.* 1988;10:111–123.

Lezak MD. Living with the characterologically altered brain injured patient. *Journal of Clinical Psychiatry.* 1978;July:592–598.

Livingston MG. Effects on the family system. In Rosenthal M, Griffith ER, Bond MR, Miller JD (eds). *Rehabilitation of the Adult and Child with Traumatic Brain Injury, 2nd ed.* Philadelphia, PA: FA Davis; 1990:225–235.

Livingston MG, Brooks DN. The burden on families of the brain injured: a review. *Journal of Head Trauma Rehabilitation.* 1988;4:6–15.

Novack TA, Bergquist TF, Bennett G. Family involvement in cognitive recovery following traumatic brain injury. In Long CJ, Ross LK (eds). *Head Trauma: Acute Care to Recovery.* New York, NY: Plenum Press; 1992:329–355.

Romano MD. Family issues in head trauma. In Horn LJ, Cope DN (eds). *Physical Medicine and Rehabilitation: State of the Art Reviews.* Philadelphia, PA: Hanley and Belfus; 1989:3(1):157–167.

Talbott, R. The brain-injured person and the family. In Wood RL, Eames P (eds). *Models of Brain Injury Rehabilitation.* Baltimore, MD: Johns Hopkins University Press; 1989:3–16.

Williams JM. Training staff for family-centered rehabilitation. In Durgin CJ, Schmidt ND, Fryer LJ (eds). *Staff Development and Clinical Intervention in Brain Injury Rehabilitation.* Gaithersburg, MD: Aspen Publishers; 1993:45–56.

Williams JM, Kay T (eds). Head Injury: A Family Matter. Baltimore, MD: Paul H. Brookes Publishing; 1991.

Family Guides

Adult Head Trauma Team. *A Family Guide to Rehabilitation of the Traumatic Brain Injury Patient.* Downey, CA: Professional Staff Association of the Rancho Los Amigos Hospital; 1979.

Deboskey DS, Hecht JS, Calub CJ. *Educating Families of the Head Injured: A Guide to Medical, Cognitive and Social Issues.* Gaithersburg, MD: Aspen Publications; 1991.

Hawley, LA. *A Family Guide to the Rehabilitation of the Severely Head-Injured Patient.* Austin, TX: Healthcare Rehabilitation Center; 1987.

Gronwall D, Wrightson P, Waddell P. *Head Injury the Facts: A Guide for Families and Care-givers.* New York, NY: Oxford University Press; 1990.

Marshall LF, Sadler GR, Bowers SA. *Head Injury.* San Diego, CA: Central Nervous System Foundation; 1985.

HISTORICAL REVIEWS

Benton AL. Historical notes on the postconcussion syndrome. In Levin HS, Eisenberg HM, Benton AL (eds). *Mild Head Injury*. New York, NY: Oxford University Press; 1989;3–7.

Boake C. History of cognitive rehabilitation following head injury. In Kreutzer JS, Wehman PH (eds). *Cognitive Rehabilitation for Persons with Traumatic Brain Injury: A Functional Approach*. Baltimore, MD: Paul H Brookes Publishing; 1991:3–12.

Boake C. A history of cognitive rehabilitation of head-injured patients, 1915 to 1980. *Journal of Head Trauma Rehabilitation*. 1989;4:1–8.

Gurdjian ES. *Head Injury from Antiquity to the Present with Special Reference to Penetrating Head Wounds*. Springfield, IL: Charles C Thomas; 1973.

Jennett B. Historical development of head injury care. In Pitts LH, Wagner FC (eds). *Craniospinal Trauma*. New York, NY: Thieme Medical Publishers; 1990:2–10.

Levin HS, Benton AL, Grossman RG. *Neurobehavioral Consequences of Closed Head Injury*. New York, NY: Oxford University Press;1982:3–48.

MEDICAL MANAGEMENT

Coma and Persistent Vegetative State

Bricolo AB, Turazzi S, Feriotti G. Prolonged post traumatic unconsciousness: therapeutic assets and liabilities. *Journal of Neurosurgery*. 1980;52:625–634.

Haig AJ, Katz RT, Sahgal V. Locked-in syndrome: a review. *Current Concepts in Rehabilitation Medicine*. 1986;3:12–15.

Plum F, Posner JB. *The Diagnosis of Stupor and Coma*. Philadelphia, PA: FA Davis; 1982.

Jennett B. Clinical and pathological features of vegetative survival. In Levin HS, Benton AR, Muizelaar JP, Eisenberg HM (eds). *Catastrophic Brain Injury*. New York, NY: Oxford University Press; 1996.

Jennett B, Teasdale G. Aspects of coma after severe head injury. *Lancet*. 1977;2: 878–881.

Teasdale G, Jennett B. Assessment of coma: a practical scale. *Lancet*. 1974;2:81–84.

Sazbon L, Costeff H, Groswasser Z. Epidemiological findings in traumatic post-comatose unawareness. *Brain Injury*. 1992;6:359–362.

Comprehensive Overviews

Becker DP, Povlishock JT (eds). *Central Nervous System Trauma Status Report*. Washington, DC: National Institute of Neurological and Communicative Disorders and Stroke; 1985.

Bontke CF, Boake. Principles of brain injury rehabilitation. In Braddom RL (ed). *Physical Medicine and Rehabilitation*. Philadelphia, PA: WB Saunders; 1996.

Cooper PR (ed). *Head Injury, 3rd ed*. Baltimore, MD: Williams and Wilkins; 1993; 137–158.

Jennett B, Teasdale GM. *Management of Head Injuries*. Philadelphia, PA: FA Davis; 1981.

Katz DI, Alexander MP. Traumatic brain injury. In Good DC, Couch JR (eds). *Handbook of Neurorehabilitation*. New York, NY: Marcel Dekker; 1994:493–549.

Kraft GH, Berrol S (eds). *Traumatic Brain Injury: Physical Medicine and Rehabilitation Clinics of North America*, Vol 3. Philadelphia, PA: WB Saunders; 1992.

Miller JD, Pentland B, Berrol S. Early evaluation and management. In Rosenthal M, Griffith ER, Bond MR, Miller JD (eds). *Rehabilitation of the Adult and Child with Traumatic Brain Injury.* Philadelphia, PA: FA Davis; 1990:21–51.

Cranial Nerves

Berrol, S. Cranial nerve dysfunction. In Horn LJ, Cope DN (eds). *Traumatic Brain Injury: Physical Medicine and Rehabilitation State of the Art Reviews.* Philadelphia, PA: Hanley and Belfus; 1989:3(1):85–93.

Murali R, Rovit RL. Injuries of the cranial nerves. In Barrow DL (ed). *Complications and Sequelae of Head Injury.* Park Ridge, IL: American Association of Neurological Surgeons; 1992:109–126.

Neuropharmacology

Cardenas DD, McLean A. Psychopharmacologic management of traumatic brain injury. In Kraft GH, Berrol S (eds). *Traumatic Brain Injury: Physical Medicine and Rehabilitation Clinics of North America,* Vol 3. Philadelphia, PA: WB Saunders; 1992:273–290.

Gualtieri CT. *Neuropsychiatry and Behavioral Pharmacology.* New York, NY: Springer-Verlag; 1991.

Ross LK. The use of pharmacology in the treatment of head-injured patients. In Long CH, Ross LK (eds). *Handbook of Head Trauma: Acute Care to Recovery.* New York, NY: Plenum Press; 1992:137–164.

Zasler ND. Advances in neuropharmacological rehabilitation for brain dysfunction. *Brain Injury.* 1992;6:1–14.

Seizures

Jennett B. *Epilepsy after Non-missile Head Injuries, 2nd ed.* Chicago, IL: William Heinemann; 1975.

Yablon SA. Posttraumatic seizures. *Archives of Physical Medicine and Rehabilitation.* 1993;74:983–1001.

MEMORY

Parenté R, DiCesare A. Retraining memory: theory, evaluation, and applications. In Kreutzer J, Wehman P (eds). *Cognitive Rehabilitation for Persons with Traumatic Brain Injury: A Functional Approach.* Baltimore, MD: Paul H Brookes; 1991: 147–162.

Glisky EL, Schacter DA. Remediation of organic memory disorder: current status and future prospects. *Journal of Head Trauma Rehabilitation.* 1986;3:54–63.

Mateer CA, Sohlberg MM. A paradigm shift in memory rehabilitation. In Whitaker HA (ed). *Neuropsychological Studies of Nonfocal Brain Damage: Dementia and Trauma.* London, England: Springer-Verlag; 1988:202–225.

Mateer CA, Sohlberg MM, Crinean J. Focus on clinical research: perceptions of memory function in individuls with closed-head injury. *Journal of Head Trauma Rehabilitation.* 1987;2:74–84.

Ritchie WR. The traumatic amnesias. *International Journal of Neurology.* 1968;7: 55–59.

Schacter DL, Crovitz HF. Memory function after closed head injury: a review of the quantitative research. *Cortex.* 1977;13:150–176.

Squire LR. *Memory and Brain.* New York, NY: Oxford University Press; 1987.

Squire LR. Mechanisms of memory. *Science.* 1986; 232:1612–1619.

Wilson BA. *Rehabilitation of Memory.* New York, NY: Guilford Press; 1987.

MILD TO MODERATE INJURIES

Alves WM et al. Understanding posttraumatic symptoms after minor head injury. *Journal of Head Trauma Rehabilitation.* 1986;1:1–12.

Barth JT et al. Forensic aspects of mild head trauma. *Journal of Head Trauma Rehabilitation.* 1986;1:63–70.

Barth JT et al. Neuropsychological sequelae of minor head injury. *Neurosurgery.* 1983;13:529–533.

Colohan ART et al. Neurologic and neurosurgical implications of mild head injury. *Journal of Head Trauma Rehabilitation.* 1986;1:13–21.

Gronwall D. Rehabilitation programs for patients with mild head injury: components, problems, and evaluation. *Journal of Head Trauma Rehabilitation.* 1986; 1:53–62.

Gronwall D, Wrightson P. Delayed recovery of intellectual function after minor head injury. *Lancet.* 1974;2:605–609.

Hoff J, Anderson T, Cole T (eds). *Contemporary Issues in Neurological Surgery: Mild to Moderate Head Injury, Vol 1.* Boston, MA: Blackwell Scientific Publications; 1989.

Levin HS et al. Neurobehavioral outcome following minor head injury: a three-center study. *Journal of Neurosurgery.* 1987;66:234–243.

Levin HS, Eisenberg HM, Benton AL (eds). *Mild Head Injury.* New York, NY: Oxford University Press; 1989.

Mattis S. Mild head trauma. In Bach-y-Rita P (ed). *Comprehensive Neurologic Rehabilitation: Traumatic Brain Injury, Vol 2.* New York, NY: Demos; 1989:41–50.

Mittenberg W, Burton DB. A survey of treatments for post-concussion syndrome. *Brain Injury.* 1994;8:429–437.

Rimel RW et al. Disability caused by minor head injury. *Neurosurgery.* 1981;9: 221–228.

Ruff RM, Levin HS, Marshal LF. Neurobehavioral methods of assessment and the study of outcome in minor head injury. *Journal of Head Trauma Rehabilitation.* 1986;1:43–52.

MOTOR SPEECH

Assessment

Barlow SM, Burton MK. Ramp-and-hold force control in the upper and lower lips: developing new neuromotor assessment application in traumatically brain injured adults. *Journal of Speech and Hearing Disorders.* 1990;33:660–675.

D'Antonio LL et al. Reliability of flexible fiberoptic nasopharyngoscopy for evaluation of velopharyngeal function in a clinical population. *Cleft Palate Journal.* 1989;26:217–225.

Faure M-A, Muller A. Stroboscopy. *Journal of Voice.* 1992;2:139–148.

Gould WJ, Korovin GS. Laboratory advances for voice measurements. *Journal of Voice.* 1994;8:8–17.

Horii Y. An accelerometric approach to nasality measurement: a preliminary report. *Cleft Palate Journal.* 1981;17:254–261.

Kent RD et al. Toward phonetic intelligibility testing in dysarthria. *Journal of Speech and Hearing Disorders*. 1989;54:482–499.

Karnell MP. *Videoendoscopy: From Velopharynx to Larynx*. San Diego, CA: Singular Publishing Group; 1994.

McHenry MA et al. Intelligibility and nonspeech orofacial strength and force control following traumatic brain injury. *Journal of Speech and Hearing Disorders*. 1994;367:1271–1283.

McHenry MA. Laryngeal airway resistance following traumatic brain injury. In Robin D, Yorkston KM, Beukelman DR (eds). *Disorders of Motor Speech: Recent Advances in Assessment, Treatment, and Clinical Characterization*. Baltimore, MD: Paul H Brookes; 1995.

Miller CJ, Daniloff R. Airflow measurements: theory and utility of findings. *Journal of Voice*. 1993;7:38–46.

Murdoch BE et al. Abnormal patterns of speech breathing in dysarthric speakers following severe closed head injury. *Brain Injury*. 1993;7:295–308.

Pannbacker M, Middleton G. Integrating perceptual and instrumental procedures in the assessment of velopharyngeal insufficiency. *Ear, Nose and Throat Journal*. 1990;69:161–175.

Read C, Buder EH, Kent RD. Speech analysis systems: an evaluation. *Journal of Speech and Hearing Research*. 1992;35:324–332.

Reich AR, McHenry MA. Estimating respiratory volumes from ribcage and abdominal displacements during ventilatory and speech activities. *Journal of Speech and Hearing Research*. 1990;33:467–475.

Shuster LI. Interpretation of speech science measures. *Clinical Communication Disorders*. 1993;3:26–35.

Theodoros D et al. Hypernasality in dysarthric speakers following severe closed head injury: a perceptual and instrumental analysis. *Brain Injury*. 1993;7:59–69.

Theodoros D, Murdoch BE. Laryngeal dysfunction in dysarthric speakers following severe closed head injury. *Brain Injury*. 1994;8:667–684.

Theodoros D, Murdoch BE, Chenery HJ. Perceptual speech characteristics of dysarthric speakers following severe closed head injury. *Brain Injury*. 1994;8:101–124.

Ziegler W, von Cramon D. Spastic dysarthria after acquired brain injury: an acoustic study. *British Journal of Disorders of Communication*. 1986;21:173–187.

Augmentative and Alternative Communication

Beukelman DR, Garrett K. Augmentative and alternative communication for adults with acquired severe communication disorders. *Augmentative and Alternative Communication*. 1988;4:104–121.

DeRuyter F, Kennedy MR. Augmentative communication following traumatic brain injury. In Beukelman DR, Yorkston KM (eds). *Communicative Disorders Following Traumatic Brain Injury: Management of Cognitive, Language and Motor Impairments*. Austin, TX: Pro-Ed; 1991:317–365.

Light J, Beesley M, Collier B. Transition through multiple augmentative and alternative communication systems: a three-year case study of a head injured adolescent. *Augmentative and Alternative Communication*. 1988;4:2–14.

Recovery and Treatment

Enderby P, Crow E. Long-term recovery patterns of severe dysarthria following head injury. *British Journal of Disorders of Communication*. 1990;25:341–354.

McHenry MA, Wilson RL, Minton JT. Management of multiple physiologic system deficits following traumatic brain injury. *Journal of Medical Speech-Language Pathology*. 1994;2:59–74.

McHenry MA, Wilson RL. The challenge of unintelligible speech following traumatic brain injury. *Brain Injury*. 1994;8:363–375.

Yorkston KM, Beukelman DR. Motor speech disorders. In Beukelman DR, Yorkston KM (eds). *Communicative Disorders Following Traumatic Brain Injury: Management of Cognitive, Language and Motor Impairments*. Austin, TX: Pro-Ed; 1991:251–315.

Workinger MS, Netsell R. Restoration of intelligible speech 13 years post-head injury. *Brain Injury*. 1992;6:183–187.

PATHOPHYSIOLOGY

Adams JH, Graham DI, Gennarelli TA. Contemporary neuropathological considerations regarding brain damage in head injury. In Becker DP, Povlishock JT (eds). *Central Nervous System Trauma Status Report*. Bethesda, MD: National Institute of Neurological and Communicative Disorders and Stroke; 1985:65–77.

Gennarelli TA. Cerebral concussion and diffuse brain injuries. In Cooper PR (ed). *Head Injury, 3rd ed*. Baltimore, MD: Williams and Wilkins; 1993:137–158.

Gennarelli TA. Initial assessment and management of head injury. In Pitts LH, Wagner FC (eds). *Craniospinal Trauma*. New York, NY: Thieme Medical Publishers; 1990:11–24.

Gennarelli TA. Mechanisms and pathophysiology of cerebral concussion. *Journal of Head Trauma Rehabilitation*. 1986;1:23–29.

Graham DI. Trauma. In Weller RO (ed). *Nervous System, Muscle and Eyes, Vol 4*. New York, NY: Churchill Livingstone; 1990:125–149.

Graham DI, Adams JH, Gennarelli TA. Pathology of brain damage in head injury. In Cooper PR (ed). *Head Injury, 3rd ed*. Baltimore, MD: Williams and Wilkins; 1993:91–113.

Mendelow AD, Teasdale GM. Pathophysiology of head injuries. *British Journal of Surgery*. 1983;70: 641–650.

Povlishock JT, Valadka AB. Pathobiology of traumatic brain injury. In Finlayson MAJ, Garner SH (eds). *Brain Injury Rehabilitation: Clinical Considerations*. Baltimore, MD: Williams and Wilkins; 1994:11–3.

PEDIATRICS

Bijur PE, Haslum M, Golding J. Cognitive and behavioral sequelae of mild head injury in children. *Pediatrics*. 1990;86:337–343.

Blosser JL, DePompei R. The head-injured student returns to school: recognizing and treating deficits. *Topics in Language Disorders*. 1989;9:67–77.

Boll TJ. Minor head injury in children—out of sight but not out of mind. *Journal of Clinical Psychology*. 1983;12:74–80.

Chadwick O et al. A prospective study of children with head injuries, II. Cognitive sequelae. *Psychological Medicine*. 1981;11:49–61.

Chadwick O et al. A prospective study of children with head injuries, IV. Specific cognitive deficits. *Journal of Clinical Neuropsychology*. 1981;3:101–120.

DePompei R, Blosser JL. Functional cognitive-communicative impairments in children and adolescents: assessment and intervention. In Kreutzer J, Wehman P (eds). *Cognitive Rehabilitation for Persons with Traumatic Brain Injury: A Functional Approach*. Baltimore, MD: Paul H Brookes; 1991:215–235.

DePompei R, Blosser JL (eds). School reentry following head injury. *Journal of Head Trauma Rehabilitation*. 1992;6(1):1–112.

Fletcher JM, Ewing-Cobbs L, Miner ME. Behavioral changes after closed head injury in children. *Journal of Consulting and Clinical Psychology*. 1990;58: 93–98.

Glang A et al. Tailoring direct instruction techniques for use with elementary students with brain injury. *Journal of Head Trauma Rehabilitation*. 1992;7: 93–108.

Hock RA. *The Rehabilitation of a Child With a Traumatic Brain Injury*. Springfield, IL: Charles C Thomas; 1984.

Jennett B. Head injuries in children. *Developmental Medicine and Child Neurology*. 1972;14:137–147.

Kraus JF, Fife D, Conroy C. Pediatric brain injuries: the nature, clinical course, and early outcomes in a defined United States population. *Pediatrics*. 1987;79:501–507.

Levin et al. Memory and intellectual ability after head injury in children and adolescents. *Neurosurgery*. 1982;11:668–672.

Levin HS, Eisenberg HM. Neuropsychological outcome of closed head injury in children and adolescents. *Child's Brain*. 1979;5:281–292.

Oddy M. Head injury during childhood: the psychological implications. In Brooks DN (ed). *Closed Head Injury: Psychological, Social, and Family Consequences*. Oxford, England: Oxford University Press; 1984:179–194.

Rosenthal M, Griffith ER, Bond MR, Miller JD (eds). *Rehabilitation of the Adult and Child with Traumatic Brain Injury, 2nd ed*. Philadelphia, PA: FA Davis; 1990.

Stover S, Zeiger HE. Head injury in children and teenagers: functional recovery correlated with duration of coma. *Archives of Physical Medicine and Rehabilitation*. 1976;57:201–205.

Ylvisaker M. Cognitive and psychosocial outcome following head injury in children. In Hoff J, Anderson T, Cole T (eds). *Contemporary Issues in Neurological Surgery: Mild to Moderate Head Injury, Vol 1*. Boston, MA: Blackwell Scientific Publications; 1989:203–216.

Ylvisaker M. Language and communication disorders following pediatric head injury. *Journal of Head Trauma Rehabilitation*. 1986;1:48–56.

Ylvisaker M (ed). *Head Injury Rehabilitation: Children and Adolescents*. San Diego, CA: College-Hill Press; 1985.

Ylvisaker M, Feeny TJ. Traumatic brain injury in adolescence. *Seminars in Speech and Language*. 1995;15:32–44.

Ylvisaker M, Feeney T, Mullins K. School reentry following mild traumatic brain injury: a proposal hospital-to-school protocol. *Journal of Head Trauma Rehabilitation*. 1995;10:42–49.

Ylvisaker M et al. School Reentry following severe brain injury: guidelines for educational planning. *Journal of Head Trauma Rehabilitation*. 1995;10: 25–41.

POSTACUTE REHABILITATION

See Rehabilitation, Community Integration

REHABILITATION

Acute

Cowley RS et al. The role of rehabilitation in the intensive care unit. *Journal of Head Trauma Rehabilitation.* 1994;9:32–42.

Ellis DW, Rader MA. Structured sensory stimulation. In *Physical Medicine and Rehabilitation: State of the Art Reviews, Vol 4.* Philadelphia, PA: Hanley and Belfus; 1990:465–477.

Farber SD. *Neurorehabilitation: A Multisensory Approach.* Philadelphia, PA: WB Saunders; 1982.

Garner R. *Acute Head Injury: Practical Management in Rehabilitation.* London, England: Chapman and Hall; 1990.

Smith GJ, Ylvisaker M. Cognitive rehabilitation therapy: early stages of recovery. In Ylvisaker M (ed). *Head Injury Rehabilitation: Children and Adolescents.* Boston, MA: College-Hill Press; 1985:275–286.

Wood RL. Critical analysis of the concept of sensory stimulation for patients in vegetative states. *Brain Injury.* 1991;5:401–409.

Wood RL et al. Evaluating sensory regulation as a method to improve awareness in patients with altered states of consciousness: a pilot study. *Brain Injury.* 1992; 6:411–418.

Behavioral Management

Edelstein BA, Couture ET (eds). *Behavioral Assessment and Rehabilitation of the Traumatically Brain Damaged.* New York, NY: Plenum Press; 1984.

Jacobs H. *Behavior Analysis Guidelines and Brain Injury Rehabilitation: People, Principles, and Programs.* Gaithersburg, MD: Aspen Publishers; 1993.

Mateer CA, Williams D. Management of psychosocial and behavior problems in cognitive rehabilitation. In Kreutzer J, Wehman P (eds). *Cognitive Rehabilitation for Persons with Traumatic Brain Injury: A Functional Approach.* Baltimore, MD: Paul H Brookes; 1991:117–126.

Wood RL. Conditioning procedures in brain injury rehabilitation. In Wood RL (ed). *Neurobehavioural Sequelae of Traumatic Brain Injury.* New York, NY: Taylor and Francis; 1990:153–174.

Wood RL, Burgess PW. The psychological management of behavior disorders following brain injury. In Fussey I, Giles GM (eds). *Rehabilitation of the Severely Brain Injured Adult.* London, England: Croom Helm; 1988:43–68.

Cognitive

See Cognitive Rehabilitation

Community Integration

Kreutzer JS, Wehman P (eds). *Community Integration Following Traumatic Brain Injury.* Baltimore, MD: Paul H Brookes; 1990:85–102.

Ylvisaker M, Gobble EM (eds). *Community Re-entry for Head Injured Adults.* Boston, MA: College-Hill; 1987.

Comprehensive Overviews in Brain Injury (General)

Goldstein G, Ruthven L. *Rehabilitation of the Brain-Damaged Adult*. New York, NY: Plenum Press; 1983.

Greenwood R et al. (eds). *Neurological Rehabilitation*. Edinburgh, Scotland: Churchill Livingstone; 1994.

Whitaker HA (ed). *Neuropsychological Studies of Nonfocal Brain Damage: Dementia and Trauma*. London, England: Springer-Verlag; 1988.

Comprehensive Overviews in Traumatic Brain Injury (or Closed Head Injury)

Bach-y-Rita P (ed). *Comprehensive Neurologic Rehabilitation: Traumatic Brain Injury, Vol 2*. New York, NY: Demos; 1989.

Brooks DN (ed). *Closed Head Injury: Psychological, Social, and Family Consequences*. Oxford, England: Oxford University Press; 1984.

Cope DN. The rehabilitation of traumatic brain injury. In Kottke FJ, Lehmann JF (eds). *Krusen's Handbook of Physical Medicine and Rehabilitation 4th ed*. Philadelphia, PA: WB Saunders; 1990:1217–1251.

Craine JF, Gudeman HE (eds). *The Rehabilitation of Brain Function: Principles, Procedures, and Techniques of Neurotraining*. Boston, MA: Houghton Mifflin; 1981.

Deutsch PM, Fralish KB (eds). *Innovations in Head Injury Rehabilitation*. New York, NY: Mathews Bender; 1994.

Finlayson MAJ, Garner SH (eds). *Brain Injury Rehabilitation: Clinical Considerations*. Baltimore, MD: Williams and Wilkins; 1994.

Fussey I, Giles GM (eds). *Rehabilitation of the Severely Brain-Injured Adult: A Practical Approach*. London, England: Croom Helm; 1988.

Giles GM, Clark-Wilson J. *Brain Injury Rehabilitation: A Neurofunctional Approach*. London, England: Chapman and Hall; 1993.

Horn LJ, Zasler ND (eds). *Rehabilitation of Post-concussive Disorders: Physical Medicine and Rehabilitation State of the Art Reviews, Vol 6(1)*. Philadelphia, PA: Hanley and Belfus; 1992.

Horn LJ, Cope DN (eds). *Traumatic Brain Injury: Physical Medicine and Rehabilitation State of the Art Reviews, Vol 3(1)*. Philadelphia, PA: Hanley and Belfus; 1989.

Levin HS, Grafman J, Eisenberg HM (eds). *Neurobehavioral Recovery from Closed Head Injury*. New York, NY: Oxford University Press; 1987.

Levin HS, Benton AL, Grossman RG. *Neurobehavioral Consequences of Closed Head Injury*. New York, NY: Oxford University Press; 1982.

Long CJ, Ross LK (eds). *Handbook of Head Trauma: Acute Care to Recovery*. New York, NY: Plenum Press; 1992.

Rosenthal M, Griffith ER, Bond MR, Miller JD (eds). *Rehabilitation of the Adult and Child with Traumatic Brain Injury, 2nd ed*. Philadelphia, PA: FA Davis; 1990.

Rosenthal M, Griffith ER, Bond MR, Miller JD (eds). *Rehabilitation of the Head Injured Adult*. Philadelphia, PA: FA Davis; 1983.

Whyte J, Rosenthal M. Rehabilitation of the patient with head injury. In DeLisa J (ed). *Rehabilitation Medicine: Principles and Practices*. Philadelphia, PA: JB Lippincott; 1988:585–611.

Wood RL (ed). *Neurobehavioural Sequelae of Traumatic Brain Injury*. New York, NY: Taylor and Francis; 1990.

Models/Paradigms

Ben-Yishay Y et al. Neuropsychologic rehabilitation: quest for a holistic approach. *Seminars in Neurology.* 1985;5:252–259.

Condeluci A. Brain injury rehabilitation: the need to bridge paradigms. *Brain Injury.* 1992;6:543–551.

Gross Y, Schutz LE. Intervention models in neuropsychology. In Uzzell BP, Gross Y (eds). *Clinical Neuropsychology of Intervention.* Boston, MA: Martinus Nijhoff; 1986:179–204.

O'Hara CC, Harrell M. The empowerment rehabilitation model: meeting the unmet needs of survivors, families, and treatment providers. *Journal of Cognitive Rehabilitation.* 1991;9:14–21.

Stanczak DE, Hutcherson WL. Acute rehabilitation of the head-injured individual: toward a neuropsychological paradigm of treatment. In Long CJ, Ross LK (eds). *Handbook of Head Trauma: Acute Care to Recovery.* New York, NY: Plenum Press; 1992:125–136.

Wood RL. Neurobehavioural paradigm for brain injury rehabilitation. In Wood RL (ed). *Neurobehavioural Sequelae of Traumatic Brain Injury.* New York, NY: Taylor and Francis; 1990:3–17.

Wood RL (ed). *Brain Injury Rehabilitation: A Neurobehavioural Approach.* London, England: Croom Helm; 1987.

Wood RL, Eames PG (eds). *Models of Brain Injury Rehabilitation.* Baltimore, MD: Johns Hopkins University Press; 1989.

SENSORY STIMULATION

See Medical Management, Coma

Appendix C

Commonly Referenced Assessment Scales

Agitated Behavior Scale (ABS)
Corrigan JD. Development of a scale for assessment of agitation following traumatic brain injury. *Journal of Clinical and Experimental Neuropsychology.* 1989;11: 261–277.

Coma/Near-Coma Scale (CNC)
Rappaport M, Dougherty AM, Kelting DL. Evaluation of coma and vegetative states. *Archives of Physical Medicine and Rehabilitation.* 1992;73:628–634.

Disability Rating Scale (DRS)
Rappaport M, Hall K, Hopkins K, Belleza T, Cope DN. Disability Rating Scale for severe head trauma: coma to community. *Archives of Physical Medicine and Rehabilitation.* 1982; 63:118–123.

Galveston Orientation and Amnesia Test (GOAT)
Levin HS, O'Donnell VM, Grossman RG. *Journal of Nervous and Mental Disorders.* 975;167:675–684.

Glasgow Coma Scale (GCS)
Jennett B, Bond MR. Assessment of coma: a practical scale. *Lancet.* 1974;1:81–84.

Glasgow Outcome Scale (GOS)
Teasdale G, Jennett B. *Lancet.* 1975;1:480–484.

Katz Adjustment Scale-Relative's Form (KAS-R)
Katz MM, Lyerly SB. Methods of measuring adjustment and social behavior in the community. *Psychological Reports.* 1963;13:503–535.

Neurobehavioral Rating Scale (NRS)
Levin HS, High WM, Goethe KE, Sisson RA, Overall JE, Rhoades HM, Eisenberg HM, Kalisky Z, Gary HE. The Neurobehavioral Rating Scale: assessment of the behavioral sequelae of head injury by the clinician. *Journal of Neurology, Neurosurgery, and Psychiatry.* 1987;50:183–193.

Orientation Group Monitoring System (OGMS)
Corrigan JD, Arnett JA, Houck LJ, Jackson RD. Reality orientation for brain injured patients: group treatment and monitoring of recovery. *Archives of Physical Medicine and Rehabilitation.* 1985;66:626–630.

Paced Auditory Serial Addition Task (PASAT)
Gronwall DMA. Paced auditory serial-addition task: a measure of recovery from concussion. *Perceptual and Motor Skills.* 1974;43:67–373.

Rancho Los Amigos Levels of Cognitive Functioning (LOCF)
Hagan C, Malkmus D, Durham P. Levels of cognitive functioning. In *Rehabilitation of the Head Injured Adult: Comprehensive Physical Management.* Downey, CA: Professional Staff Association of Rancho Los Amigos Hospital; 1979.

Sensory Stimulation Assessment Measure (SSAM)
Radar MA, Ellis DW. The Sensory Stimulation Assessment Measure (SSAM): a tool for early evaluation of severely brain-injured patients. *Brain Injury.* 1994;8:309–321.

Western Neuro Sensory Stimulation Profile (WNSSP)
Ansell BJ, Keenan JE. The Western Neuro Sensory Stimulation Profile: a tool for assessing slow to recover head injured patients. *Archives of Physical Medicine and Rehabilitation.* 1989;70:104–108.

Index